BACK REHABILITATION

Low back pain affects most of us at some time, and exercise is key to both its prevention and treatment. Critically appraising work from several approaches to produce an integrated, practical approach suitable for day-to-day clinicians and personal trainers, this essential guide looks at the science and practice of designing and teaching the best exercise programmes for this common condition. Learn:

- Vital client assessment skills
- Which exercises to use and why
- The most effective teaching methods
- How to structure and progress a full back pain management programme

Aimed at student therapists and clinical exercise teachers, as well as trainers planning exercise programmes for subjects recovering from low back pain, *Back Rehabilitation* is essential reading for therapists and exercise academics and professionals of all types.

Christopher M. Norris is a Chartered Physiotherapist (MCSP) who runs his own physiotherapy practice, Norris Health, in Cheshire, UK. He earned an MSc in exercise science from the University of Liverpool, UK, and a PhD on spinal rehabilitation from Staffordshire University, UK. He also holds postgraduate certification in occupational health, orthopaedic medicine, and medical education. He is a certified strength and conditioning coach and a qualified teacher of both yoga and Pilates.

BACK REHABILITATION

Core Stability Re-examined

Third Edition

Christopher M. Norris

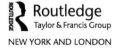

NEW YORK AND LONDON

Designed cover image: MarianVejcik

Third Edition published 2023
by Routledge
605 Third Avenue, New York, NY 10158

and by Routledge
4 Park Square, Milton Park, Abingdon, Oxon, OX14 4RN

Routledge is an imprint of the Taylor & Francis Group, an informa business

First edition published 2015

ISBN: 978-1-032-43215-1 (hbk)
ISBN: 978-1-032-43214-4 (pbk)
ISBN: 978-1-003-36618-8 (ebk)

DOI: 10.4324/9781003366188

Typeset in Bembo
by codeMantra

CONTENTS

FIGURES

TABLES

PREFACE

Core stability was a leading popular method of exercise in the 1990s, linked to muscle imbalance and posture-based exercise interventions. Pioneering research initially led to its use by physiotherapists for rehabilitation of low back conditions. It quickly spread into popular culture, its use paralleling the rapidly increasing development of commercial gyms, and exercise classes. Gradually, research emerged which confirmed that the method, although effective, was no better as a treatment of back conditions than other forms of exercise and its clinical usage began to diminish.

The advent of social media has divided the exercise world into two distinct camps. Core stability is still popular in gyms and exercise classes with terms such as 'maintain neutral position' and 'engage your core' frequently used. In the clinical world there has been a steadily increasing volume of criticism of the method, and it is often demonised in popular social media posts.

This book is the Third Edition of the text *Back Stability* (Human Kinetics 2000, 2008). It has expanded to further combine knowledge from the healthcare, exercise science, and coaching fields. Importantly the book critically appraises scientific work within these fields and adds to this practical experience gained by the author from treating patients over a 40-year period.

Back Rehabilitation introduces the 3Rs approach, a clinical framework to guide therapists, exercise professionals, and users when applying progressive exercise therapy for the low back.

Back Rehabilitation aims to present scientific material in a readily accessible form and makes extensive use of tables, line drawings, and photographs together with definition boxes and points-to-note. In addition, it includes clinical cases throughout the text to illustrate important points and has a whole chapter on patient case histories to guide therapists and exercise professionals.

Back Rehabilitation, Third Edition, takes classical methods of core stability, adapts them, and uses them as part of a progressive exercise programme within a biopsychosocial (BPS) healthcare model. Using the 3Rs approach the book combines early exercise interventions traditionally used within physiotherapy to treat medical conditions, with those popular in healthy recreational exercise users. The approach takes users further and applies knowledge traditionally held in the domain of elite sport to the sphere of rehabilitation.

Back Rehabilitation, Third Edition, provides a complete pedagogical resource for therapists, exercise teachers, athletes, and casual exercise users.

ACKNOWLEDGEMENTS

Models: Lore Hare, Abi Blythe, Emily Wilkinson, Hildi Carruthers, Chris Norris.

1

NATURE OF THE PROBLEM

If you are reading this book, chances are that you either have back pain, know someone who has, or treat people with the condition. Back pain is a universal problem, one that is particularly important in the increasingly sedentary Western world. We can all recall someone with this problem, because as many as 80% of people in the Western world will suffer at least one disabling episode of low back pain (LBP) during their lives. The cost is tremendous, both financially and in terms of personal suffering. In the UK, the health service spends more than £1 billion annually on this condition alone (Smith et al. 2014). Direct costs include inpatient hospitalisation, outpatient physiotherapy, primary care appointments, medication, radiology, and community care. Indirect costs due to lost production and informal care may be ten times higher (Maniadakis and Gray 2000). Most people with LBP recover within 6 weeks, but 5–15% of individuals progress to permanent disability, accounting for up to 90% of total expenditure for this condition. Consider this for a moment. Many individuals suffer with their back on a more or less permanent basis. It reminds them throughout their daily lives that the condition is still there. Their job and daily routine, hobbies, and family life are all affected by this condition. Sometimes it is in the background, while at other times it is a dominant feature. Unfortunately, recurrence of back pain after an initial episode is common. More than 60% of those suffering an acute episode of LBP will experience another bout within a year, and 45% of these will have a second recurrence within the following four years. Bad enough that the condition is so painful and so present in day-to-day life, but once it eases, it often comes back.

> **Keypoint:**
>
> As many as 15% of people with low back pain progress to permanent disability, and 60% suffer from a recurrence of pain within one year.

DOI: 10.4324/9781003366188-1

LBP is a common clinical condition, which has traditionally been said to present as an acute (<6 weeks), sub-acute (6–12 weeks), or chronic (>12 weeks) incident, where focus is on duration of symptoms. The terms acute (lasting a few days to a few weeks) and persistent (greater than this) are also commonly used.

Prevalence of Chronic Low Back Pain (CLBP) in individuals between 20 and 59 years is 19.6% rising to 25.4% in those older (Meucci et al. 2015). Both pain and disability are described as part of this condition, with CLBP reported as the leading cause of years lived with disability (Hurwitz et al. 2018). Relapse of the condition is common, with as many as two thirds of individuals having a recurrence within 12 months of initial onset (da Silva et al. 2019). This is a horrendous statistic. Not only is LBP a potentially crippling condition, but once it has eased it often comes back again and again. Non-specific LBP is low back pain not attributable to a known cause and represents up to 95% of cases (Bardin et al. 2017). Despite extensive research in this area, disability levels have so far failed to improve (Tousignant-Laflamme et al. 2017). In fact, disability caused by CLBP has increased by more than 50% since 1990, particularly in low- and middle-income countries with limited healthcare resources and a general shift towards a more sedentary lifestyle (GBD 2017). Whatever we are doing in the therapy and exercise teaching worlds, it is not good enough and things need to change.

Definition:

Non-specific low back pain (NSLBP) is low back pain not attributed to a known cause, and accounts for 95% of cases.

Guidelines

Clinical practice guidelines for the management of non-specific LBP in primary care recommend history taking and physical examination to identify red flags which may indicate a possible serious pathology requiring onward referral. Neurological testing is used where radicular syndrome is suspected, with imaging used only if a more serious pathology is suspected. This type of assessment can categorise LBP into non-specific LBP, radiculopathy, or specific LBP. Neurological examination may include straight leg raise (SLR), and assessment of strength, sensation, and reflexes. Imaging is discouraged for routine usage.

Definition:

Radiculopathy occurs when a nerve root is compressed resulting in sensory (numbness, tingling) or motor (weakness, changed reflexes) changes in the limbs.

Red flags

A red flag is literally a warning of danger. In an examination, the term red flag is used to indicate that a sign or symptom may suggest the presence of a more sinister pathology, and therefore requires additional information from medical investigations or onward referral. Importantly a red flag is not a diagnosis, and this should not be implied to a person. During examination of LBP there are four main areas of concern: Cauda equina syndrome, spinal fracture, cancer, and infection (see Chapter 5).

General recommendations for the management of non-specific LBP are non-pharmacological and non-invasive with advice to stay active and to use patient education and exercise therapy (O'Connell et al. 2016). Reassurance of a favourable prognosis, advice on returning to normal activities, and the avoidance of bed rest are all suggested. The use of nonsteroidal anti-inflammatory drugs (NSAIDs) and weak opioids is indicated for short periods only. Exercise therapy and advice are important with secondary referral where there are red flags, radiculopathy, or no improvement after four weeks.

In the NICE (National Institute for Health and Care Excellence) guidelines on the treatment of LBP, exercise is a key treatment modality, with manual therapy and psychological therapies only to be considered as part of a treatment programme which includes exercise (NICE 2016). The focus is on self-management of LBP (with or without sciatica) at all steps of the treatment pathway. The guidelines emphasise that no one exercise type is superior to another, the choice of exercise intervention should consider patient needs, preferences, and capabilities. Psychological interventions are recommended where psychosocial factors (yellow flags) are identified at assessment and limit recovery.

Keypoint:

In the NICE guidelines on the treatment of LBP, *exercise* is a key treatment modality.

Exercise and psychological interventions

Exercise types used in the management of CLBP include (but are not limited to); aerobic exercise, strength/resistance exercise, coordination/stabilisation exercise, motor control approaches, Mind-body exercise such as Pilates or yoga. All have been shown to effectively reduce pain and disability (compared to passive or no intervention), but no differences have been found between the different exercise modalities (Malfliet et al. 2019). Where time is a limiting factor to compliance with home exercise programmes, walking interventions may be used as they have been shown to improve pain, quality of life, disability, and fear avoidance to a similar degree as exercise in patients with CLBP (Vanti et al. 2019).

> **Keypoint:**
>
> No difference has been found in general between different exercise approaches used in the management of CLBP.

In addition, reductions of pain and/or disability resulting from exercise therapy have been shown to be unrelated to musculoskeletal improvements such as mobility, trunk extension strength, trunk flexion strength, and back muscle endurance (Steiger et al. 2012). This may suggest that changes in psychological factors may be more important drivers of improvement in pain or disability related to CLBP.

Focussing on a single method of treatment or a single exercise therapy approach (monodisciplinary treatment) is generally less effective than combining exercise therapy with behavioural/psychological approaches (multidisciplinary treatment). Long-term follow up (one year) showing better improvement, measured as sick-leave days (Roche-Leboucher et al. 2011), and reducing disability, fear-avoidance beliefs, and pain, and enhancing patient quality of life (Monticone et al. 2013).

Psychological interventions when used in isolation can be effective in the management of CLBP but have shown equal results to active exercise interventions (Hoffman et al. 2007). The use of pain neuroscience education (PNE) and cognition targeted exercise has been shown to reduce central sensitisation and improve disability (maintained for 12 months) when used as a monodisciplinary approach (Malfliet et al. 2018). PNE aims to reconceptualise pain relating it to an alteration of central nervous system processing ('software' metaphor) rather than a direct result of tissue damage ('hardware' metaphor) explaining the usual lack of significant findings on imaging. In this way, PNE aims to reduce the threat value of pain to reduce kinesiophobia and disability in the short term especially (Malfliet et al. 2019). Both PNE and exercise therapy show strong evidence of benefit on pain and function in musculoskeletal conditions, compared to only moderate benefit (modest effect sizes) for non-steroidal anti-inflammatory drugs (NSAIDs) and opioids (Babatunde et al. 2017).

> **Definition:**
>
> *Kinesiophobia* is a debilitating fear of movement or activity which results from a feeling of vulnerability due to pain or injury.

Exercise therapy may be given in a form which creates a bridge between psychological and physical interventions to emphasise a biopsychosocial (BPS) model of patient management and this methodology is used throughout the 3Rs approach (see below) but especially in the *Reactive phase*. Cognition targeted exercise focusses on stopping an exercise/activity at a specific time (time-contingent) rather than as the result of discomfort or pain (symptom-contingent). Such an approach relies heavily on establishing a therapeutic alliance between the patient and therapist, the latter acting as instructor rather than taskmaster.

Graded activity and graded exposure may also provide a BPS link. Graded *exposure* introduces activities which a patient fear's (e.g., flexion or lifting) in a hierarchical fashion (least feared progressing to most feared) to gradually increase confidence and capability. Graded *activity* is more physical in its aims, as it progresses components of an exercise (e.g., strength, range of motion, aerobic fitness) applying overload with the aim of achieving tissue adaptation. Graded exposure has been shown to be more effective than graded activity in decreasing catastrophising in the short term (Lopez-de-Uralde-Villanueva et al. 2016).

> **Definition:**
>
> *Catastrophising* is viewing a situation as considerably worse than it actually is.

Use of scans in patients with low back pain

Despite the tremendous increase in the number of back pain sufferers in the past three decades, popular understanding about the nature of back pain has remained somewhat static. It is commonly believed that back pain results from a structural injury or fault that must be corrected to reduce pain and restore full function. According to this viewpoint, normal function is impossible—or even dangerous—until the defective structure has changed. In common parlance people often feel that their back has 'gone out' and needs to be 'put back in'.

Although it is true that many people with LBP exhibit structural changes, computed tomography (CT) scans reveal positive findings in up to 50% of normal, asymptomatic people (Jensel et al. 1994). It is the same with radiographic (X-ray) changes in the lumbar spine: As many people without pain show evidence of disc degeneration as do those with pain (Nachemson 1992).

The purpose of an X-ray is often to identify an abnormality, or a structural change or pathology of bone. Studies have shown that more than 75% of spinal X-rays present no useful clinical information. In a study of 1,095 lumbar X-rays, 46% were normal or had incidental findings (findings that were not directly related to a condition) and a further 32% had radiological findings of questionable clinical significance (Scavone et al. 1981). Typical changes on lumbar radiographs often associated with long-standing back pain are largely unrelated to eventual outcome. Symptoms such as pain and weakness often improve despite x-rays remaining the same. In the case of LBP structure often does not dictate function.

Degenerative changes, disc narrowing, and the presence of osteophytes (bone spurs) are all common diagnoses given out freely to worried people, but these do not correlate with the presence of LBP (Craton 2006). X rays have little place in the diagnosis of long-term (chronic) back pain, to the extent that the European Guidelines for the Management of Chronic Non-specific Low Back Pain (NSLBP) do not recommend radiographic imaging for chronic non-specific LBP persons and NICE (2016) recommend that imaging (CT, MRI, X-ray) should not be used routinely (in a non-specialist setting) for people with LBP with or without sciatica.

Studies with cadavers have shown no correlation between structural changes in the lumbar spine and a history of low back pain, and large disc lesions with nerve compression (often a common diagnosis) may be totally asymptomatic (Saal 1995).

Imaging has also been shown not just to increase direct healthcare costs, but to increase general healthcare interventions such as medication, injections, and surgery and to lead to a greater mean work absence compared to non-imaging groups (Lemmers et al. 2019).

Keypoint:

Structural changes in the spine are as likely in asymptomatic people as in those with low back pain and loss of function.

It is not just current back pain which has been the focus of imaging findings, but development of pain in later life (Sääksjärvi et al. 2020). In a study of military recruits aged 20 with LBP, MRI was used to determine degenerative changes of the lumbar discs (L4-L5 and L5-S1). Those who were found to have early disc degeneration were not linked to pain or disability in later life. In other words, the structural changes found in youth were not a predictor of poor outcome when older.

Overuse of imaging not only fails to improve patient outcomes but may cause harm. The patient's interpretation of imaging results (terms such as 'wear and tear', 'degeneration', 'ageing', for example) may decrease perception of personal health leading to catastrophising and fear-avoidance behaviour (Flynn et al. 2011). Three main areas of harm have been identified with the inappropriate use of imaging for LBP (Table 1.1). Unhelpful advice may be given by clinicians through misinterpretation of results, and further unnecessary investigations

TABLE 1.1 Potential harm caused by inappropriate imaging for low back pain

- Misinterpretation of results by clinicians resulting in unhelpful advice or further unrequired testing
- Misinterpretation of results by patients driving catastrophising, fear avoidance, and low self-efficacy
- Side effects of radiation exposure

Source: Data from Darlow et al. (2017).

ordered. Psychological factors such as fear, avoidance of activity, and low expectations of recovery may occur where results or explanations are misconstrued by patients. Finally, exposure to radiation itself is not without potential harm (Darlow et al. 2017).

Disturbingly, despite guidelines to the contrary, imaging use for LBP has not reduced. In a systematic review of 45 papers detailing over 4 million imaging requests over a 21-year period Downie et al. (2020) found one if four patients presenting to primary care and one in three presenting to the emergency department received imaging for LBP. Interestingly a study of family doctors in Canada (Pike et al. 2022) looked at the reason for over-imaging for NSLBP and found several barriers to reducing imaging. These included (i) the belief in negative consequences if imaging was not done (fear that they may miss something serious), (ii) patient demand and social influences (the patient felt they needed a scan because it was always done), (iii) organisation within the healthcare system (the system encourages unnecessary imaging and the family doctors may not have access to allied health practitioners), (iv) time and resources (the doctors may not have enough time to examine patients fully or to counsel them).

> ### CASE NOTE
> A fifty-two-year-old female experienced first episode low back pain referred into the right leg (posterior thigh to the knee) after four hours gardening. The pain was so intense that she called an ambulance and was taken to the local accident and emergency (A&E) department. In the ambulance she received gas and air (nitrous oxide and oxygen) and was examined at the hospital where red flags were cleared, and she was told that she had likely pulled muscles in her back and put pressure on a nerve. She received pain killers and was discharged. That night she was unable to sleep, instead sitting in an armchair. The next night she was able to get into bed, but her sleep was disrupted. Her leg pain had begun to settle but as she had a medical insurance policy with her work, she decided to ask for a scan and she received an x-ray of her lumbar spine at a private imaging centre. Her x-ray report noted some disc narrowing in her lower lumbar spine. She presented for physiotherapy six weeks following the incident and had been inactive since that time. She had pain to flexion which eased with repetition and all other spinal movements were full. Her straight leg raise (SLR) was full and painless, and examination of the hips and pelvis was unremarkable. The patient was given a rehabilitation programme of progressive exercises and she commented that she did not know she was able to exercise her spine given that she had narrow discs and still had local pain.

Non-neural back pain

LBP may arise from several structures or pathologies other than the nerve root (Table 1.2). Nociceptive drivers have been identified to some extent in the intervertebral disc, facet joint, and vertebral endplate. Although the disc is often said to be the source of pain, investigations have largely failed to accurately identify the source of discogenic pain, and spontaneous regression of disc prolapse is seen. Modic changes to the vertebral end plate have been shown to cause pro-inflammatory changes which may allow microbial infiltration or an autoimmune reaction inducing nociceptive stimulation (mechanical or chemical). However, their contribution to pain remains uncertain (Hertvigsen et al. 2018). Facet joint anaesthesia can cause temporary pain reduction; however, no association has been found between radiographic osteoarthritis of facet joints and LBP (Kalichman et al. 2008).

> **Definition:**
>
> *Modic changes* are lesions within the body marrow of the vertebral body, seen on MRI scan. They include bone marrow oedema, hypervascularisation, fatty deposits, and subchondral bone sclerosis.

Specific pathologies may also be associated with spinal pain. Vertebral fracture either through direct trauma to the healthy skeleton or minimal trauma in an osteoporotic person may cause pain. In the latter this may have a significant health impact due to prolonged rest and can increase mortality risk (Schousboe 2016). Red flags for fracture with the highest probability for detection are older age, prolonged use of corticosteroid drugs, severe trauma, and presence of contusion

TABLE 1.2 Low back pain—where does the pain come from?

Source		
Nociceptive contributor	• Intervertebral disc • Facet joint • Vertebral endplate	• Imaging & clinical findings vary • Temporary relief using facet joint injection • Modic changes may cause pro-inflammatory response
Pathology	• Vertebral fracture • Axial spondyloarthritis • Malignancy • Infections • Cauda equina syndrome	• Symptomatic minimal trauma fracture due to osteoporosis • Chronic inflammatory disease of axial skeleton which may be visible on x-ray (ankylosing spondylitis) • Vertebral metastases in 3–5% of people with cancer • Spinal infection—bacterial or disease related • Cauda equina compression through disc herniation

Data from Hertvigsen et al. (2018).

or abrasion, with the likelihood of fracture greater where multiple red flags are present (Downie et al. 2013). Metastatic cancer may also cause spinal pain, with 3–5% of people with cancer developing metastases. A past history of malignancy is the most reliable indicating clinical sign at first contact, with breast, lung, prostate, thyroid, and gastrointestinal solid tumours (adenocarcinomas) most commonly metastasising (Downie et al. 2013).

> **Definition:**
>
> An *adenocarcinoma* is a cancer which forms in glandular tissue lining internal organs that release substances to the body.

Axial spondyloarthritis (AxSpA) is a chronic inflammatory disease affecting the axial skeleton. It may affect the spine and sacroiliac joints where structural damage can be seen. Previously termed ankylosing spondylitis it can give pain prior to the development of structural damage (non-radiographic spondyloarthritis). Typical presentation is of morning stiffness (> 30mins) which improves with exercise (but not rest), and night pain in the second half of the night. There is often a family history of inflammatory conditions, and HLA-B27 may be positive with raised CRP and ESR in a blood test.

> **Definition:**
>
> *HLA-B27* is human leukocyte antigen B27 which is a protein found on the surface of white blood cells. *CRP* is C-reactive protein a marker of inflammation in the body. *ESR* stands for Erythrocyte sedimentation rate and is an indirect measure of the degree of inflammation in the body.

Spinal infections such as osteomyelitis (bone inflammation), spondylodiscitis (infection of the spinal disc) epidural abscess, and (less commonly) facet joint infection may give intense spinal pain. Infection may be caused by bacteria (pyogenic infection) from inside or outside the body, or from diseases such as tuberculosis (TB) or brucellosis. People who are immunosuppressed are at greater risk of spinal infections.

Non-structural causes of back pain

At least three sources of back pain do not originate directly in the sufferer's body: iatrogenic, forensic, and behavioural (Zusman 1998).

Iatrogenic factors (brought on by the practitioner) include labels of disability and the consequences of subsequent deconditioning through prolonged rest. For example, a label such as *prolapsed disc* is far more threatening to a person than *simple back pain,* even though the total amount of pain experienced by the person may be the same in both cases. Labels that imply disease or disability, such as *arthritis or wear and tear,* also suggest severe conditions even though a mild form of the pathology may be present. Such labels are likely to reinforce rest or reduction in general activities. Alternatives such as *slight roughening* or *normal ageing* are often less threatening. Although avoiding activities that place stress on the back can be important in the early stages of back pain (reactive phase, see Chapter 6), and limited rest has its place, prolonged bed rest has been shown to be counterproductive and this has been known for some time. In an early study, Deyo and colleagues (1986) compared two days of bed rest with two weeks of bed rest. They found both periods to be equally effective in terms of pain reduction, but the two-week period led to significant negative effects attributable to immobilisation (such as weakening and stiffness around the spine) that were not present in the two-day period.

Forensic factors (those associated with legal proceedings) contribute significantly to chronic back pain. In a study of 2,000 back pain sufferers (Long 1995), involvement in litigation was the only factor that accurately predicted that a person would not rapidly return to work. Disability resulting from legal proceedings varies between countries, and the definition of disability due to LBP is influenced by social norms, local healthcare approaches, and legislation (Maniadakis and Gray 2000). In low-income and middle-income countries social support is negatively impacted by CLBP as it is a drain on resources. However, in high income countries healthcare approaches to LBP have been shown to contribute to the overall burden by increasing overtreatment (Deyo et al. 2009).

Behavioural factors include factors such as perceived disability and the anticipation of pain. People often fail to take part in daily activities because they believe they are physically incapable of doing the task—although structural changes in their spines do not bear out this belief. Perceived disability is often associated with a mistaken fear of reinjury (Vlaeyen et al. 1995). Frequently the anticipation of pain rather than pain itself is enough to limit activity and create protective behaviours. The physical changes brought about by the fear of pain can be measured on surface electromyography (sEMG). Main and Watson (1996) applied experimental noxious stimuli to the upper trapezius of normal people and those with back pain. Normal people showed the expected reflex increase in sEMG activity in the trapezius muscles. Those with back pain, however, showed the reaction not in the upper trapezius but rather in the lumbar region—suggesting that the people viewed any pain as an inherent part of their back condition even when the pain was occurring in another part of their bodies.

Keypoint:

Perceived disability and the anticipation of pain contribute significantly to loss of function.

Psychology of low back pain

Let's look at the psychological factors involved in back pain. Pain and disability are not the same thing; pain is simply a person's symptom, whereas disability results from restricted activity, often as a result of CLBP. Pain can be considered to consist of a number of aspects, *nociception, pain, pain behaviour, and suffering* (Table 1.3). *Nociception* is the detection of a reaction by specialised peripheral sensors in the tissue which relay information to the dorsal horn of the spinal cord. These sensors (transducers) respond to mechanical, thermal, or chemical stimulation which is sufficient to damage cells. The signals for nociception can be blocked by anaesthesia designed to prevent axonal depolarisation, and by descending modulation from the brain. In a normal state, the response to nociception is *pain*. However, changes to the peripheral nerves, spinal cord, or brain can lead to the report of pain in the absence of noxious stimuli, a classic example being phantom limb pain in a person with an amputated limb.

Suffering is a negative affective response generated by the brain as a response to pain, but also by psychological states such as fear, anxiety, stress, or loss. *Pain behaviour* is an affective response which is attributed to pain such as facial expressions, guarding, limping, and avoidance.

Definition:

An *affective response* is a psychological state demonstrated by an individual including emotions, mood, and body language.

Effects of pain

Generally, in CLBP, nociception and pain have less effect than do suffering and pain behaviour. The effect of pain is therefore greater than the pain itself. This may not have been the case when the back pain originally occurred, but over time the effect of the injury and pain itself have become secondary to the suffering and physical changes that the injury has caused. In CLBP, then, if we focus

TABLE 1.3 Aspects of pain

Nociception	Process by which noxious stimuli are communicated through the nervous system
Pain	An unpleasant sensory and emotional experience associated with actual or potential tissue damage
Pain behaviour	A learned or conditioned response attributed to pain.
Suffering	A negative emotional response of unpleasantness and/or aversion to a perception of potential harm.

Source: Data from Loeser (1980, 2006).

all our treatment on pain reduction, we will fail to address a very large part of the person's condition.

> **Keypoint:**
>
> Focussing treatment on pain reduction alone fails to address the whole of a person's condition.

Pain is both a sensory and an emotional experience. It is more than an indication of simple tissue damage, and if treatment focusses on tissues alone, the emotional aspect of pain may go unaltered. Nociceptive signals pass from receptors in the body tissues to the brain, where the signals are experienced or felt. However, in their journey from sensor to brain, the signals are always modulated or changed slightly by the nervous system before they reach conscious awareness and are felt. It is impossible to separate pain sensation, then, from the emotional effect of pain: The two are permanently intertwined. The International Association for the Study of Pain (IASP) has defined pain as "an unpleasant sensory and emotional experience associated with, or resembling that associated with, actual or potential tissue damage" (IASP 2022). This definition has important considerations shown in Table 1.4.

Within this definition, pain is seen as a psychological and emotional state rather than simply a physical stimulus. Even if tissue damage is not present, pain may still be experienced. Additionally, pain is very much a personal experience, and the IASP definition emphasises the belief that tissue damage may occur. This is especially important to the concept of fear of movement.

> **Definition:**
>
> *Nociception* is the process of communicating information about noxious (harmful) stimuli through the nervous system.

TABLE 1.4 Considerations of pain

- Pain is always a personal experience which is influenced by biological, psychological, and social factors.
- Pain and nociception are different phenomena. Pain cannot be inferred solely from activity in sensory neurons.
- A person learns the concept of pain through their life experiences.
- A person's report of an experience as pain should be respected.
- Although pain usually serves an adaptive role, it may have adverse effects on function and social and psychological wellbeing.
- Verbal description is only one of several behaviours to express pain; inability to communicate does not negate the possibility that a person experiences pain.

Data from IASP (2022).

Why is chronic low back pain disabling?

Disability is simply a restriction of activity. The World Health Organization (WHO) defines disability as "any restriction or lack (resulting from an impairment) of ability to perform an activity in the manner or within the range considered normal for a human being" (WHO 1980). There are three aspects to disability (Table 1.5), with disability referring to difficulty in any of the areas. *Impairment* is a problem with a body function or alteration in body structure. In the case of a person suffering CLBP this may be a drop foot, for example, producing an antalgic gait, or muscle wasting as a result of pain or enforced inactivity.

Definition:

An *antalgic gait* is an abnormal pattern of walking secondary to pain. This may present as a limp with the stance phase of walking shortened relative to the swing phase.

Activity limitation occurs when a person has difficulty carrying out an action or activity. For example, a person with CLBP may have a limited bending ability making it difficult for them to tie their shoelaces or put their socks on. *Participation restriction* is a problem with involvement in an area of life, for example, being unable to play for a sports team because of low back pain.

Both personal and environmental factors may interact to contribute to disability. *Personal* factors such as motivation or self-efficacy may limit how much a person is willing to do and how they participate in the activities of daily living (ADL). Equally *environmental* factors produced by the world in which the person functions may contribute to disability, acting as facilitators (positive) or barriers (negative).

What is of interest is how CLBP leads to disability. It is often assumed that pain lasting for a prolonged period will inevitably lead to disability purely because of time. However, clinically this is not what we see. It is common to see a person who demonstrates high levels of disability with very little pain as well as a person who has high levels of pain with very little disability. The combination of pain with lack of activity over time can lead to a preoccupation with physical symptoms and a change in the person's belief about the meaning of his or her pain. People can learn to avoid activities that they believe will cause or exacerbate pain (pain behaviour) and to rely on passive coping strategies rather than active ones.

TABLE 1.5 Areas of change to human functioning due to disability

Impairment	*Problems in body function or alteration in body structure*
Activity limitation	Difficulties in executing activities
Participation restriction	Problem with involvement in an area of life

Source: Data from World report on disability. WHO (2011).

Passive coping strategies see people handing over responsibility for their care to something external (e.g., therapist, back support, medication) with the attitude that there is nothing they personally can do to help themselves. They often engage in negative self-talk, using phrases like "I can't get comfortable with this back" or "I couldn't do that because of my back". They tend to avoid activities and situations that they believe will cause or exacerbate pain, even if they have not tried these activities. This may also be encouraged or reinforced by a therapist or trainer even if unwittingly. Phrases such as "be careful of your back" or "engage your core" prior to an exercise imply fragility. When using active coping strategies, people take part in their own care. They often use exercise, seek treatment, and adapt their lifestyle to continue with daily activities.

Models of healthcare

Healthcare models have evolved over the last century, from the traditional *biomedical* model towards a more holistic BPS approach (Engel 1977), and this has particular significance in the management of LBP. The BPS model stresses the importance of a complex interaction between biological (e.g., genetic, structure, chemical), psychological (e.g., mood, behaviour), and sociological (e.g., family, environment, culture) factors when treating a patient. This approach is broader and less reductionist than the standard biomedical model which directly links structure to pathology (e.g., a lumbar disc causing pain) seeing the body alone as responsible for symptoms. The biomedical model traces back to the 16th century and the work of Rene Descartes, with the view that the body and mind are separate (Cartesian dualism). The biomedical model remains dominant in the public understanding of illness, and frequently encourages isolated pathological diagnosis in healthcare, often reasoning that a patient's symptoms are driven by a single structural factor. However, the BPS model underlies person-centred care, and may better demonstrate the true breadth of a disability (Wade and Halligan 2017). The BPS model consists of three overlapping components which may be considered a mixture of science on the one hand and humanities on the other, broadly differentiated into 'numbers' and 'description'.

TABLE 1.6 Biomedical and biopsychosocial models in low back pain

Biomedical model	Biopsychosocial (BPS) model
• Tissue causes pain in a predetermined way	• Interaction between biological,
• Pain messages travel from tissue in specialised pain neuron to input into defined brain regions	• psychological and social factors
	• Pain as a brain output to protect body from further harm
• Pain intensity describes amount of tissue damage	• PNS senses environment, interpretation of signals as threat by CNS
• Site of pain defines site/type of tissue damaged	• Information assessed by brain compared to past experiences
• Target tissue with modality and pain will reduce	• All regions of brain play role in pain experience—pain neuromatrix (cerebral signature)

Note: PNS—peripheral nervous system, CNS—central nervous system.

In relation to LBP, essential features comparing the biomedical and BPS models are highlighted in Table 1.6. From a biomedical perspective, the view is of a single tissue causing pain in a predetermined way. In this view greater pain means greater harm, pain intensity describing the degree of tissue damage. Further, the site of pain defines the site of damage, and so treating this area alone should give rise to a healing response. The BPS model in contrast, rationalises pain as an output or series of signals from the brain designed to protect the body from further harm, which may be either real or perceived. The nervous system senses the environment (both external and internal) and the brain interprets the signals received by comparing the information to past experiences, social norms, and beliefs. For example, if you stepped on a stone when on a beach, you may simply look down and notice what is happening. However, if you had previously been cut by a rusty can while walking on a beach, your reaction to a sudden sharp sensation on your foot is likely to be exaggerated. You would likely flinch, pull away from the area, and perhaps break out into a cold sweat. All these reactions are greater than those which occurred when you simply thought you were stepping on a stone, not because of the intensity of tissue stress or damage, but because of your interpretation of what you are feeling. Interpreting the noxious signal (nociception) as being more harmful than it actually is. Many regions of the brain play a role in the pain experience and are collectively described as a pain neurosignature, being part of the neuromatrix theory proposed by Melzack (1990).

Definition:

A *neurosignature* is a neural pattern made up of a group of memories and/or emotions which is activated by a particular stimulus, but which may activate independently of the original stimulus.

TABLE 1.7 Interacting factors in low back pain

Physical	Cognitive	Psychological	Lifestyle	Social	Co-morbidities
Maladaptive posture & movement patterns	Beliefs	Fear	Inactivity	Socioeconomic status	Obesity
Pain behaviour	Catastrophising	Anxiety	Sleep disturbance	Family	Chronic fatigue
Deconditioning	Hypervigilance	Depression	Life stress	Work	Irritable bowel syndrome
	Self efficacy			Culture	Inflammatory disorders
	Coping strategies				Peripheral sensitisation

Source: Data from O'Keefe et al. (2015), O'Sullivan (2017).

Several BPS factors may interact in patients with LBP (Table 1.7). Physical influences include items such as alteration to movement patterns, maladaptive postures, and general deconditioning. Cognitive factors include beliefs which the person has about their condition, which have led to catastrophising, hypervigilance, and poor self-efficacy (see Chapter 5). Thoughts that pain relates to tissue condition (hurt equals harm), the back is naturally fragile, something has 'slipped out', that discs are 'worn' will all limit recovery and must be addressed. Psychological influences include emotional response such as fear, anxiety, and depression, and these may drive associated lifestyle changes such as sleep disorders and chronic stress responses. The social domain reflects influences from work, and home/family especially, and this may be either positive (support) or negative (judgemental). Finally, comorbidities may be important with some (such as obesity) influencing back pain and being modifiable, and others (such as chronic fatigue, irritable bowel syndrome) being related to back pain but less directly modifiable.

The 3Rs approach

The approach to back rehabilitation used in this book is called the 3Rs (Norris 2020). The approach provides a clinical framework for practitioners and exercise teachers to prescribe exercise to those recovering from LBP at any stage of their condition. The 3Rs approach represents a structured care pathway incorporating pain management, patient education, and physical conditioning. It aims to present holistic therapeutic management within a BPS framework. As such, the emphasis is on whole person management rather than tissue specific treatment. The three phases of the 3Rs approach (see Chapter 6) represent a progression over time (temporal) and of activity grade (functional), and broadly adhere to the healing timescale of pathology. As normal healing progresses, pain and inflammation subside and recovery ensues, with patients typically returning to some level of function without rehabilitation. Usually, symptoms even out over time and return to average/normal—a phenomenon known as *regression to the mean*. However, the nature of LBP is such that function is often reduced and recurrence of symptoms is typical. The 3Rs approach aims to increase a patient's capacity by improving function and lessening the likelihood of injury recurrence.

Definition:

Regression to the mean (RTM) occurs when data evens out through natural variation.

References

Babatunde, O.O., Jordan, J.L., Van der Windt, D.A., Hill, J.C., Foster, N.E., and Protheroe, J. (2017). Effective treatment options for musculoskeletal pain in primary care: A systematic overview of current evidence. *PloS One* 12(6): e0178621.

Bardin, L.D., King, P., and Maher, C.G. (2017). Diagnostic triage for low back pain: A practical approach for primary care. *Medical Journal of Australia* 206(6): 268–273.

Craton, N. (2006). Diagnostic triage in patients with spinal pain. In C. Liebenson, Ed., *Rehabilitation of the spine* (2nd ed). Philadelphia: Lippincott, 197–218.

da Silva, T., Mills, K., Brown, B.T., et al. (2019). Recurrence of low back pain is common: A prospective inception cohort study. *Journal of Physiotherapy* 65(3): 159–165.

Darlow, B., Forster, B.B., O'Sullivan, K., et al. (2017). It is time to stop causing harm with inappropriate imaging for low back pain. *British Journal of Sports Medicine* 51: 414–415.

Deyo, R.A., Diehl, A.K., and Rosenthal, M. (1986). How many days of bed rest for acute low back pain. *New England Journal of Medicine* 315: 1064.

Deyo, R.A., Mirza, S.K., Turner, J.A., et al. (2009). Overtreating chronic back pain: Time to back off? *Journal of the American Board of Family Medicine* 22: 62–68.

Downie, A., Hancock, M., Jenkins, H., et al. (2020). How common is imaging for low back pain in primary and emergency care? Systematic review and meta-analysis of over 4 million imaging requests across 21 years. *British Journal of Sports Medicine* 54: 642–651.

Downie, A., Williams, C.M., Henschke, N., et al. (2013). Red flags to screen for malignancy and fracture in patients with low back pain: Systematic review. *British Medical Journal* 347: f7095.

Engel, G.L. (1977). The need for a new medical model: A challenge for biomedicine. *Science (New York, N.Y.)* 196(4286): 129–136.

Flynn, T.W., Smith, B., and Chou, R. (2011). Appropriate use of diagnostic imaging in low back pain: A reminder that unnecessary imaging may do as much harm as good. *The Journal of Orthopaedic and Sports Physical Therapy* 41(11): 838.

GBD 2016 Disease and Injury Incidence and Prevalence Collaborators. (2017). Global, regional, and national incidence, prevalence, and years lived with disability for 328 diseases and injuries for 195 countries, 1990–2016: A systematic analysis for the Global Burden of Disease Study 2016. *Lancet* 390(10100): 1211–1259.

Hertvigsen, J., Hancock, M.J., Kongsted, A., et al. (2018). What low back pain is and why we need to pay attention. *Lancet* 391(10137): 2356–2367.

Hoffman, B.M., Papas, R.K., Chatkoff, D.K., et al. (2007). Meta-analysis of psychological interventions for chronic low back pain. *Health psychology: Official Journal of the Division of Health Psychology, American Psychological Association* 26(1): 1–9.

Hurwitz, E.L., Randhawa, K., Yu, H., et al. (2018). The global spine care initiative: A summary of the global burden of low back and neck pain studies. *European Spine Journal: Official Publication of the European Spine Society, the European Spinal Deformity Society, and the European Section of the Cervical Spine Research Society* 27(Suppl 6): 796–801.

IASP. (2022). https://www.iasp-pain.org/resources/terminology/#pain accessed 18/02/2022.

Jensel, M.C., Brant-Zawadzki, M.N., and Obuchowki, N. (1994). Magnetic resonance imaging of the lumbar spine in people without back pain. *New England Journal of Medicine* 2: 69.

Kalichman, L., Li, L., Kim, D.H., et al. (2008). Facet joint osteoarthritis and low back pain in the community-based population. *Spine* 33: 2560–2565.

Lemmers, G.P, W, v. L., Westert, G.P., et al. (2019). Imaging versus no imaging for low back pain: A systematic review, measuring costs, healthcare utilization and absence from work. *European Spine Journal* 28(5): 937–950.

Loeser, J.D. (1980). Perspectives on pain. In Turner P., Ed., *Clinical pharmacology and therapeutics*. London: Macmillan, 313–316.

Loeser, J.D. (2006). Pain as a disease. In Cervero, F., and Jensen, T.S., Eds., *Handbook of clinical neurology*. London: Elsevier. Chapter 2.

Long, D.M. (1995). Effectiveness of therapies currently employed for persistent low back and leg pain. *Pain Forum* 4: 122.

López-de-Uralde-Villanueva, I., Muñoz-García, D., Gil-Martínez, A., et al. (2016). A systematic review and meta-analysis on the effectiveness of graded activity and graded exposure for chronic nonspecific low back pain. *Pain Medicine* 17: 172–188.

Main, C.J., and Watson, P.J. (1996). Guarded movements: Development of chronicity. *Journal of Musculoskeletal Pain* 4: 163–170.

Malfliet, A., Ickmans, K., Huysmans, E., et al. (2019). Best evidence rehabilitation for chronic pain part 3: Low back pain. *Journal of Clinical Medicine* 8(7): E1063.

Malfliet, A., Kregel, J., Coppieters, I., et al. (2018). Effect of pain neuroscience education combined with cognition-targeted motor control training on chronic spinal pain: A randomized clinical trial. *JAMA Neurology* 75: 808–817.

Maniadakis, N., and Gray, A. (2000). The economic burden of back pain in the UK. *Pain* 84: 95–103.

Melzack, R. (1990). Phantom limbs and the concept of a neuromatrix. *Trends in Neurosciences* 13(3): 88–92.

Meucci, R.D., Fassa, A.G., and Faria, N.M. (2015). Prevalence of chronic low back pain: Systematic review. *Revista de Saude Publica* 49: 73.

Monticone, M., Ferrante, S., Rocca, B., et al. (2013). Long-lasting multidisciplinary program on disability and fear-avoidance behaviors in patients with chronic low back pain: Results of a randomized controlled trial. *Clinical Journal of Pain* 29: 929–938.

Nachemson, A.L. (1992). Newest knowledge of low back pain. *Clinical Orthopaedics* 279: 8.

NICE. (2016). *Low back pain and sciatica in over 16s: Assessment and management*. London: National Institute for Health and Care Excellence.

Norris, C.M. (2020). Back rehabilitation – The 3R's approach. *Journal of Bodywork and Movement Therapies* 24(1): 289–299.

O'Connell, N.E., Cook, C.E., and Wand, B.M., et al. (2016). Clinical guidelines for low back pain: A critical review of consensus and inconsistencies across three major guidelines. *Best Practice & Research: Clinical Rheumatology* 30: 968–980.

Pike, A., Patey, A., Lawrence, R., et al. (2022). Barriers to following imaging guidelines for the treatment and management of patients with low-back pain in primary care: A qualitative assessment guided by the theoretical domains framework. *BMC Primary Care* 23(1): 143.

Roche-Leboucher, G., Petit-Lemanac'h, A., Bontoux, L., et al. (2011). Multidisciplinary intensive functional restoration versus outpatient active physiotherapy in chronic low back pain: a randomized controlled trial. *Spine* 36: 2235–2242.

Sääksjärvi, S., Kerttula, L., et al. (2020). Disc degeneration of young low back pain patients: A prospective 30-year follow-up MRI study. *Spine* 45(19): 1341–1347.

Saal, J.A. (1995). The pathophysiology of painful lumbar disorder. *Spine* 20: 180–183.

Scavone, K.P., Latshaw, R.F., and Rohrar, G.V. (1981). Use of lumbar spine films: Statistical evaluation at a university teaching hospital. *Journal of the American Medical Association* 246: 1105–1108.

Schousboe, J.T. (2016). Epidemiology of vertebral fractures. *Journal of Clinical Densitometry* 19: 8–22.

Smith, B.E., Littlewood, C., and May, S. (2014). An update of stabilisation exercises for low back pain: A systematic review with meta-analysis. *BMC Musculoskeletal Disorders* 15: 416.

Steiger, F., Wirth, B., de Bruin, E.D., et al. (2012). Is a positive clinical outcome after exercise therapy for chronic non-specific low back pain contingent upon a corresponding improvement in the targeted aspect(S) of performance? A systematic review. *European Spine Journal* 21: 575–598.

Tousignant-Laflamme, Y., Martel, M.O., Joshi, A.B., et al. (2017). Rehabilitation management of low back pain – It's time to pull it all together! *Journal of Pain Research* 10: 2373–2385.

Vanti, C., Andreatta, S., Borghi, S., et al. (2019). The effectiveness of walking versus exercise on pain and function in chronic low back pain: A systematic review and meta-analysis of randomized trials. *Disability and Rehabilitation* 41: 622–632.

Vlaeyen, J.W.S., Kole-Snijders, A.M.J., Boeren, R.G.B., and van Eek, H. (1995). Fear of movement/reinjury in chronic low back pain and its relation to behavioural performance. *Pain* 62: 363–372.

Wade, D.T., and Halligan, P.W. (2017). The biopsychosocial model of illness: A model whose time has come. *Clinical Rehabilitation* 31(8): 995–1004.

WHO. (1980). *International classification of impairments, disabilities, and handicaps*. Geneva: World Health Organisation.

WHO. (2011). *World report on disability*. Page 5. Malta: World Health Organization.

Zusman, M. (1998). Structure-oriented beliefs and disability due to back pain. *Australian Journal of Physiotherapy* 44: 13–20.

2

STRENGTH AND CONDITIONING IN REHABILITATION

Principles of training

There are a variety of underlying principles to training. When we train, the body will change in predictable ways, with some variety between individuals depending on variables such as exercise history and medical conditions. Table 2.1 shows some commonly quoted exercise principles which we will look at in more detail below.

Response and adaptation

When a subject exercises, the body changes in two important ways (Norris 2013). The first is immediate and is called the exercise *response*. Increased heart and breathing rate, sweat response, and blood flow change are all examples of a short-term exercise response which a user will be aware of themselves. When the exercise session stops, these processes gradually slow down and the body returns to its normal physiological level. If the exercise bout is repeated, the same changes occur, but over a period of time a person's body becomes better at coping with the exercise. Sweat response is lessened, heart and breathing rates lower and exercise can be maintained for longer periods. The longer-term changes represent an exercise *adaptation* which may not be directed visible, but which can be measured.

> **Definition:**
>
> A *response* is the immediate effect of exercise on the body, while *adaptation* represents longer term and more enduring body changes.

DOI: 10.4324/9781003366188-2

TABLE 2.1 The principles of training

Principle	Meaning
Individuality	Each person will respond differently to a stimulus (physical or mental)
Specificity	SAID principle (Specific Adaptation to Imposed Demand). Change (adaptation) will match (be specific to) demand imposed by an exercise
Adaptability	Over time body will become accustomed (accommodate) to a physical stress and will plateau
Overload	Stress imposed must be greater than that which is normally used to
Progression	As adaption occurs, stress must increase to continue to challenge the body
Recovery	Time to recover for adaption to occur—overreaching may progress to overtraining if insufficient recovery allowed.
Reversibility	Performance improvements will be lost if physical stress is taken away or recovery insufficient

Source: Adapted from Norris (2019).

Supercompensation

To achieve a training effect (adaptation), the body must be *overloaded*, that is, exposed to a physical stress which is greater than that encountered in everyday living. The reaction to this training stress is *catabolism*, the breakdown of metabolic fuels or tissues. When muscle is the tissue being studied, the phenomenon is called *Exercise Induced Muscle Damage* (EIMD). Following this catabolic response, the tissues react by adapting and becoming better suited to coping with the imposed stress; this adaptation is known as *anabolism* and involves tissue changes and growth. With training, the anabolic effect is excessive, causing the tissues to grow stronger, a process called *supercompensation*.

> **Keypoint:**
>
> *Catabolism* is the breakdown of body tissues; *anabolism* is the build-up of tissues or products.

General adaptation syndrome

Adaptation to exercise (a physical stress) can be understood through the principles of the General Adaptation Syndrome (GAS) first described by the Hungarian endocrinologist Hans Selye in the 1930s with reference to psychological stress. Plotting time against resistance to stress Figure 2.1a the GAS consists of three phases. The first is the alarm phase as the body reacts by preparing its 'fight or flight' mechanisms releasing hormones such as adrenalin and cortisol, two of the

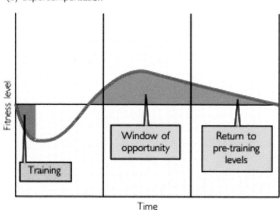

(a) General Adaption Syndrome (GAS)

(b) Supercompensation

FIGURE 2.1   General adaptation syndrome (from CGET). (a) General adaption syndrome (GAS). (b) Supercompensation.

so-called stress hormones. This first phase of the GAS is negative because the physiological state of the body decreases. Phase two is the resistance phase when the body tries to cope with the imposed stress, so this phase is positive. The final phase is exhaustion (again negative) when the body has depleted its coping mechanisms and may suffer from conditions such as high blood pressure or ulcers, for example. The key to the GAS is that the body can either positively adapt (called *Eustress*), for example, becoming stronger through weight training or negatively adapt (called *Distress*), for example, by overtraining.

Keypoint:

Eustress is positive adaptation of the body (e.g., becoming stronger). *Distress* is negative adaptation (e.g., overtraining).

The GAS is modified slightly when the imposed stress is exercise. The initial physical stress (exercise) is an overload which is at a higher level than that normally encountered. This stress causes body reactions which are physiological, biomechanical, and psychological in nature. Immediately after training, fatigue in all three areas causes the body to be less able to react to an imposed stressor. For example, following heavy weight training muscles feel exhausted and the mind lacks motivation (Figure 2.1b). The body gradually recovers, a process which may take one or two days and even up to a week if the imposed stress is very great (running a marathon, for example). As the body adapts, pre-exercise levels are restored, but the adaptation continues (supercompensation) so that the body becomes better equipped to cope with the imposed stress. During this period further exercise causes the whole cycle to be repeated but this time as the starting point (fitness level) is higher, the compensation is greater. For this reason, the period of supercompensation is often referred to as the *window of opportunity*. Two keypoints emerge from this process. The first is that the body must be given the opportunity to adapt with adequate rest and good nutrition, for example. The second is that the next training period must occur during the window of opportunity. Clearly, if the next training period occurs too soon the body will not have finished adapting, but if it occurs too late, the body will have returned to pre-training fitness levels.

Keypoint:

Following training, the body must be given time to recovery for maximal tissue adaptation to occur.

The overload is made up of four factors described by the simple pneumonic FITT, standing for *Frequency, Intensity, Time, and Type.* Together, these variables make up the training volume representing the total amount of exercise/work performed as shown in Table 2.1 For example, heavy weight training is clearly harder than light jogging (exercise type), while slow walking is easier than fast walking (intensity). Performing a trunk curl exercise every hour throughout the day is harder than performing it every other day (frequency) and performing 10 reps is easier than 100 reps (duration). Performing the trunk curl every day for 3 sets of 10 reps gives a larger training volume than performing it 3 times each week for 2 sets of 12 reps.

Keypoint:

Training volume is the total amount of work performed during an exercise by combining the training variables frequency, intensity, time, and type.

As the body habituates (gets used to) the training stimulus, the stimulus must increase or progress. Failing to change the stimulus can lead to the subject's fitness gains plateauing. As an example, a subject may be able to lift a 10 kg for 10 repetitions (reps) before fatigue. If they practise this action three times per week, after one or two weeks they will be able to perform a greater number of repetitions before fatigue sets in. If they can perform 15 or 16 reps, to continue to practise 10 reps with the same 10 kg weight will not stimulate continued adaptation. The overload needs to progress, and they may lift 12 kg for 10 reps, for example. As we will see later, increasing the resistance (weight in this case) is only one way of progressing. Changing the action, altering the timing or rest period, changing the type of muscle work are all examples of progressing an overload.

> **Keypoint:**
>
> To continue to gain benefits from training, the body must be subjected to a progressive overload.

Fitness-fatigue model

The GAS model is expanded and modified slightly in the Fitness-Fatigue or two-factor model (Bannister 1991). Here, an emphasis is placed on the different physiological responses to varying training stresses. Strength-based athletes will see changes in muscle cross sectional area (CSA), contractile protein, and metabolic changes, for example, while endurance-based athletes will likely experience changes in both cardiopulmonary and muscular factors such as capillary density, mitochondrial density, and oxygen consumption (Chiu and Barnes 2003). Following training, as with the GAS model the response may be either positive or negative. The fitness after effect (positive) and fatigue after effect (negative) interact to result in a performance change at both short and long term.

When we talk about fatigue, what exactly do we mean? Fatigue is both physical and mental. We can talk about fatigue due to muscle damage, but also that due to neural changes both centrally within the central nervous system (CNS) and peripherally. CNS changes would include things like lack of motivation, while peripheral changes can refer to things such as motor unit recruitment or muscle synchronisation changes.

> **Definition:**
>
> A *motor unit* consists of a single neuron and the muscle fibres it supplies and is the basic functional unit of skeletal muscle. *Muscle synchronisation* is the firing of motor units at the same time.

However, neural changes can also be positive of course. Muscle post-activation potentiation (PAP) is a short-term increase in force production following light training. A typical example would be the increase in vertical jump height seen by performing a set of light (bodyweight) squats prior to vertical jump testing. The effect is to 'remind' the leg muscles how to work most effectively.

As mentioned above, the GAS model is an adaptation of a model originally designed to illustrate changes due to psychological stress. These changes are largely instigated by the hypothalamic-pituitary-adrenal (HPA) axis and underlie the fight or flight response. The fitness-fatigue model is an adaptation of this to better suit the changes typically seen following physical training such as strength work which may not necessarily be only a result in HPA axis changes.

Definition:

The hypothalamic-pituitary-adrenal (HPA) axis refers to the interaction between the *hypothalamus*, and *pituitary* glands located above the brainstem, with the *adrenal* glands found on top of the kidneys.

Reversibility

Failure to overload tissue sufficiently will result in loss of the benefits gained as part of the training adaptation, a process called *detraining*. Training effects are not permanent. The motor system adapts to the level (overload) and type (specificity) of stress that is imposed on it. If the stress is removed, and training ceases, the motor system will again adapt to the new, now lower, level of stress, and detraining will occur. This transient nature of training adaptation is known as the *reversibility* principle.

Definition:

The *reversibility principle* describes the gradual loss of training effects when the training overload is reduced, a process referred to as detraining.

However, sometimes athletes especially, can believe that even a single training session dropped, or day lost will result in detraining, and this is far from the truth. Detraining must be differentiated from *tapering*. Tapering involves a gradual reduction in training volume prior to a competition to give a physical and psychological break from the physical and mental demands of continuous training. Tapering allows muscle to repair micro-damage (EIMD see above) caused through intense training (eccentric actions especially) and to replenish energy stores.

Detraining sees the loss of the effects of training, but in a much slower rate than injury or immobilisation. The detrained athlete will show muscle wasting (atrophy) and this will be more noticeable in those who are highly trained because they obviously have more to lose. Atrophy is accompanied by reductions in muscle strength and endurance. Endurance begins to reduce after two weeks due to a reduction in oxygen usage capacity. Loss of cardiorespiratory endurance is greater over a similar period than strength which requires only minimal stimulation to maintain it, while flexibility losses occur quite quickly (see Norris 2019).

The reversibility principle has important clinical implications. If the body is not subjected to physical stress, detraining will occur and if enforced rest is imposed due to pain or pathology, disuse atrophy will typically result. Failure of the muscular system to support joints can change joint loading, increasing strain on the non-contractile tissues (ligaments, joint capsule) integral to a joint. This altered loading may drive inflammation and/or pain by irritating pain sensitive structures. The result can be pain from deconditioning rather than pathology itself.

Definition:

Detraining typically refers to a lack of physical stimulus greater than normal daily actions, while *deconditioning* is a lack of stimulus above a resting level.

CASE NOTE

A forty-six-year-old male complained of low back pain made worse through bending. He had a history of bending while gardening six months ago and woke with severe pain the next morning. His pain was into his right leg travelling into the buttock and back of his leg to knee level. At the time all movements seemed painful, but after 4 days his leg pain had eased, and he was able to sleep without being disturbed by pain. His pain gradually subsided and after 1 month it had gone to general movements throughout the day. Now, he reported pain following a weekend doing DIY where he was painting at low levels. On examination, he was only able to bend forwards to knee level before he experienced low back pain, which he scored as 7/10. On closer inspection, spinal flexion occurred mostly at high lumbar and thoracic regions, with a flat appearance to the lower lumbar region. All other spinal movements were painless, and his neurological examination was unremarkable. When encouraged to perform repeated bending actions (lumbar and hip flexion) he was able to gradually bend further to mid shin, and his pain intensity lessened to 4/10 on a pain scale. It was hypothesised that his original spinal pathology had now cleared, and his symptoms and movement limitation was due to deconditioning, most notably stiffness to lumbar flexion and weakness of the hip and spinal extensor muscles. The subject was encouraged to use controlled flexion of the spine, initially bending using a rolling action (modified Pilates rolldown) from standing to below knee level. This was performed for 5 repetitions, followed by tall standing (standing upright for 30–60s) and then a second set of 5 reps bending. The two sets of 5 reps bending were repeated in the morning and evening and the subject was encouraged to focus on bending the spine as though curling the trunk around a beachball. After 7 days the subject's motion range had increased, flexion occurred throughout the lumbar spine and pain in the back eased with repetition. He was given a supervised progressive exercise programme focussing on whole body exercise with spinal flexion incorporated into the programme. After 1 month, at following-up, the patient reported he was pain free and able to participate in all his normal activities without limitation.

Individuality

Training responses are not equal between individuals, in the same way that treatment effects are largely patient specific. Changes which relate to a specific person represent individuality. Each person reacts slightly differently to training stimuli due to differences in growth rate (genetically determined), and regulation of the cardiovascular and respiratory systems, for example. In addition, muscular growth and performance differs markedly due to cellular growth rate and metabolic variation.

Individuality explains why when two people begin a gym programme, one may progress quite rapidly (high responder) while the other may struggle to make gains (low responder). The main reason for individuality is hereditary. The principle of individuality underlies successful exercise prescription. Variation in tissue adaptation, neural, cardiopulmonary, and endocrine changes, and psychology dictate that subjects will often respond differently to similar exercise bouts.

Definition:

Individuality is the familial and/or genetically determined aspect of an exercise response or adaptation.

With physical training then, we are trying to challenge the body to gain a positive response. However, sometimes the balance between training and recovery is lost and the result is negative. When this occurs, we call it *overtraining*, or officially an overtraining syndrome (OTS).

After a training bout some fatigue is desirable, and this acute (short term) fatigue leads to an increase in performance. However, if the training volume is too great, or the recovery period between training bouts too brief, subjects will see a temporary reduction in performance, a feature called *overreaching*. A brief reduction in performance occurs which requires a longer recovery period—typically between 5 and 10 days. If recovery is not adequate and further training continues, the progression is to overtraining. Recovery in this case may take many months.

Typical symptoms of overtraining include changes to performance, alteration in physiological measures (respiration, sleep disturbance, change to eating patterns), psychological changes (mood change, depression), impaired immune function (increase rate of respiratory infection), and changes to blood biochemistry (hormone level changes, changes to muscle and blood chemistry). For more details on OTS, see Norris (2019) pages 63–65.

Keypoint:

Symptoms of overtraining can include reduced performance, sleep disturbance, change in eating patterns, alteration in mood states, impaired immune function, and changes in blood biochemistry.

Components of fitness

What do we mean by the term fitness? People often talk about getting fit after a prolonged period of inactivity or keeping fit if they have an inactive job. After an injury such as a broken leg, we may lose fitness through enforced rest, but what does this all mean? Physical fitness can be viewed as a set of attributes that relate to the ability of a subject to perform physical activity, it is really the ability of a person to function efficiently and effectively in demanding situations and is usually closely related to health.

Fitness can be thought of as a continuum from optimal fitness at one side through average fitness to complete lack of fitness and eventually death. The exact components of fitness required to make an individual optimally efficient and effective will be determined largely by the physical activity to be performed and the function required.

Fitness may be subdivided into two types. Task (performance) related fitness is that required for sport, general everyday functions, and occupation (work). Health related fitness includes components which are associated with some aspect of health and wellbeing. Physical training will improve fitness but may not always enhance health. Extreme development of any one of the fitness components, on its own, can upset the delicate balance between the components, and may be detrimental to health. For example, excessive development of flexibility can lead to hyper flexibility and, when strength lags behind, may progress to a reduction in joint stability. Excessive development of strength and hypertrophy may reduce range of motion, leaving a subject 'muscle bound'.

The benefits of exercise are numerous. However, as we have seen above there is a fine balance between training sufficiently hard to gain the effects of overload, but not so hard that the subject overreaches (OR) in the short term or eventually progresses to OTS.

Keypoint:

Task related fitness is that required for sport, everyday function, and occupation. *Health related* fitness includes components associated with some aspect of health and wellbeing.

Fitness components

The fitness components may be conveniently remembered as 'S' factors (Table 2.2). The term *stamina* is used to encompass both cardiopulmonary and local muscle endurance. Cardiopulmonary endurance is associated with a reduced risk of coronary heart disease, but also obviously the most important fitness component in endurance (aerobic) sports such as marathon running. Local muscle endurance is a factor in any sustained activity, especially joint stability or stopping a joint giving way and is the focus of anaerobic metabolism. *Suppleness* (flexibility) and *strength* are concerned with the health of the musculoskeletal system, to maintain both range of movement and joint integrity. The term suppleness used here embraces both flexibility methods such as static (hold), dynamic (moving), and PNF (muscle reflexes) stretching types. Loaded stretching (moving to end range and maintaining the position with bodyweight or resistance) can be seen as forming a bridge between stretching and strength. In addition, suppleness is a blanket term which includes agility (speed, agility, and quickness or SAQ).

Definition:

Agility is an all-encompassing term reflecting rapid direction change, including acceleration and deceleration. It will be influenced by co-factors such as balance, strength, coordination, and skill.

The strength fitness component encompasses muscle contraction and strength types (isometric, concentric, eccentric) used in different strength training methods.

Speed (rate of movement) and power (rate of doing work) are both needed in later stage rehabilitation. *Skill* training is important, not just for sports specific actions, but for the skill of individual movements such as gait re-education or lifting, for example. *Structure* refers to body composition. Variance in body

TABLE 2.2 'S' factors of fitness

'S' factor	Interpretation
Stamina	Cardiovascular and local muscle endurance
Suppleness	Range of motion, static and dynamic flexibility. Agility
Strength	Concentric/eccentric/isometric
Speed	Acceleration & deceleration/Power
Skill	Movement quality/sensorimotor training
Structure	Body composition/anthropometry
Spirit	Psychological fitness/psychosocial aspects of injury
Specificity	Task & sport related requirements

Source: Adapted from Norris (2017).

composition between subjects (for example, limb length) has an important bearing on exercise choice in strength and conditioning (S&C) particularly. Body fat percentage and its relationship to obesity is an important health consideration for cardiopulmonary health and joint loading.

The term *specificity* in sports training means matching training adaptations to sporting requirement. It is more easily understood using the SAID pneumonic standing for Specific Adaptation to Imposed Demand. The change taking place in the body of a subject (*adaptation*) as a result of training (the *imposed demand*) will be determined by the type of training, which is used, and will be *specific* to it.

Specificity certainly applies to strength and power development, but also to the energy systems used while exercising. A particular cardiopulmonary training programme will cause specific training adaptations. Aerobic fitness developed on a cycle ergometer, for example, will differ slightly from that obtained while running. It is important, therefore, that any training matches as accurately as possible the action which the subject will use in a sport in terms of joint range, muscle work, energy system, and skill.

Keypoint:

Specificity of training means that exercise must mirror the actions used subsequently in sport.

The term *spirit* covers the psychological effects of exercise, and several psychological characteristics have also been shown to change as a result of regular exercise. Enhancement of self-confidence, self-esteem, self-efficacy, and body image are seen, together with reductions in anxiety, depression, stress, and tension (Norris 2019).

Definition:

Self-esteem is the degree to which individuals feel good (positive) about themselves. *Body image* is the perception of one's own body and general physical dimensions. *Self-efficacy* is the strength of a subject's belief in their ability to complete tasks and reach goals.

Exercise may create psychological changes in several ways. Exercise participation distracts the subject from stress. Comparisons between exercise, meditation, and distraction show similar reductions in state anxiety, but the effect resulting from exercise appears to last longer and may be important in chronic pain states as well as within the general population. Depression is also affected by exercise. Reductions in noradrenaline (norepinephrine) and serotonin are associated with depressed states in humans, and these same chemicals have been shown to increase with long-term exercise.

As with physical changes, psychological changes due to exercise can be both positive and negative. Exercise addiction, or exercise dependence, is the physiological or psychological dependence on regular exercise. Subjects who are addicted to exercise show symptoms of withdrawal and often uncontrollable craving for a particular exercise type at the expense of other training.

Keypoint:

Subjects who are *addicted* to exercise often show symptoms of withdrawal (mood state change) and cravings for a type of training at the expense of other daily activities.

The experience of exercise for a subject, and the way in which this fits into the rest of his or her life, is one factor which determines whether an exercise becomes addictive. An individual's need for exercise can be either positive or negative. Positive addiction exists when a subject receives some psychological or physical benefit from an activity and can control the activity. The negatively addicted subject is controlled by the activity and will experience severe negative effects (withdrawal) with a missed exercise bout.

Balancing the fitness components

The human body keeps its internal environment balanced through a process of *homeostasis*. Injury or change of use can disrupt this homeostasis leading to a range of mostly biochemical changes.

Definition:

Homeostasis is the process of self-regulation by which a biological system maintains equilibrium by adjusting to conditions it is exposed to.

Excessive (supra-physiological) loading on tissue will cause adaptation through a training response providing there is sufficient time for recovery, as we have seen. A sudden imposition of extreme force, however, may exceed the load capacity of tissue, leading to negative changes which may be termed maladaptation. Similarly, repetitive small forces which occur too frequently may not allow sufficient time for tissue to adapt to the new loading level, in both instances *injury* may result. At the other extreme, too little (sub-physiological) loading, for example, through prolonged rest, also disrupts homeostasis leading to changes such as muscle atrophy and bone mineral loss, reflecting *deconditioning* as mentioned above.

The region of loading between under and over usage has been described as an 'envelope of function' and represents the area of load acceptance (Dye 2005).

Where loading exceeds the capacity of a bodypart, the action can be envisaged as occurring outside the envelope of function, and the tissues may be irritated giving rise to symptoms such as pain and swelling. At this stage reducing or changing loading may restore homeostasis, with a view to later increasing tissue capacity with progressive rehabilitation and elevating the upper limit of the functional envelope (See also Chapter 6).

The aim of rehabilitation is to increase the capacity of the injured tissue, and to offload it by enhancing the strength of surrounding muscle. Tissue capacity may be built with progressive overload, which may be either simple or complex (Cook and Docking 2015). Simple loading targets the specific tissue (for example, the medial collateral ligament of the knee), while complex loading targets the tissue within the context of the whole limb or body region (for example, a squat action). The load chosen for rehabilitation must accurately reflect the type of load the tissue may be placed under during any functional action in daily living or sport. Training specificity of this kind is vital to increase tissue capacity relevant to the subjects' actions (patient centred) rather than increasing capacity to fulfil pre-determined goals (therapist centred).

Progressing and regressing exercise

One of the fundamental principles of exercise is that tissue must be overloaded to enhance its performance. As the tissue adapts and improves, exercise must get harder to continue to offer an adequate challenge. This graduated increase in difficulty is called exercise *progression*. When practicing a rehab programme however, a subject may react poorly to an exercise, and require a reduction in tissue loading called exercise *regression*.

> ### Definition:
>
> *Progressing* an exercise makes it harder, *regressing* an exercise makes it easier.

Most people think of progressing a weight training exercise (resistance) by increasing the weight lifted, and of progressing running (endurance) by running further or faster. In fact, there are several ways to vary exercise intensity (Table 2.3) and we will look at some of the most common below.

Leverage

The first method of progression and one which is often obvious from general life experience is leverage. When you move any part of your body the effective weight of the body part is greatest as the limb gets closer to the horizontal and lessens as it gets further away from the horizontal. Takes as an example a good morning exercise (see Chapter 9). When standing upright leverage is minimal as the body is vertical. If we angle the body forwards to 45 degrees leverage has increased reflected by the vertical distance between the original body line and the centre of the trunk. Note that the leverage is calculated as the horizontal distance rather than simply the length of the spine. As the user angles their body further forwards towards the horizontal, although their spine is obviously the same length the leverage effect is increasing and so the force they would have to produce from their spine and hip muscles must be greater (Figure 2.2).

TABLE 2.3 Aspects of exercise progression

Aspect	Meaning
Leverage	Short/long lever arm. Matching to ROM
Stability	Stable/less stable/unstable
Energy system	Aerobic/anaerobic
Momentum	Acceleration/deceleration in relation to load
Friction	Greater/lesser
Speed of movement	Link to momentum, reaction time, agility
Complexity	Simple or complex task in relation to motor learning
Gravity	Gravity neutral/gravity resisted/gravity assisted
Muscle work	Isometric/concentric/eccentric
Range of motion	Total range and position within range
Starting position	Ease of use and stability
Resistance	Weight, resistance band thickness, machine cam shape

ROM—range of motion.

Source: After Norris (2013).

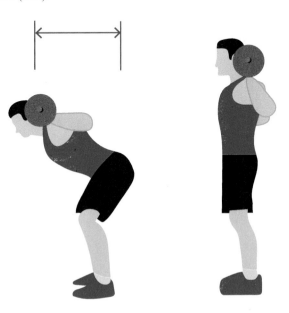

FIGURE 2.2 Leverage during exercise.

A muscle is strongest at its mid-range position (see below). If the point of maximum leverage corresponds to inner or outer range, it can be difficult for a client with weak muscles to move into this range. If they can move into the range, they may need to use a weight that is so light the rest of the range is not taxed. In many modern weight training machines this situation is overcome by using accommodating resistance. This uses a Cam (irregular shaped rotating part of a machine) to alter the resistance to match the force output of the moving joint. Although this can be helpful there are two disadvantages. First, the machine will only suit a single joint, so, for example, a trunk extension machine can't be used for squats, whereas using a free weight such as an Olympic bar both exercises may be performed using the same equipment. Second, an accommodating resistance machine must be adjustable enough to suit different sizes and shape of user. If it is not, the changing resistance may not match the body requirement of each individual user, only a theoretical average user.

Muscle work

Muscle contraction can be concentric (lifting), eccentric (controlled lowering), or isometric (holding). Broadly speaking, concentric actions accelerate (for example, standing up from sitting in a chair) and eccentric actions decelerate (sitting down into the chair). Strength ability (how much you can lift) reduces from eccentric to isometric and finally concentric. Using a chin-up exercise (Chapter 9) as an example, when a user can't perform any more reps, have then step onto a bench and hold themselves with their elbows bent to 90 degrees. This action (isometric hold) may be possible even though they could not lift their bodyweight anymore (concentric). Finally, the user can no longer hold themselves, they may be able to perform 1 or 2 extra reps if their training partner lifts them up and they lower their bodyweight slowly (eccentric). This is a frequently used technique in bodybuilding known as a 'forced repetition', and the lowering (eccentric) portion of the movement is referred to as a 'negative rep'.

The three types of muscle work also have an important place within rehabilitation. Isometric actions in rehab can be used to hold a joint firm and prevent excessive motion. They are the stabilising actions which protect a joint. Building up the amount of time that a client can maintain an isometric contraction (holding time) is often important when re-educating stability following injury. For example, core stability targets the central portion of the body (pelvis and lower back) and has a place in rehab following back injury. After a knee injury stability exercise such as standing on one leg and moving the body without the knee giving way are effective. Eccentric actions are important because they often represent periods when the muscle is controlling movement of a joint as the body is lowering. It is during this type of movement that joints can feel at risk, so training eccentric actions help to prevent this while giving the client confidence. As an example, someone with knee pain often finds it far easier to go upstairs than to come down. Coming down is an eccentric action and each step takes longer than when going up. We can train this action by progressing the lowering action using a step down from a shallow step (stand on a book), then a larger step (wooden yoga brick) and finally a single step on a staircase. In the elderly, eccentric actions also have an important part to play. When sitting down into a low chair, lack of eccentric control (leg and hip muscles) can cause a subject to drop into the chair suddenly. If the chair slides backwards, a fall may result. Rather than simply using a walking aid, strength training to include eccentric control is vital for seniors.

Concentric actions are often the hardest to retrain when a muscle is very weak and, they can be a source of demotivation for clients. To retrain the actions, begin with eccentric actions and follow with assisted concentric. For example, following knee injury which effects a person's ability to lift correctly, a client may find it difficult to straighten their leg in a sitting position (sitting leg extension). Straighten their leg for them and then ask them to lower it slowly, building up the time of lowering (3 seconds, 5 seconds, 10 seconds). Next, ask them to lift (knee extension) while the therapist or trainer supports the lower leg, taking some of its weight. Gradually ease off the lifting pressure as the subject can support more of their own limb weight. This type of active assisted action is the rehab equivalent to the forced reps used by bodybuilders mentioned above.

Keypoint:

Active assisted movements involve a client trying to perform an action which their coach or therapist helps them with. It is the rehab equivalent to a forced rep commonly used in bodybuilding.

Gravity

As we have seen above gravity effects are associated with leverage in exercise. Gravity can also prove useful in the early stages of rehab when it can be utilised to free off a stiff joint or to ease back pain. A useful way to begin a shoulder exercise that would otherwise be stiff and painful is to allow the arm to hang freely while performing a shoulder exercise—this is called a pendular movement as the arm is swinging freely. Hanging from a high bar and allowing gravity to stretch the spine can relieve compression and pain on the lower back and apply traction to de-load the spinal tissues.

The position of the body can also govern how gravity effects it. Gravity obviously acts vertically, so, in standing, gravity is acting directly through the length of the spine as a compression force. When we lead forwards, gravity is now acting at an angle to the spine creating shearing forces and turning forces (torsion).

Definition:

A *shearing* force acts at an angle to the body pushing one part in one direction, and another part of the body in the opposite direction. *Torsion* is a turning force acting on an object due to an applied force. *Compression* force acts through the body when two adjacent bodyparts are aligned to each other.

Compression, shearing, and torsion forces are resisted by soft tissues including muscle to offload joints. However, in an acute stage of an injury often compression is better tolerated than shearing. For example, using a spinal rotation exercise early on in a client's rehab programme is likely to be more comfortable in standing (spine vertical) rather than angled forwards at the hip (spine at 45° to the vertical). The standing position imposes mostly compression forces on the spine while the forward leaning action will also impose shearing and torsion forces.

Stability

Stability becomes more important in balance exercises. For example, standing on one leg (single leg standing) is important during the rehabilitation of lower limb injuries, but will also challenge the trunk musculature which stabilises the spine. Stability is harder when the base of support is narrower. This means that a standing exercise performed with the legs apart is easier in terms of stability than one performed with the legs together, and this in turn, is easier than one performed standing on one leg. In addition, the width of the base of support must be broader in the same direction as the movement which an athlete is carrying out (Figure 2.3) PHOTOS A/B/C/D/E. When an athlete is moving their arms from side to side (shoulder abduction), stability is improved by widening the base of support in this direction of movement by standing with the feet apart. Where the action is forwards and back (shoulder flexion/extension), to become stable if lifting a heavier weight, the base of support must

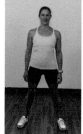 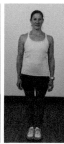 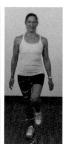 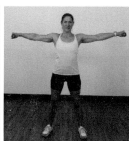 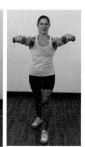

FIGURE 2.3 Stability during exercise.

now be widened in this direction by placing one foot forwards and one back. In each case the area of the base of support is the same, but the direction in which it is widened changes. Stability can also be challenged by making the base of support moveable. Using a balance board effectively moves the floor beneath the client's feet, challenging stability. Balance boards and cushions may be used as can 'D' rolls. Where movement occurs in only one direction (D roll) there is less challenge to stability than when movement can occur in several directions (balance cushion). In each case, an exercise performed in standing on a floor will be made more difficult (challenging stability) by performing the same action on an unstable or 'wobbly' surface.

Range of motion

Range of motion is how far a person is able to move a joint. Normally, throughout the day we only use a limited amount of movement at our joints because we rarely open (extend) or close (flex) the joint fully. This middle part of the joint's movement is called *mid-range*. When we fully open a joint we are moving and stretching the muscles acting over the joint to *outer range*. When we fully close a joint and shorten the muscles, we are moving within *inner range*.

> **Definition:**
>
> At *end-range* a joint is fully open, and at *inner-range* it is closing. *Mid-range* is between these two extremes and is the range used most often in daily living.

The key during rehab is both to use full range movements during training, and to match the movement range with that used in the activities your subject will return to. With low back pain (LBP), there is often a tendency to avoid bending forwards. This is understandable to an extent, as flexion is often an action which may have caused pain in the first place. However, once a subject is pain free and their back has recovered, it is important to use full range movements and that includes maximum flexion in a controlled manor.

Momentum and friction

Momentum is important when performing faster actions particularly. Momentum builds up if you move your arm quickly, for example, meaning that it is difficult to stop moving suddenly. The heavier a limb is, the more momentum it will have, because momentum is the product of mass times velocity, and is often termed mass in motion. If you keep your arm straight and swing it from the shoulder, it has a certain momentum. Perform the same action holding a dumbbell and the momentum is dramatically increased because the mass (limb and dumbbell combined) has increased.

Keypoint:

Momentum can be viewed as mass in motion. It is the product of mass times velocity and is measured in kilogram meters per second (kg.m/s).

Momentum can be important at the very start of rehab and at the very end. At the start, a very stiff joint can often be freed up by using very gentle pulsing action. At the end of rehab, the ability of muscle to work quickly enough to control momentum is important when performing cutting drills (changing direction rapidly) in sport, for example. An exercise can therefore be progressed by performing it faster or using a load and stopping the action or changing direction rapidly to increase the effect of momentum.

Friction may be used to both progress and regress an exercise. Often the resistance setting on home-user static cycles is friction based using either mechanical or electromagnetic braking and increasing the friction setting makes the cycle harder to pedal. Friction can also be used for sliding. Slide training actions can be performed using a pair of thick socks on a shiny surface, or specially designed slide pads. In this case friction is reduced to allow free movement, for example, side-to-side leg actions (abduction).

The friction of a tyre pulled over a sports pitch significantly increases the difficulty of running. The advantage of using this type of resistance over a machine is that the tyre pull makes the action more functional (it closely resembles the action used in sport). Using a sled or prowler (Figure 2.4) is a common action in many gyms. These may be pushed or pulled, and weight added to make them heavier. They rely on friction as resistance to the horizontal motion of the machine.

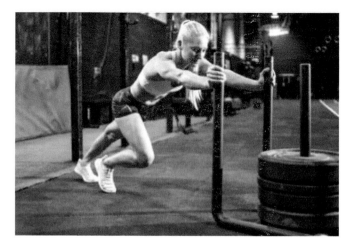

FIGURE 2.4 Prowler exercise.

Definition:

Friction is the resistance force that one surface or object has as it rubs over against another. It is measured in newtons (N).

Designing resistance training programmes

Needs analysis—what does your client really require?

Prior to designing a programme for a subject, we need to determine their requirements. Depending on the instructor's background (therapist, trainer, or coach) this will normally consist of a needs analysis and some type of physical assessment (see Chapter 5). Assessment may be made of a pathology (therapist), movement skill (trainer), or sport technique (coach) and there will be considerable interaction between these three.

Having assessed the subjects' requirements and questioned them on their current exercise practice, it is useful to assess movement skill either using a test battery or formative assessment throughout the subjects training. Aims and objectives are then determined, and a training plan formulated.

The needs analysis looks at both the subject and the task/activity to be performed. Information gained about these two areas serves as a foundation for designing an individualised programme—that is a programme aimed directly at the client, rather than one which is 'off the shelf'. Exercise history and current fitness level give a starting point in terms of skills which the subject possesses, and within this area we should consider injury history and any exercise adaptations required as a result of previous injury or any medical conditions. For example, if a client has a history of an ankle sprain, we may expect some asymmetry in range of motion and/or strength at the ankle and perhaps an alteration in gait pattern when walking or running. We would aim to build in some rehabilitation exercise targeting these areas as part of our general exercise programme. Equally, non-musculoskeletal (MSK) factors may be important and can represent co-morbidities. High blood pressure (hypertension), obesity, degenerative or inflammatory arthropathies, or neurological conditions are all examples of conditions which can benefit from exercise, but which may require exercise adaptations.

Definition:

A *co-morbidity* is the existence of an additional disease or medical conditions in a client, other than the primary area of interest.

Tests of neuromuscular skill level may be relevant and can form part of a functional screen targeting the skill base of the task or sport to be performed. For example, a manual worker with a history of LBP may require screening for lifting and bending actions which mimic their working environment (height/weight/complexity), while a trail runner may need screening of lower-limb alignment in single-leg squat to reflect hill descent on uneven ground. Movement analysis forms an important part of the preparation and gives information on joint movements and muscle work especially. From this the physiological requirements of the task/sport can be implied, and a programme planned accordingly, with specific aims and objectives.

Definition:

An *aim* is what is intended to be achieved (the 'what' of the programme). *Objectives* are the steps required to achieve them (the 'how' of the programme).

An example of needs analysis is shown in Table 2.4 for an inactive female aiming to run a 5k (couch to 5k).

TABLE 2.4 Example needs analysis

Athlete/Subject	*Task/Sports*
Exercise history • The subject regularly walks her dog three miles per day and walks two miles to work three times per week. • She exercises using an aerobic exercise video twice each week and performs a variety of home exercises (mostly abdominal based) on the days when not using the video.	**Movement analysis** • The subject wishes to take part in a 5k charity run and return to playing competitive (club level) badminton
Current fitness level • Aerobic fitness was assessed using the Cooper **12-minute** run test on a treadmill • Power was assessed using a counter movement jump (CMJ)	**Physiological requirements** • A 5k run requires a moderate aerobic fitness level and adequate leg strength and flexibility. • Badminton requires shoulder and spine range of motion, and general speed and power actions.
Neuromuscular skill level • Neuromuscular skill level was determined using a test battery shown in table 3.	**Injury risk** • Overhead reach, low reach, and lunge actions with a badminton racquet will all place stress on the low back and shoulder. • Lunging actions at speed stress the lower limb, with particular emphasis on the calf & Achilles.

Source: After Norris (2019).

TABLE 2.5 Formulating a resistance training programme

Program design variable	Meaning
Needs analysis	Requirements of the user
Exercise selection	Which exercises to pick
Training frequency	How often should they exercise
Exercise order	Which exercises go first and which last
Training load & repetitions	How heavy, and how many
Volume	Combination or reps/sets/weight
Rest & recovery	Between set rest/between workout rest/recovery strategy

Source: After Haff and Triplett (2016).

Following a need analysis, programming can begin. There are many ways to formulate a resistance training programme, and users and trainers often have their favourites. A logical format has been proposed by the National Strength and Conditioning Association (NSCA) which is shown in Table 2.5 which forms a useful starting point.

Exercise selection

Multijoint or single joint

Resistance exercises are commonly grouped into either *Multijoint* or *single joint* movements. Multijoint (core), as the name suggests, move several joints at once and so recruit large areas of muscle mass. Typically, these would be exercises such as squat or deadlift or many of the Olympic lifts such as snatch or clean or their derivatives. Whole body multijoint movements are often referred to as *Primary lifts*, and their component actions as *Assistance lifts*. Single joint (isolation) movements will focus on a movement at one joint. Single joint actions may also be referred to as *Auxiliary lifts* when they are chosen to develop a subject's ability to perform a primary lift (Curtis 2021). For example, single joint exercises such as an arm curl (biceps) or seated arm extension (triceps) action focus on movement at the elbow while the shoulder is held relatively still. A multijoint action such as a shoulder press (military press) will also work the triceps, but in conjunction with movement at the shoulders (Deltoid and Pectorals) while a pull up action sees movement at the elbow, shoulder, chest, and forearm to work flexor muscles at each area. Multijoint actions will work muscles in different planes and angles of pull to offer a more complete muscle stimulation (Schoenfeld and Fisher et al. 2021).

Exercise equipment

Resistance may be offered by several means. The most obvious method is to use weights, but resistance tubes/bands may be incorporated into both gym-based and home exercise programmes. Hydraulic (oil) or pneumatic (air) resistance is often used both for training and rehabilitation. Friction or electromagnetic resistance is often used on cardiopulmonary machines such as static cycles or cross-trainers but will also feature in actions such as a tyre pull or sled-based training. Water may be used for both resistance and buoyancy, effects which may be manipulated using floats or fins.

Where weight is used to provide resistance both free weights (barbell and weight disc) and machines (multistack blocks and pin) are commonly available, and both have advantages and disadvantages. Free weight usage is typically cheaper, and equipment may be used for several actions. In addition, free-weight actions are typically more complex requiring a greater amount of skill with an additional focus on balance and coordination. Machine actions tend to focus on one or two movements and as such a greater variety of machines is required (at greater cost) to offer a full body workout. They generally require less complex movements and often aim to protect the user from unplanned actions. They can be more suitable for less experienced users. The cost of less movement variation is that anatomical and biomechanical considerations require machine adjustment in several axes and planes to suit a variety of users. Machines which fail to offer this level of variation will only suit an average user, not each individual user.

Balanced exercise practice

Where an exercise can emphasis a single action or bodypart, it is possible to miss out part of the body in a workout and fail to give a balanced programme. Table 2.6 lists a useful overview of exercise types which can guide programme design, which is typically categorised into seven fundamental movements. Brace (isometric muscle action to maintain body alignment) is sometimes added to guide programme design and referred to as an 'anti' movement such as anti-extension (abdominal action) or anti-rotation (core work). This categorisation can act as a useful checklist for whole body training over a programme in any single week.

In addition to exercise variety, favouring a single movement over another can be useful to change muscle focus across a joint or bodypart. For example, where

TABLE 2.6 Balanced exercise practice

Movement	Consideration	Example
Push	Pushing from the upper body	Bench press, shoulder press
Pull	Pulling from the upper body	Chin up, lat pull
Squat	Bending at the hips, knees, & ankle	Barbell squat
Lunge	Unilateral leg bend at hips, knees & ankle	Single leg squat
Hinge	Flex at hips, keeping knees & spine straight	Good morning, deadlift
Rotate	Twisting at the hip, shoulder, or spine	Pulley wood chop
Gait	Moving the whole body	Sled or loaded carry

one muscle in a group action is weaker or tighter, asymmetrical strengthening or stretching is often prescribed as part of a corrective exercise approach.

Definition:

Corrective exercise uses an understanding of anatomy, kinesiology, and biomechanics to change movement compensation or tissue imbalances with the aim of enhancing movement quality (adapted from NASM 2022).

Although rehabilitation programmes often use isolation actions with the aim of specific tissue adaptations (for example a knee-to-wall action aiming to increase ankle dorsiflexion range following ankle sprain) the traditional corrective exercise approach is often criticised as it can focus on normal anatomy and/or alignment implying that only this will provide optimal performance. This belief fails to allow for individual differences and adaptability which underlies optimal function without optimal alignment.

Training frequency

Resistance training is typically practised two or three times per week on non-consecutive days for beginners to allow adequate recovery between workouts. This type of exercise usually selects a series of exercises to work the whole body at each session. More experienced users frequently use a *split routine* where certain body regions are worked at each session, and more training days are used. For example, a popular split is to work out four times per week with the upper body worked on two days and the lower body on two days. Other examples of split routines are shown in Table 2.7.

TABLE 2.7 Split routine examples

Sun	Mon	Tues	Wed	Thurs	Fri	Sat	Times per week
REST	Lower body	Upper body	REST	Lower body	Upper body	REST	4
REST	Chest	Lower body	Back	REST	Chest	Lower body	5
	Shoulders			Traps		Shoulders	
	Triceps			Biceps		Triceps	
Chest	Lower body	Shoulders	REST	Chest	Lower body	Shoulders	6
Back		Arms		Back		Arms	

Source: Adapted from Haff and Triplett (2016).

Training frequency will also be affected by the type and intensity of exercise, a more intense workout requiring greater recovery. In running for example, greater distances must be practised less often to allow recovery between training bouts. This will also be affected by the competitive season. When training for a marathon, distance will gradually ramp up as the race approaches, meaning the training frequency must reduce. Early season work may for example comprise 4–6 session per week but as competition approaches (pre-season and in-season) the session number would reduce to 3–4 and eventually 1–3 per week as mileage increases.

Training frequency can also be used to incorporate exercise throughout the day during rehabilitation where time is short, or a subject is less able or willing to use a traditional exercise programme. This is the concept of exercise breaks or *exercise snacking*. The guidelines for physical activity published by the World Health Organization (WHO) recommend 150–300 minutes of moderate activity or 75–150 minus of vigorous activity or any combination of the two (Bull et al. 2020). Previously the minimum duration of exercise was ten minutes, but this has now been deleted from the guidelines as even short bouts of exercise show benefits on health and disease. Circuit training typically uses short periods of exercise to one bodypart immediately followed by another bodypart, or a period of active recovery. In HIIT (High Intensity Interval Training) the intensity of exercise is increased, and the duration reduced meaning that the overall exercise period is shorter. With exercise snacking, the concept is modified. Rather than being consecutive, the exercise bouts are strung out through the day with effects still being significant (Little et al. 2019).

Definition:

Exercise snacking is a method of structuring exercise into short bursts of activity strung out throughout the day.

Exercise order

The order in which exercises are performed during a workout is often determined by the effect one exercise has on the next. Frequently exercises involving a greater number of bodyparts and more muscle mass (multijoint) as practised before those working smaller body areas (single joint). Typically, multijoint power actions such as Olympic lift and their derivatives, squats, and deadlifts are used first as they require a high level of skill which can easily degrade with fatigue. Additionally, multijoint actions require high levels of energy expenditure so leaving them until later in a programme when a subject is fatigued may risk exercise performance degrading.

Where less experienced users are working, alternating upper and lower body exercises gives an opportunity for recovery and forms the basis of a circuit training approach. This type of approach may progress to HIIT (see above) which uses short but intense periods of anaerobic exercise followed by periods of less intense actions for active rest (active recovery). This type of training initially involved 20 seconds of intense (170% VO2 max) exercise followed by 10 seconds of rest for 4 minutes in total with Olympic speedskaters and was referred to a Tabata training after the first author of the paper describing the technique (Tabata et al. 1996). Although this intense type of training is useful for experienced athletes, its intensity must be modified for less fit individuals.

Definition:

Active recovery involves performing low level exercise to maintain blood flow through a body area with the aim of removing metabolic waste products and replenishing energy supplies.

Alternating exercise may also be used with opposite (antagonist) actions such as push and pull. Again, this gives the opportunity for active recovery, but also forms the basis of more advanced programmes where it is called a superset or compound set. *Supersets* involve work two opposing muscle groups (agonist and antagonist), for example, biceps and triceps in the arms, while *compound sets* work the same muscle group with two exercises performed in sequence, for example, a barbell arm curl followed by dumbbell arm curls for the elbow flexor muscles.

Training load, repetitions, and volume

Load (defined as the sum of the forces acting on the body) is simply the amount of weight lifted, but can also be calculated for bands, springs, and other forms of resistance. *Repetitions* are the number of movements of an exercise, for example, the number of times a weight is lifting. Load and repetitions are inversely related, as the load in increased, the number of repetitions (reps) which can be performed reduces. Often load is recorded as a proportion of how much can be lifting in a single repetition or 1RM (rep max). Although this can be a useful method of expressing how a load affects a subject in terms of training intensity, the method for calculating a 1RM can be complex and more usually 3RM or 5RM is used and the 1RM calculated from this using widely available estimation tables and smartphone apps.

Alternative methods of expressing training intensity include reps in reserve (RIR), momentary muscular failure (MMF), and rating of perceived exertion (RPE) scales. *RIR* is a measure of how many more reps could be performed prior to failure. *MMF* simply means that a user can't perform any more reps because the force output produced by the working muscle has reduced so much that is now equals the load being lifted. *RPE* is a measure how hard a subject feels they are working; it is a subjective measure of exercise intensity.

Keypoint:

Reps in reserve (RIR), momentary muscular failure (MMF), and rating of perceived exertion (RPE) are all methods of expressing exercise intensity.

Rep number range and proportional load is typically used to work for different aims. Maximum strength typically requires lower reps (2–5) and higher weight (80–95% 1RM) while muscle size (hypertrophy) uses higher reps (6–10) and therefore lower weight (70–80% 1RM). Endurance is worked using rep range above 15 and resistance in the region of 50–60% 1RM. Hypertrophy can still be produced using lower intensity and higher reps, providing training volume (reps x weight) is matched (Schoenfeld and Fisher et al. 2021).

Rest and recovery

When we train, the body is subjected to loads which stress tissues and as we have seen this causes microscopic damage (see above). The tissue adapts to the load providing sufficient recovery is given, and homeostasis is maintained. Where a load exceeds the body's capacity to adapt or insufficient recovery is given, performance may suffer. Reduction in performance because of training is called over-reaching (see above). Where this training impairment progresses further, overtraining results. Overtraining also results in a reduction in performance, but clinical symptoms such as a change in mood, reduction in immunity, poor sleep, and increase susceptibility to injury may be seen (Norris 2017, Norris 2019).

Rest periods between exercise sets should be sufficient to allow recovery and avoid reducing performance on the subsequent set, but not too long to reduce *potentiation*. Higher load training typically requires longer periods of rest. Recommendations of 2–5 mins rest between sets for Strength training, and 0.5–1.5 mins for hypertrophy have been quoted (Haff and Triplett 2016), but individuals should monitor their own response, with heart rate and breathing rate reducing to comfortable levels.

Definition:

Potentiation (post activation potentiation or PAP) is the increase in muscle force development following a previous contraction of the same muscle.

Acute to chronic workload ratio

Load imposed on a tissue is often monitored using a variety of laboratory devises such as dynamometry or EMG which are not readily available to most subjects in the gym environment of clinic. This type of monitoring measures what happens to a subject from the outside (external load measurement) and may quantify training using sets & reps, poundage lifted, for example. Measurement from within the subject (internal load measurement) assesses physiological and psychological responses to an activity using heart rate, RPE or psychological inventories. While external load gives an understanding of the work completed, internal load determines whether training is creating an appropriate stimulus for optimal biological adaptation. Internal load monitoring is generally more sensitive than external measures in determine both acute and chronic changes to a subject's individual wellbeing (Soligard et al. 2016).

> **Definition:**
>
> *External load measurement* measures load imposed on the body from outside by quantifying load, reps, sets, for example. *Internal load measurement* measures the effect of this load on the load by using physiological or psychological measures.

There is a high correlation between the results of external measurement and the use of an RPE as an internal measure. The RPE is a 10-point scale where the client uses their body sensations to create a perception of how hard they are working. RPE is a measure of exercise intensity at a specific time point and is extended to sessional RPE (sRPE) by multiplying the total time of an exercise session (minutes) by the exercise intensity (RPE score). For example, a 30-minute workout at an RPE intensity of 5/10 would give a sRPE value of 150 units, whereas a slightly longer but more intense workout of 40 minutes at 7/10 would give a sRPE of 280 units, clearly illustrating the difference between the two exercise sessions.

Adding the sRPE values up over a continuous seven-day period gives a value called the acute workload and taking the average of these over a four-week period gives a value for chronic workload. The ratio of these two values, known as the acute to chronic work ratio (ACWR) can be an important determinant of injury risk. If, for example, your sRPE values for a week came to 2,100, and your average to 2,500, your ACWR is 1.19.

ACWR and injury

The ACWR is a useful model of the relationship between changes in training loads. Where chronic load increases slowly but progressively to high levels, and acute load is low, subjects can adapt to the changing workload and the risk of injury is low. However, if acute load exceeds chronic load injury risk is increased, as tissue adaptation may not be sufficient. In general, the body adapts more effectively to relatively small increases or decreases in training volume rather than large fluctuations. High training loads which have been brought about by controlled progression offer a protective effect against injuries by mediating the effect of load on adaptation and increasing tissue capacity. Where the ACWR exceeds

1.5, that is, the load is one-and-a-half times greater than the average during the last four weeks, the likelihood of injury more than doubles.

> **Keypoint:**
>
> The body adapts more effectively to small increases or decreases in training volume rather than large fluctuations.

Research has shown that a 'sweat spot' exists within the centre of the ACWR values, between 0.8 and 1.3 (Gabbett 2016). Values below 0.8 represent undertraining, and those above 1.3 overtraining, and both make indirect (non-contact) injury more likely.

Consideration of both physical (sports/work) and mental loads (psychological well-being) is important when using exercise therapy and sports training. Stress imposed on the body will cause a short-term reaction and a longer-term adaptation (positive) or maladaptation (negative). The effect of training on the body will depend on both training intensity and recovery periods, with positive and negative effects represented as the overtraining continuum. With light training and adequate recovery, acute fatigue is initially seen, followed by functional and non-functional overreaching as training intensity increases and recovery reduces. OTS sees a reduction in sports performance and body function, with subclinical tissue damage, and eventually clinical symptoms. This process is reversed when adequate recovery is given, and tissue remodelling is allowed. Homoeostasis is restored with an increased fitness level and improved sports performance. Maladaptation can be triggered by poor load management interacting with psychological stressors.

In sports, competition may represent a rapid increase in load, and an increased frequency of matches or events has been shown to lead to an increase in injury rates in many studies. In addition, psychological variables such as negative life events, daily hassles, and sports-related stress may increase vulnerability to injuries. As we have seen in Chapter 1 (Table 1.7), the interaction between psychosocial and physical factors is equally important in LBP subjects.

References

Bannister, E.W. (1991). Modelling elite athletic performance. In Mac Dougall, J.D., Wenger, H.A., and Green, H.J., Eds., *Physiological Testing of the High-Performance Athlete*. Champaign, IL: Human Kinetics, 90–93.

Bull, F.C., Al-Ansari, S.S., Biddle, S., et al. (2020). World Health Organization 2020 guidelines on physical activity and sedentary behaviour. *British Journal of Sports Medicine* 54: 1451–1462.

Chiu, L.Z.F., and Barnes, J.L. (2003). The fitness-fatigue model revisited. *Strength and Conditioning Journal* 25(6): 42–51.

Cook, J.L., and Docking, S.I. (2015). "Rehabilitation will increase the 'capacity' of your …insert musculoskeletal tissue here…." Defining 'tissue capacity': A core concept for clinicians. *British Journal of Sports Medicine* 49: 1484–1485.

Curtis, J. (2021). *Strength training. Level 4 Strength and Conditioning course notes.* www.strengthandconditioning.com.

Dye, S. (2005). The pathophysiology of patellofemoral pain – A tissue homeostasis perspective. *Clinical Orthopaedics and Related Research* 436: 100–110.

Gabbett, T.J. (2016). The training-injury prevention paradox: Should athletes be training smarter and harder? *British Journal of Sports Medicine* 50: 273–280.

Haff, G.G., and Triplett, N.T. (2016). Essentials of strength training and conditioning (4th ed). Champaign, IL: Human Kinetics.

Little, J.P., Langley, J., Lee, M., et al. (2019). Sprint exercise snacks: a novel approach to increase aerobic fitness. *European Journal of Applied Physiology* 119: 1203–1212.

NASM. (2022). What is corrective exercise. https://www.nasm.org/continuing-education/fitness-specializations/corrective-exercise-specialist/what-is-corrective-exercise accessed 23rd January.

Norris, C.M. (2013). *The complete guide to Exercise therapy.* London: Bloomsbury.

Norris, C.M. (2017). Injury, tissue capacity and load management. In *Touch* Spring (edition 158): 10–15.

Norris, C.M (2019). Treatment note 2.1 Overtraining syndrome. In *Sports and soft tissue injuries* (5th ed). London: Routledge, 63–65.

Schoenfeld, B., Fisher, J., et al. (2021). Resistance training recommendations to maximize muscle hypertrophy in an athletic population: Position stand of the IUSCA. *International Journal of Strength and Conditioning* 1(1): 94–103.

Soligard, T., Schwellnus, M., Alonso, J.M., et al. (2016). How much is too much? (Part 1) International Olympic Committee consensus statement on load in sport and risk of injury. *British Journal of Sports Medicine* 50(17): 1030–1041.

Tabata, I., Nishimura, K., et al. (1996). Effects of moderate-intensity endurance and high-intensity intermittent training on anaerobic capacity and VO(2max). *Medicine and Science in Sports and Exercise* 28(10): 1327–1330.

3

TEACHING EXERCISE

In this chapter we look at how to teach exercise. Teaching exercise (coaching) will often determine how an exercise is performed and will have important implications for exercise effectiveness in rehabilitation. Often therapists and trainers place great emphasis on which exercises to pick (exercise selection), and how to change these exercises to make them harder (progression) or easier (regression). What is less emphasised in the therapy world, however, is how an exercise is taught, and this is the focus of this chapter.

Learning skilled movements

What is a motor skill?

A motor skill is demonstrated by a person's ability to exert voluntary control over a movement. It involves a variety of body regions to perform a specific task—it is literally the body's capacity to manage the process of movement. Learning how to do this is called motor learning, and this must be differentiated from motor performance. Performance gives a measurable *outcome*, whereas learning is a (relatively permanent) change in *behaviour*.

> **Definition:**
>
> A *motor skill* is an act which involves the use of the body's muscles to perform a specific task.

Acquiring a motor skill involves information processing (Figure 3.1), in many ways similar to the process a computer uses. This view is often termed the

DOI: 10.4324/9781003366188-3

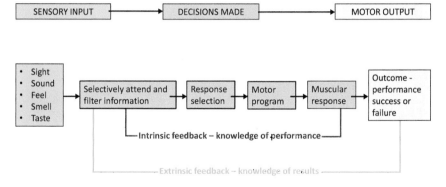

FIGURE 3.1 Information processing model.

'black box' model of information processing. Information is input (sensory information such as touch, vision, hearing), the information is processed, and an output (movement) results. The three stages are classically referred to as stimulus identification, response selection, and response programming (Whiting 1969). Inherent in this model is the process of feedback which can be used to modify performance. Feedback may be intrinsic (within the body) or extrinsic (from the environment).

Processing of information may occur in parallel (at the same time) or in series (one after another). In general, simple properties may be processed in parallel, but more complex features are processed in series, the processing of a second feature having to wait for the completion of the previous one. The hold-up period is classically referred to as the *information processing bottleneck* (Broadbent 1958). The time taken to input and then process information is called the *reaction time*, while the time taken from selecting the required movement to carrying it out is called *response time*. The amount of time it takes to make a decision will increase with the greater number of choices available, a relationship called Hick's Law.

Definition:

Hick's Law states that the more choices users face, the longer it will take them to make a decision.

The process of carrying out motor skills (motor control) begins by identifying a task to be performed and gathering sensory information. At any one time a person is being bombarded with information, and determining which information is important to us involves a process of *reception* (receiving a stimulus, for example, light entering the eye) and *perception* (transporting a signal from the eye to the brain). Determining which signals to ignore and which to notice involves a process of *selective attention*.

Once a signal has been selected, it is processed by the central nervous system (CNS) and an outcome determined. Movements are then carried out (muscle coordination) and sensory feedback is supplied to the CNS to determine how successful the process has been in achieving the movement goal (knowledge of results or KR) or to refine the movement (knowledge of performance or KP). Information about the motor skill may be stored for future performance of the same task to form a *motor programme*.

Definition:

A *motor programme* is a series of commands (sub-routines) organised within the central nervous system (CNS) in a sequence to perform a movement. The programme is stored in long term memory (LTM).

In general, motor programmes are *hierarchical* (some are more important than others), *sequential* (they are performed in a specific order), and they are made up of *sub-routines* (small components which combine to form the whole programme).

Motor control theory

We can see if a person has achieved an action by looking at their performance. However, the process they have gone through to achieve this (motor learning) is less obvious. For this reason, there are several theories of motor control (Table 3.1), which will only be briefly overviewed. Importantly each theory is related in some way, and not all theories will fit in with a coach's teaching style or a subject's learning style. Rather than sticking rigidly to one style, a 'what works best' approach is usually better if it brings the results which are aimed at (Massi and Jeffreys 2021).

At a very basic level, movement can be seen as controlled by reflexes involving sensory reception and motor activation (stimulus-response) via the spinal cord. These fundamental (primitive) reflexes include the stretch reflex (facilitatory) and golgi tendon organ (inhibitory) reflex, both originally described by the work of Sherrington (1906) which underlie our most basic movements. They are most readily seen in babies and young children, and in neurological disorders, but occur in all actions, for example, stepping on a drawing pin (withdrawal reflex). Although important, reflexes are not considered a basic unit of motor behaviour and cannot explain novel movements which occur without a prior sensory stimulus.

Definition:

A *facilitatory* reflex increases neural activity, an *inhibitory* reflex reduces neural activity.

TABLE 3.1 Motor control theories

Motor control theories	Author	Date	Overview	Clinical & training implications
Reflex Theory	Sherrington	1906	• Movement is controlled by stimulus-response. • Reflexes are the basis for movement and are combined into actions to create behaviour.	• Use sensory input to control motor output • Stimulate good reflexes and inhibit undesirable (primitive) reflexes • Rely heavily on Feedback
Hierarchical Theories	Adams	1971	• Cortical centres control movement in a top-down manner. • Sensory feedback is needed and used to control the movement.	• Identify & prevent primitive reflexes • Normalise tone and facilitate desired movement patterns • Use neuro-developmental Sequences
Dynamic Systems Theory	Bernstein	1967	• Movement emerges to control degrees of freedom. • Patterns of movements self-organise. • Functional synergies are developed through practice and experience.	• Movement is an emergent property from the interaction of multiple elements. • Understand the physical & dynamic properties of the body.
Motor Programme Theory	Schmidt	1976	• Adaptive motor programmes (MPs) and generalised motor programmes (GMPs) control actions with common characteristics. • Higher-level MPs store rules for generating movements.	• Abnormal Movement may be reflex linked or include abnormalities in higher-level motor programmes. • Retrain movements important to a functional task, do not re-educate muscles in isolation
Ecological Theories	Gibson & Pick	2000	• Person/task/environment interact to influence motor behaviour and learning • Motivation to solve problems and accomplish a movement goal facilitates learning.	• Help subject explore multiple ways to achieve a functional task by discovering the best solution for them.

Source: Data from: https://www.physio-pedia.com/Motor_Control_and_Learning. Accessed Jan 2022, Shumway-Cook and Woollacott (2017), Massis and Jeffreys (2021), Schmidt and Lee (2011).

The nervous system is organised hierarchically (brain, spinal cord, peripheral nerves) and top down or hierarchical theories were pioneered by Adams (1971) with reference to the *closed-loop theory* of motor control. In this theory, an action is carried out using a pre-structured programme with central control. Information about how the action was performed and what it achieved is used to modify the action before it is repeated and correct for any errors. Using the closed-loop theory for learning requires repeated performance of the same action with errors simply reinforcing incorrect learning if the error does not result in movement modification. Importantly changes are dependent on there being sufficient time to alter the input and make any changes required.

Several other motor control theories exist, including *Dynamic systems theory* (DST) which views the body as a mechanical system with several degrees of freedom which need to be controlled (Bernstein 1967). Control is obtained through CNS hierarchy acting on muscle synergies and joint actions, to self-organise the body systems in response to environmental conditions. There is a reduction in emphasis on the CNS and an increased importance placed on physical explanations for movement, with the system always seeking stability.

Schema theory (Schmidt 1975) is one of the most used theories and proposes the formation of a generalised motor programme (GMP). This consists of a set of motor commands or template that is retrieved from long term memory (LTM) and then adapted to each specific task requirement. For example, when teaching an athlete to perform a zigzag run, their brain would retrieve the GMP for a running action and simply modify it rather than learning a zigzag run as a novel action. The GMP contains two types of information (Fairbrother 2010). The first type is related to aspects of the schema which do not change between performances of similar actions. In our run, foot contact and knee lift will occur in some fashion whether we run straight, side to side or zigzag. The second information type is that which will change between each performance such as range of motion, force, and speed, for example, which will vary depending on the type of run we are completing.

The *ecological theory* proposed by Gibson and Pick (2000) views interaction between the task, the environment, and the individual as the basis for motor control. Learning is driven by the need to solve a motor problem to achieve a desired movement goal. The brain and body work together based on what the brain views as possible.

Stages of motor learning

The practical implications of the motor learning models are the most important factor with reference to training and rehabilitation. Subjects often pass through distinct but interrelated stages as they practise. A three-stage model (first proposed by Fitts and Posner 1967) is commonly used and has implications for coaching and exercise practice (Table 3.2).

During the *first stage* (Cognitive) the aim is understanding what is required for an action. The process is cognitive (thinking) rather than motor (doing) in nature, and hence the title of this learning stage. The subject is learning what to do (and importantly, what not to do), and how to do it. Environmental cues which later will go unnoticed are important to this early stage of learning. They provide an important frame of reference for building the new skill. For example, when learning a new dance step, a person will often focus attention on the foot position, which they later take for granted.

In this stage, movements will be poorly coordinated. The subject must concentrate intensely and will therefore tire easily. The therapist can assist by

TABLE 3.2 Stages of motor learning

Stage of learning		
Stage (I)—understanding	*Stage (II)—effective movement*	*Stage (III)—automatic action*
Understanding what is required from action	Refine action	Less attention required
Environmental cues important	Able to recognise own mistakes	Movement seems to 'run by itself'
Movements poorly coordinated	Movements more consistent and efficient	Speed of movement increased
Demonstration and movement cueing important	Energy expenditure lower	
Practical implication		
Split complex movement sequences into simple components	Correct movement pattern when/if it erodes	Distract athlete to ensure less attention is used
Increase movement awareness by cueing	Stop if athlete becomes fatigued	Progress speed of movement while maintain accuracy
Use palpation and passive movement to facilitate learning	Link simple actions together into sequences	Increase repetitions
Slow precise actions	Reduce environmental cues	Alter environment cues
Progress only when athlete can perform action independently of therapist	Increase repetitions as endurance improves	Perform multiple actions
	Require athlete to recognise their own mistakes (self-monitoring)	

From: Norris (2019).

providing clear instructions and feedback. Complex actions should be split up into more simple components (see below). Demonstration of the movement is important, and the athlete will need constant coaching and correction of the skill to prevent them practising mistakes and reinforcing undesirable technique. Cueing is important in the cognitive stage of motor learning as it helps to paint a mental picture of an action in terms which a subject can easily understand.

The *second stage* of learning (associative or motor) is the stage of effective movement, when the subject will try to make the motor programme more precise and refine the action. It is as though the original clumsy action is 'whittled down' or 'sculpted' to a smoother defined movement. Through practice, the subject is now able to recognise mistakes, and so self-practice (unsupervised) can now be allowed, and a home exercise programme (HEP) developed.

The dependence on visual and verbal *external* cues (stage I) now gradually gives way to the reliance on proprioceptive and kinaesthetic *internal* information. Movements become more consistent, and the subject can work on the finer details of an action. As the action becomes more efficient, energy expenditure is reduced because the subject does not have to work as hard to produce the action. Environmental cues are used for timing and as anticipation develops, movements become smoother and less rushed.

Keypoint:

As a motor skill becomes more efficient, energy expenditure is reduced, and movements become smoother.

The individual movement sequences used in stage I are now linked together to give a longer skill sequence. The actions must still be slow and precise, with progression made only when the movement sequence is correct.

The *third stage* (automatic or autonomous) sees the action appearing to 'run by itself' and become automatic or 'grooved' in the vernacular. This may take months or years in some cases and is seen in elite athletes with sports skills. Movements in this stage demand less attention to perform and so the subject can undertake other actions at the same time. The speed of the movement may be increased, and functions such as muscle reaction time become important. Here, the body is challenged (for example, knocking it off balance) and the subject must react quickly with appropriate changes in posture and movements. This type of final training is used with balance balls and gym balls, for example.

The three stages may also be represented in terms of degrees of freedom described in DST detailed above. Remember DST viewed the body as a mechanical system with several degrees of freedom which needed to be controlled by the body self-organising. In the first stage (cognitive) the required action must be simplified and so the degrees of freedom are reduced. In stage two (motor) movement can be varied increasingly so the degrees of freedom are increasing.

In the autonomous (stage 3) stage more degrees of freedom are available and so other actions can be carried out because the primary action has been learnt so well it does not require focussed attention.

> **CASE NOTE**
> A 60-year-old female presented with hip pain following a fall. Following physiotherapy management her pain levels had reduced sufficiently to begin exercise, and a sit-to-stand (STS) exercise was chosen. Following the injury, she was nervous about sitting without holding onto something, and was unable to stand from a chair without rocking forwards and backwards several times to build momentum. Initially the STS was demonstrated to her with the therapist showing a face on and side on view. The need to draw the feet back and lean forwards was emphasised with the cue 'nose over your toes' to facilitate *understanding* (stage 1). The exercise was begun by having her hold the therapists' hands and initially sit down onto the chair and then stand up during which the therapists gently pulled her hands forwards to encourage anterior bodysway. As she began to *understand* (stage 2) what was required the hand position was changed so she touched but could not grip the therapists' hands. Finally, no hand contact was made, she simply reached forwards towards the therapists' hands which were held up in front of her. Over several treatment sessions leg strength was built up and confidence gained until the patient was able to perform the STS action independently. Finally, to demonstrate *automatic* (stage 3) action a soft foam ball was thrown towards her (initially using a 3-2-1 count), and she would stand up to catch the ball. Finally, the count was dropped, and she had to predict when the ball would arrive having been thrown towards her, and when she would need to stand.

How do we learn a physical action?

As has been mentioned above, we can measure what has been learnt but it is more difficult to determine *how* we learnt it. What should we do to help a person learn? Learning methods have been distilled down to main six types (Table 3.3). *Explicit* learning is traditional coaching where a coach gives an instruction, and the subject performs the described action. It can be especially useful at the start of a coaching programme where the user has little idea of what is required of them. *Implicit* learning involves performing one action and learning about another without realising it. For example, passing a football may be used to enhance single leg balance in an older person. *Physical practice* is simply repeating an action until it is learnt, but in this context the action is chosen by the subject. *Mental practice* (imagery) involves picturing an action to get it clear in the mind and is usually done in a relaxed state. This type of learning can have good results where someone is fearful of performing an action, for example. *Observation* is typically seen in young children where they see an older sibling perform an action and try

TABLE 3.3 Learning methods

Method	Description
Explicit	Being taught what to do
Implicit	Doing one action and learning about another without being aware
Physical practice	Subject chooses what they want to do
Mental practice	Imagining a skill being learnt
Observation	Imitating the action of another person
Trial & error	Try several methods of performing an action and decide which works best.

Source: Data from Massis and Jeffreys (2021).

to copy it, and this may be enhanced in adults using video playback. *Trial and error* occurs when someone performs an action in several ways and decides which works best. In the therapy world this is especially useful as it leads to shared decision-making where the subject and the therapist both have an input into what is done and how it is done.

Effective exercise teaching

We have seen that learning motor tasks involves processing sensory input and creating a habitual link between actions to form a motor programme of some type. We now focus on the teaching (coaching) aspect of exercise. Once we have selected an exercise for a subject, how do we help them achieve a satisfactory performance?

Simplifying movements

Exercise teaching will often begin with a demonstration of the exercise, either in its entirety (whole task) or split up into smaller components (part task) (Hasher 1971, Wightman and Lintern 1985). Teaching the exercise in a single unit, called whole task training is generally more suitable for simple tasks, whereas splitting the task up into several components to perform part-task training is often more suited to complex tasks. The overall aim of this type of training is to improve learning efficiency and make learning a task easier.

Three types of part-task training are typically used—Segmentation, Fractionation, and Simplification (Table 3.4).

> **Keypoint:**
>
> Part-task training may be practised using *segmentation, fractionation,* or *simplification.*

TABLE 3.4 Part-task training

Segmentation	Fractionation	Simplification
A procedure that *partitions* **on temporal (timing) or spatial (position) dimensions.**	Splits a task up into components (sub-tasks), where two or more subtasks are executed *simultaneously*.	A procedure in which a difficult task is made easier by *adjusting* one or more of the task characteristics.

Source: Data from Wightman and Lintern (1985).

Segmentation may be used where an action can be logically divided because the components have a definite start or finish. The individual components (sub-tasks) each have an identifiable end point and so may be practised separately and in any order. For example, a tennis serve could be divided into an overhead throw of the ball, the overhead swing of the racquet, and finally a step forward while bringing the racquet head down. When teaching a group, it would be possible to teach the overhead throw separately focusing on throw height and angle, for example. *Fractionation* is better used when the part tasks are carried out at the same time (simultaneous execution of sub-tasks). For example, in a push-press lift in the gym (pressing the bar overhead from the sternum, see Chapter 9) the knees must bend to absorb the shock of the bar as it descends. Both actions must occur at the same time but may be emphasised separately. *Simplification* is making a complex task easier by taking one aspect of it away. For example, a squat action in the gym using a free weight bar may be simplified by performing the same action on a Smith frame, a unit which allows the bar to move vertically but not forwards or back for a great distance.

Once several sub-tasks have been learnt, they may put back together (integrated). Often two or three sub-tasks will be combined and practised. Once learnt, more sub-tasks may be combined until the whole task is practised in its entirety.

Demonstrating movements

'A picture paints a thousand words' is an adage frequently used in education. Talking about or describing an exercise using instructions alone is often far less effective than simply demonstrating the movement. Movements may be demonstrated as a whole to give a general overview of an action, or in parts. Often it is useful to demonstrate the whole movement first and then demonstrate the component to be practised again. Demonstration should be used from multiple angles to facilitate viewing. Using a front on, side or, or back towards stance to demonstrate an action in an exercise class, for example, is a common and effective exercise teaching method.

The use of vision to cue (see below) an exercise is a vital part of teaching, but what if you can't personally perform the action yourself? This will often occur when teaching, as an elite athlete, for example, would often be able to perform an action better than a coach. Using another subject to demonstrate the action or showing a video of the exercise technique are both useful alternatives.

Video is also extremely valuable for technique analysis and feedback both following an action and during its execution. Use of smartphones and tablets make this type of feedback easily accessible, and several apps are available to augment movement analysis using slow motion replay and grid overlays.

Cueing

A cue is a signal which prompts a subject to engage in a specific action. It is a trigger to encourage movement in a certain way. Cues may be visual (seeing), verbal (spoken), auditory (hearing), or tactile (feeling) and often a combination of cues works best, a technique called *multisensory cueing*.

> ### Definition:
>
> *Multisensory cueing* is the use of cues targeted at several body senses.

If we take a hip hitch (standing leg shortening) movement as an example, although this action is familiar to an instructor, it is most likely completely new to a subject being taught. If the action is demonstrated too quickly, it will be difficult for the subject to work out what is required for successful performance of the exercise. Lots of different parts of the body are moving, in quite subtle ways. If the instructor is dressed in shorts the subject can see the movement clearly, so *visual cues* are being given. Slowing the action down and splitting it up to using part-task training makes learning easier. For example, beginning by focussing just on the pelvis, using this single point of focus to the exclusion of all others is helpful. As an instructor, demonstrate by pointing directly at your own hip and pelvis, telling the subject that your pelvis is lifting, and you are keeping your leg straight. The action is in the frontal plane so placing your back against a wall will emphasise this. In addition, when your subject practises, using a back to wall starting position reduces the chance of them twisting by rotating the lumbar spine or moving around the weight bearing hip. By removing these actions, we are using *simplification*, a type of part-task training (see above).

As the pelvic action (side flexion) occurs, we must make sure that the leg on the non-weight bearing side (the one which is being pulled up or hitching) stays straight so that the leg shortening action we are aiming for occurs using pelvic movement and is not an apparent (but false) shortening using knee flexion. We begin by focussing attention on the two actions separately (*Fractionation* part-task training). Once each individual movement (pelvic side flexion and leg bracing) is learnt and can be reproduced, the two can be combined (integrated) into a single hip hitch movement.

Tactile cueing (touch) may be used to focus attention on each bodypart in turn. The instructor can place one hand on the pelvic rim (iliac crest) to encourage drawing it upwards. Using the flat of the hand rather than gripping is better as subjects are often ticklish, and make sure you ask the subject's permission before touching as the pelvis is an intimate body area. It is often useful for the subject to also use their own hand for self-practice as again it focusses the mind on one action. Once the subject can reproduce the pelvic lift accurately, change from tactile to *verbal cueing*. Remove your hand, stand back, and use a single word instruction such as 'lift' or 'pull' for simplicity. Tactile cueing may again be used to ensure that the knee remains locked. This may take the form of pressing into the thigh muscles (quadriceps) to ensure knee bracing. Touching, gripping, shaking, and taping are all useful forms of muscle facilitation which are used in neurological physiotherapy and transfer well to exercise instruction.

Definition:

Muscle facilitation is a method of encouraging muscle contraction by increasing sensory stimulation to the muscle.

Once each action is mastered separately, the two are combined (integrated) and the subject can move away from the wall to practise the hip hitching action unsupported.

In addition to our visual and tactile cues, we can also use *verbal or auditory cues*. Verbal cues use words to describe the exercise, and both the choice of words and the way they are expressed can be important. Auditory cues use sounds such as a metronome for timing/pace or clapping the hands to signal the beginning or change point of an exercise.

Cueing is clearly giving information to a subject, and that information can be classed as feedback. If it is given at the same time as the action is performed, it is termed *concurrent*, but if it is given at the end of a performance, it is called *terminal* feedback. Examples of terminal feedback would be talking about a subject's performance, what they got right and what they got wrong. Use of video analysis to view the performance, often in slow motion and focusing on specific sections of an action are popular methods of termination feedback when teaching motor skills.

Keypoint:

Concurrent feedback is given as an exercise is being performed. *Terminal* feedback is given when an exercise has been completed.

Using verbal cues

Verbal cues are instructions about performing an exercise. However, the choice of which words to use and how many words to use at one time is important. Cues may be classified as internal (related to the body) or external (related to the environment). For example, when straightening the leg an internal cue might be 'tighten your quads' or 'pull your kneecaps up' while an external cue might be 'push your foot into the floor' when standing or 'press the back of your knee against the floor' when lying. In general, better results are usually obtained with external cues (Wulf et al. 1998).

> **Keypoint:**
>
> _Internal_ cues are related to a subject's body, _external_ cues are related to the environment in which the subject is exercising.

When constructing verbal cues, they must be differentiated from exercise instructions. An instruction is one or two whole sentences describing a movement, for example, when teaching bench press exercised

> Press the barbell from your chest towards the ceiling until your arms are straight. Lower under control.

When cueing the same movement, one or two action words or short phrases (usually less than 5–6 words) may be used such as

> push the barbell through the ceiling.

Choosing which words to use becomes easier if you aim for a noun (naming word), verb (doing word), and preposition (linking word). The noun would be the point in space where you are aiming during an exercise. In the case of the bench press, it is the ceiling (push the bar through the ceiling) or in the case of a squat, it may be the floor (press your feet into the floor). The verb is to push or press in these cases and the choice of verb is important as it must suggest action. _Punch_ your hand through the ceiling is stronger than _press_ your hand through the ceiling, for example. These words also indicate high degrees of action whereas the choice of words such as _move_ or _reach_, are less active and may be appropriate where a subject is too aggressive in their actions. The preposition provides the link between noun and verb and suggests the direction of the movement _towards_ the ceiling. Other directional words which are opposites to each other include towards/away, from/to, out of/into, off/on, for example (Winkelman 2021).

It is also useful to compare the action to a movement which is more familiar to a subject and to use a metaphor or analogy. An analogy is a word or expression which compared one thing to another, while a metaphor is a figure of speech that describes an action (or object) in a way that isn't literally true but helps explain the idea. In the case of exercise cueing, the two are often used interchangeably. For example, we might use the expressing 'back as flat as a tabletop' when performing an action in kneeling or when performing a birddog action in kneeling and straightening and arm and leg 'as though tightening a string running from your hand to your heel'.

> **Definition:**
>
> An *analogy* is a word or expression which compares one thing to another. A *metaphor* is a figure of speech that describes an action (or object) in a way that isn't literally true but helps explain the idea.

Once we have decided which words to use, we must determine if the cue has worked, and the action is performed by the subject as we intended. If it has not, we need to modify the cue and say *less* or *more* or even say it *differently*. Using a kneeling leg extension exercise as an example we may cue the action by saying

> Press your heel to the wall behind you.

If the subject does not lock their knee, we expand the cue (*say more*) to

> Straighten your leg to press your heel towards the back wall.

Once they have achieved the correct action, our cue is used more for motivation as the subject performs several repetitions and so we can maintain their focus but *say less* such as

> Heel to back wall.

Where the subject does not understand the action, we can split it up (part-task training) and use a separate cue for each stage of the action, for example, and *say it differently*

> "Lock your leg out keeping your toes on the floor" and then
> "Lift your straight leg" and finally when these actions are achieved
> Form a straight line between your shoulder, hip and heel.

Constraints based coaching

We saw with cueing that it can be a very hands-on approach where we use tactile cues to touch a subject and may even deliberately move a subject into position (adjustment). A constraints-based approach is really the opposite, it is very hands off and has its basis in DST (see above). The subject is challenged to find their own solution to a movement, rather than being given specific step-by-step instructions of a stylised ideal movement. The constraints are boundaries within which the subject can move, and they may be physical or metaphorical. The boundaries are manipulated to encourage the subject to find the best movement solution, by self-organising during the performance of an action.

Constraints are classified into three categories (Newell 1986), those relating directly to the *individual*, those related to the *environment* in which the subject is exercising, and those related directly to the *task* being performed (Figure 3.2).

Constraints based on the individual *performer* may be both structural and functional. Structural constraints could be associated with body proportions (anthropometry) but may also be due to pathology. For example, the way a person bends down to the floor may be different if they have longer or shorter legs but would also be different if they had one knee which was stiffer than the other due to an old injury. Functional constraints associated with the performer might be due to psychological factors. These could include confidence in a limb, fear of movement, motivation, or skill level, for example. Clearly some performer related constraints we have control over, while others we do not. However, an awareness of this type of constraint is helpful when guiding exercise.

Environmental constraints come from outside the body and are usually physical in nature but may also be cultural or sociological. Items such as training surface, gravity, friction would be considered as well as cultural norms. For example, the height of a hurdle to step over is physical, but an older patient dressed in a skirt may not be comfortable lifting their leg high. Both constrain a movement and should be considered in exercise performance.

Task constraints are often the most easily brought to mind for therapists and exercise professionals. These could be physical in nature and related to equipment, goals, or other people, for example. But they may also be verbal in nature and related to cueing or instructions. For example, when performing a squat using the therapist's hand in front of the subject's shoulder can be a useful constraint to avoid excessive forward angulation of the trunk. Equally, the cue 'weight over your heels' may achieve the same aim.

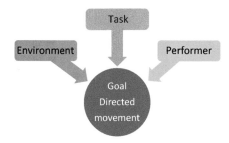

FIGURE 3.2 Constraints based learning.

Using an example of an Olympic lift will serve to illustrate the approach. When performing a Snatch, the aim is to keep the bar close to the bodyline throughout the lift. If the bar travels too far forwards, leverage is introduced as the distance between the bar and centre of gravity of the body increases, effectively making the bar act as though it were heavier. Placing a pole in front of the subject encourages them to keep the bar close to the body by constraining forward movement of the bar. The same effect may be achieved by using the instruction 'lift your t-shirt with the bar' (Figure 3.3 photo a, b, c).

CASE NOTE

A 35-year-old female was recovering from low back pain and had progressed to using her local gym. She decided to join a yoga class at the gym but had problems using the triangle pose. She felt unstable in the position and was not able to perform the exercise to the same standard as others in the class. When demonstrating the exercise, she practiced quickly and performed the initial part of the exercise well (standing with the feet apart) but got confused when turning her feet. When she tried to turn her body, she began to wobble causing her to step forwards and out of the pose. To teach the exercise it was divided into three parts (segmentation), and a chair was used to reduce motion range and enhance balance (constraints-based coaching). In *part one* of the pose the subject stood with her feet apart and practiced turning her leading leg fully (90°) and her trailing leg partially (45°). Initially, this was performed to instruction (verbal cueing). To encourage further movement of the leading leg the instructor passively moved the leg (tactile cueing) with the client's permission. Once the leg distance and foot turn was achieved, a chair was used to encourage side bending into the triangle pose position (*part two*). The client was instructed to place her flat hand on the chair seat as she bend sideways rather than placing her hand on her leg. Once a stable position was achieved with practice, the pose was

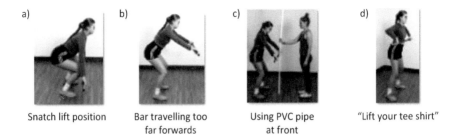

| a) | b) | c) | d) |
| Snatch lift position | Bar travelling too far forwards | Using PVC pipe at front | "Lift your tee shirt" |

FIGURE 3.3 Example of using a constraints based approach.

progressed to performing the triangle without the chair, and the arm reach upwards (*part three*) was added.

How should we practise?

How we structure a learning session (therapy or coaching period) is important to give a subject the best chance for successful learning, and some types of practice will be more suitable for certain tasks. We could simply practise repeatedly. This type of set up (termed *massed practice*) is good for learning tasks quickly but does not ensure retention—that is, remembering the skill over a long person so it can be reproduced at will. Splitting a session up by dividing the practice period with short rest periods (termed *distributed practice*) takes longer but is generally better for more complex tasks and gives better retention. It is especially useful for subjects who tire easily or who have a limited focus or concentration.

Another way of splitting things up to aid focus is to distinguish between *constant* and *variable* practice. Constant practice means to repeat the same action without changing it, variable practice as the name suggests varies the condition slightly. If we take a box squat as an example, we could simply perform three sets of ten reps, each of the same action. To vary the action, but still to keep it as a box squat we could vary box height, or foot width (narrow, wide, average) or weight (light weight for ten reps, heavy weight for three reps). Constant practice in general is better in the early stages of learning as it leads to rapid skill acquisition. Variable practice is better once the skill has been learnt and has the advantage of increasing adaptability; changing the action slightly to suit different conditions. Where an open skill is being practised (one which is heavily influenced by the environment) variable practice is often better. With closed skills (ones which focus more on the body to the relative exclusion of the environment) are often better learnt through constant practice.

> **Definition:**
>
> An *open* skill is affected by the environment, and *closed* skill is largely unaffected by the environment.

When we want a subject to learn a skill, teaching it to them is the obvious choice. However, using instructions or cueing (*guidance practice*) is only one method. We could simply ask the subject to work out for themselves how to do the task (*discovery practice*). Finding solutions to be able to perform an action can often be effective but is generally slower and often more suitable in later stages of skill learning.

Motivation to learn

We have looked at theories of motor learning, but what makes individual subjects want to learn, and can we enhance this desire? The answer to this question was dealt with in the OPTIMAL approach, an acronym for *Optimising Performance Through Intrinsic Motivation and Attention for Learning* (Wulf and Lewthwaite 2016). This approach uses motivation and attention to facilitate learning, through goal-action coupling.

> **Definition:**
>
> *Goal-action coupling* combines what the learner wants to do (the goal), with how a skilled movement can be used to achieve this (the action).

A central tenet of the OPTIMAL approach is to enhance a subject's *self-efficacy*, their confidence in their own ability to perform an action. This is often determined by past experiences and understanding a subject's past experiences can create training situations to build self-efficacy. There are three components to the approach. First, the therapist or coach should improve or enhance the subjects' *expectations* about their future success. Second, allowing individuals to exert some control over their environment (*autonomy*) is important. Finally, using cueing which has an *external focus* has been found to enhance learning (Table 3.5).

When subjects have a good experience or a positive outcome of an action, it is thought to stimulate the release of dopamine in the brain (a neurotransmitter) which is part of a pleasure and reward system facilitating learning and behaviour. To assist with the expectation of a positive result, we can provide results which suggest that the subject's performance is better than average. In addition, observing others in a class situation, for example, can also give a favourable expectation of success—especially if others have similar problems/pathologies and are further along the rehabilitation timeline. Goal setting and rewards are important, with goals being achievable so that rewards can be given frequently. Expectations may also be enhanced when a subject is working alone (home practice). Prior

TABLE 3.5 OPTIMAL theory of motor learning

Aspect	Coaching
Enhanced expectancy	• Suggest subjects' performance is better than average
	• Use goal setting & rewards
Support Autonomy	• Involve subject in decision making
	• Give the subject choice
External focus of attention	• Aim focus at effect of subjects' action
	• Avoid emphasis on subjects' body or sensations

Source: Wulf and Lewthwaite (2016). https://www.physio-pedia.com accessed February 2022.

to the session they should agree a standard to be achieved, and a reward which is meaningful to the subject. This may be a brief rest, sip of drink or mark in a record book, for example. The aim is to link or 'code' the performance with success.

Definition:

Coding refers to the method in which a memory is stored in the brain.

It is also important not to reinforce failure (code it with experience) by dwelling on it or punishing failure in any way.

Focussing on person-centred care is important within therapy and giving the subject control over their environment and task is important. If the subject can make a choice, they will be more in control of the situation. Creating autonomy by giving a subject choice may be achieved simply by asking them what they want to do, to make them integral to the decision-making process. Full autonomy is not given (subjects can't just do anything!), but autonomy is guided. For example, if three actions are to be performed, subjects may choose the order in which they are performed. This type of process can reduce stress and enhance self-efficacy. Additionally, variability can strengthen the learning process. Mixing up practice in this way (contextual interference) has been shown to worsen practice performance but strengthen retention (Magill and Hall 1990).

Using an external focus of attention (aimed at the effect of an action) rather than an internal focus (aimed at the body and body sensations), leads to more effective motor learning. An example of external focus would be focussing on a bat or target when swinging, for example rather than focussing on the arm swing or elbow angle. External focus is thought to allow processing with less conscious control, encouraging greater variability and shorter reaction times.

Practicalities of teaching exercise

One of the first things we must be concerned with when teaching an exercise is not to cause an injury. First, do no harm (Primum non nocere in Latin) is a central tenant of many of the caring professions, and health and safety should be our main concern prior to and during exercise teaching.

Health and safety

There are several health and safety considerations during exercise practice (Table 3.6). The exercise environment usually has unfamiliar equipment, which is constantly moving, and so the risk of something falling or someone being hit is heightened. It is important to predict if an action may put a user or another at risk and avoid or modify the action accordingly. This requires self-monitoring by individuals and close supervision by the coach. Obviously, this becomes more important with less experienced users or children. Fresh air flow to lessen the impact of respiratory infections and to ensure a more pleasant working environment with respect to body smells is also important. Finally, exercise equipment (especially in commercial gyms) is often complex with several moving components so it must be regularly checked, and faults reported.

Exercise classes and gyms can become fashion emporia, and whilst this can enhance a person's self-image, some find it intimidating. It is important that users feel comfortable, both physically to enhance freedom of movement and psychologically so they do not feel self-conscious or pressured into wearing something which they are not happy with.

Fluids and food are often a subject of debate with protein featuring highly in bodybuilding and isotonic drinks in running. However, simply taking regular

TABLE 3.6 Health and safety considerations during exercise practice

Feature	Explanation
Working environment	• Ensure area is clear of obstacles or trip hazards • Allow fresh air flow • Ensure comfortable temperature for exercising
Clothing	• Wear comfortable clothing • Wear clothing which does not make you self conscious • Ensure clothing does not restriction motion range • Ensure clothing will not restrict blood flow during exercise
Fluids & food	• Keep hydrated during exercise • Replace body fluid which is lost through sweating • Generally, do not eat during exercise unless you have a medical condition which requires this
Body awareness	• You may feel mild soreness during exercise but not intense pain • Notice any changes in your body (skin colour, joint alignment)
Monitor exercise intensity	• Be aware of any changes in your heartrate or breathing • Stop exercising if you feel dizzy, notice vision changes, or experience headaches
Equipment safety	• Check equipment before use • Report equipment faults to a supervisor
Start & finish	• Warm-up at the beginning of exercise and cool down at the end. • Take instruction on appropriate contents of a warm-up/cool down
Other users	• Be always aware of other users • Be considerate and polite • Do not tolerate bullying, sexism, or racism—report it to a supervisor

water in to replace sweat is probably all that is required at normal exercise intensities.

Being aware of your own body is vital during exercise, and something which improves with exercise longevity. Assessing changes and monitoring exercise intensity and technique is important. This is increasingly emphasised in exercise styles which work on whole body techniques such as Pilates, dance, and yoga.

Beginning and finishing an exercise or an exercise class can be important. Although warmup has not been shown to either enhance performance or reduce the likelihood of injury, many athletes and coaches feel better using a warmup. Some of this will be ritualistic, but sometimes it is about changing body awareness from the levels used in daily living to that used during exercise.

A simple pneumonic to work with when planning a warm-up is RAMP, a 3-phase approach standing for *Raise, Activate, Mobilise, and Potentiate* (Jeffreys 2007). In the phase 1 (raise), the aim is to increase metabolic rate and to choose actions to be used later in a sport or exercise workout. Using this as a basis for cardiopulmonary work makes the warm-up more functional from the outset. In phase 2 (activate and mobilise), the aim is to increase range of motion using functional patterns likely to be used later in sports such as squat, lunge, and press actions, for example. The focus is on dynamic rather than static stretch to move through a range of motion, and any weakness in movement patterns can be addressed at this stage prior to loading the body further. Phase 3 (potentiate) includes sports specific activities which gradually increase in intensity. The aim here is to use the actions to be performed later, but at a lower level. If we take a bench press action as an example, heart and breathing rate can be raised and blood flow improved to the upper body by performing light upper body calisthenics. Performing pushing actions (forward and overhead) targets the body areas to be used in the bench press (shoulders, arms, and chest). Performing the bench press with an empty bar for the first set potentiates the movement, rehearsing aspects such as grip width, motion range and body alignment before weight is added for subsequent sets.

Cool down normally means reducing intensity gradually and monitoring the athlete. However, some athletes like to practise stretching, shaking, or even foam rolling actions claiming that they reduce post-workout soreness.

References

Adams, J.A. (1971). A closed-loop theory of motor learning. *Journal of Motor Behaviour* 3(2): 111–150.

Bernstein, N.A. (1967). *The co-ordination and regulation of movements.* Oxford: Pergamon Press.

Broadbent, D. (1958). *Perception and communication.* London: Pergamon Press.

Fairbrother, J.T. (2010). *Fundamentals of motor behavior.* Champaign, IL: Human Kinetics.

Fitts, P. M., and Posner, M. I. (1967). *Human performance.* Cole, Belmont, CA: Brooks, 5, 7–16.

Gibson, E.J., and Pick, A.D. (2000). *An ecological approach to perceptual learning and development*. Oxford: Oxford University Press.

Hasher, L. (1971). Retention of free recall learning: The whole-part problem. *Journal of Experimental Psychology* 90(1): 8–17.

Jeffreys, I. (2007). Warm-up revisited: The ramp method of optimizing warm-ups. *Professional Strength & Conditioning* 6: 12–18.

Magill, R.A., and Hall, K.G. (1990). A review of the contextual interference effect in motor skill acquisition. *Human Movement Science* 9(3): 241–289.

Massis, M., and Jeffreys, I. (2021). Skill acquisition and motor learning. In Jeffreys, I. and Moody, J. Eds., *Strength and conditioning for sports performance* (2nd ed). London: Routledge, 22–32.

Newell, K.M. (1986). Constraints on the development of coordination. In Wade, M.G. and Whiting, H.T.A., Eds., *Motor development in children aspects of coordination and control*. Leiden: Martinus Nijhoff, 341–360.

Norris, C.M. (2019). *Sports and soft tissue injuries* (5th ed). London: Routledge.

Schmidt, R.A. (1975). A schema theory of discrete motor skill learning. *Psychological Review* 82(4): 225–260.

Schmidt, R.A., and Lee, T.D. (2011). *Motor control and learning. A behavioural emphasis* (5th ed). Champaign. IL: Human Kinetics.

Sherrington, C.S. (1906). *The integrative action of the nervous system*. New Haven, CT: Yale University Press.

Shumway-Cook, A., and Woollacott, H. (2017). *Motor control. Translating research into clinical practice* (5th ed). Philadelphia, PA: Wolters Kluwer.

Whiting, H. (1969). *Acquiring ball skill*. London: Bell Publishers.

Wightman, D.C., and Lintern, G. (1985). Part-task training for tracking and manual control. *Human Factors: The Journal of Human Factors and Ergonomics Society* 27: 267–283.

Winkelman, N. (2021). *The language of coaching*. Champaign, IL: Human Kinetics.

Wulf, G., et al. (1998). Average amplitudes of the internal-focus, external-focus, & control groups during practice and retention of a ski simulator. *Journal of Motor Behaviour* 30(2): 169–179.

Wulf, G., and Lewthwaite, R. (2016). Optimizing performance through intrinsic motivation and attention for learning: The OPTIMAL theory of motor learning. *Psychonomic Bulletin & Review* 23(5): 1382–1414.

4

ANATOMY OF THE SPINE

The gross anatomy of the lumbar spine includes vertebral bones and joints, ligaments, spinal discs, facet joints, and (as part of the pelvis) the sacroiliac joint (SIJ). Although none of these structures moves in isolation, it is clearer to describe them individually. First however, let's take a brief look at how the human spine developed through evolution.

Evolution of the human spine

We can trace our spine back through evolution over 400 million years to ray-finned fish, whose skeleton included a vertebral column of rigid bones protecting the spinal cord. These fish had fins which were not directly connected to the spine, but were bony rays covered with skin and supported by muscles, the fore fins attached to the skull (Galbusea 2018). The first amphibians transitioned from aquatic to terrestrial life and the need to support bodyweight demanded an adaptation seeing the pelvic girdle developed for the hind limbs. The fore fins moved backwards, detaching from the skull and the shoulder girdle developed as did the neck, allowing improved vision. This classic design of tetrapod (four-limbed animal) has remained in mammals.

Fish vertebrae have a similar design to that of mammals, in that they have a vertebral body (called the centrum) and a neural arch enclosing the spinal cord. Zygapophyseal joints are present, but intervertebral discs are not. Instead, a cartilage like notochord runs the length of the spine. The intervertebral disc of mammals developed to distribute weight-bearing stresses to the vertebral endplates, with the nucleus pulposus (disc centre) developing directly from the fish notochord.

Evolution from a predominantly horizontally carried spine to a vertical one was brought about by the upright posture exhibited in primates, but also in animals such as kangaroos, penguins, and ostriches. Bipedalism (using two feet for

DOI: 10.4324/9781003366188-4

Evolution of the Spine

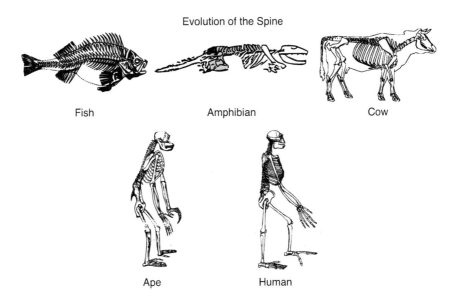

| Fish | Amphibian | Cow |

| Ape | Human |

FIGURE 4.1 Evolutionary development of human spine.

locomotion) is found in several primates and in humans. Further limb adaptation occurred as a result of chimpanzee-human divergence (7–10 million years ago) and included elongation of the femur and alteration in muscle insertion to speed up gait which was better suited to life on grasslands. Final adaptation to modern humans included increased pelvic width, larger muscle lever arms, and an S-shaped spine. Locomotor efficiency was improved by increasing stride length using pelvic motion in the transverse plane rather than hip flexion in the sagittal plane (Gruss et al. 2017). In addition, the human pelvis is shorter and broader than that of the ape, with the hip and knee held extended rather than flexed (Figure 4.1). The configuration of pelvis and S-shaped spine reduces the energy expenditure required to maintain an upright posture.

Vertebral bones and joints

The adult human vertebral column contains 33 vertebrae. Five vertebrae are fused to form the sacrum and four are fused to form the coccyx. The remaining 24 movable vertebrae are divided among the cervical (7), thoracic (12), and lumbar (5) regions (Figure 4.2 and Figure 2.1). Any two neighbouring vertebrae make up a spinal segment Figure 4.2.

The two vertebrae within a spinal segment are attached (articulated) by both joints and ligaments. There are three joints (making up an articulating triad), consisting of the disc, which forms the joint between the bodies of adjacent vertebrae, and the two facet joints (also called zygapophyseal or apophyseal joints),

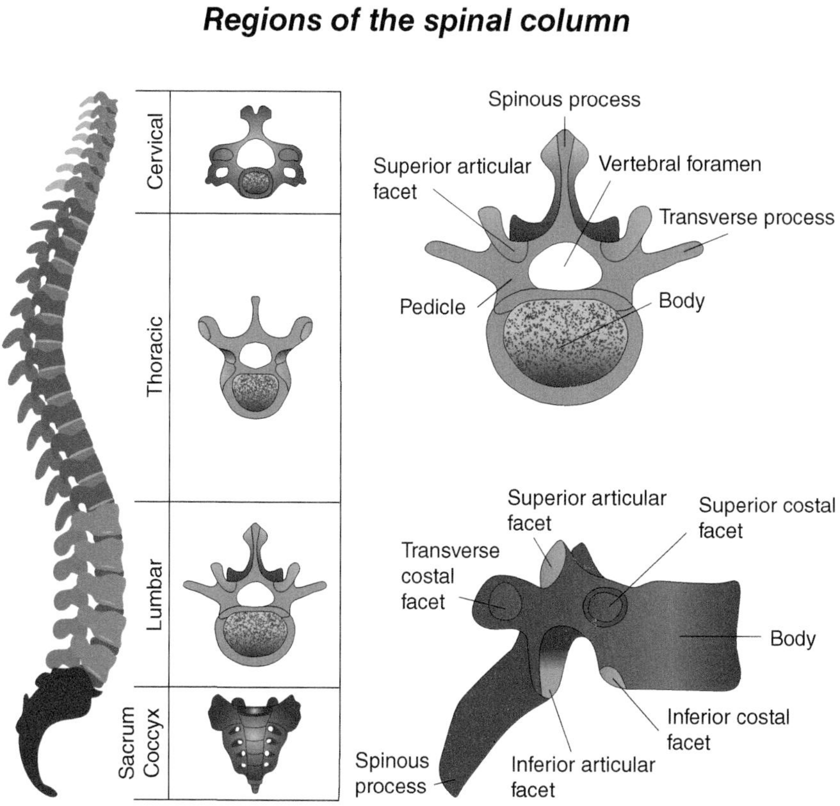

Regions of the spinal column

FIGURE 4.2 Regions of the spinal column.

where the inferior articular processes on either side of the upper vertebra come together with the superior articular processes on either side of the lower vertebra.

> **Keypoint:**
>
> A *spinal segment* contains two adjacent vertebrae, articulating with each other through the intervertebral disc and two facet joints. The articulations form a triad.

The disk and its associated facet joints are intimately linked both structurally and functionally. Degeneration of the intervertebral disc because of injury can lead to degeneration of the neighbouring facet joints. As we shall see later, the ligamentous support to both structures is continuous.

Mechanically, we can compare the spinal segment to a simple leverage system, with the facet joints forming a fulcrum. The posterior tissues (ligamentous and muscular) and the anteriorly placed disc resist both compressive and tensile

TABLE 4.1 Ligaments of the spinal segment

Neural arch	Facet joint	Vertebral body
Interspinous (between SPs)	Facet joint capsule	Anterior longitudinal (front of VB)
Supraspinous (covering SP)	Ligamentum flavum (reinforcing capsule)	Posterior longitudinal (back of VB)
Intertransverse (between TPs)		

SP—spinous process. TP—transverse process. VB—vertebral body.

forces. The ligaments themselves may be categorised into three interrelating functional groups as shown in Table 4.1.

Ligaments

The neural arch ligaments consist mainly of the ligamentum flavum and the interspinous ligament, with the supraspinous and intertransverse ligaments providing additional support (Figure 4.3). Although these four ligaments are traditionally described as separate structures, they are merged at their edges and act functionally as a single unit.

> **Definition:**
>
> The *neural arch* is the curved rear (posterior) section of the vertebra which arises from the vertebral body and encloses the spinal cord.

On dissection, when the bony components of the neural arch are removed, the neural arch ligaments can be seen to maintain their continuity (Willard 1997). The lateral fibres of the ligamentum flavum are continuous with the facet joint capsule and form the rear wall of the spinal canal. The anterior border of the interspinous ligament is a continuation of the ligamentum flavum, whereas the posterior border of this ligament is thickened into the supraspinous ligament. If the boundary joining the interspinous and supraspinous ligaments is cut, the tensile stiffness is reduced by 40% (Dumas et al. 1987), illustrating the importance of their dual structure. The supraspinous ligament actually merges with the thoracolumbar fascia (TLF), which, in turn, connects with the deep abdominal muscles at the side of the body (see below). The force generated by the deep abdominal muscles therefore can be transmitted through the TLF, via the supraspinous ligament, directly into the ligamentum flavum—preventing this ligament from buckling towards the spinal cord.

The interspinous ligament merges with the supraspinous ligament and then with the TLF, forming the interspinous–supraspinous–thoracolumbar (IST) ligamentous complex. The IST complex attaches the fascia of the back to the lumbar spine (Figure 4.4). The importance of this system is that tension developed in the extremities is transmitted to the vertebral column, making the seemingly distant limb musculature important to the rehabilitation of spinal function. The intertransverse ligament, although small, becomes more important caudally as it expands into the iliolumbar ligament.

Keypoint:

Tension from the extremities is transmitted through the back fascia directly to the spine.

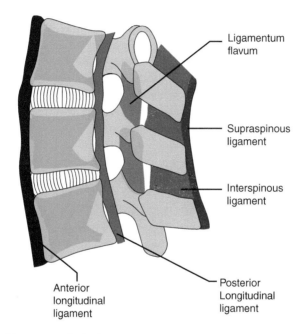

FIGURE 4.3   Ligaments of spinal segment.

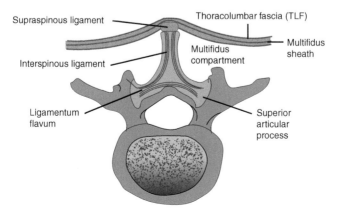

FIGURE 4.4   IST ligamentous complex.

The capsule of the facet joint is reinforced posteriorly by the multifidus muscle and anteriorly by the ligamentum flavum. It is surrounded by fascia, which itself is continuous with that covering the ligamentum flavum and the investing fascia of the vertebral body. The facet joint capsule therefore can be seen as a bridge of connective tissue between the ligaments of the neural arch and those of the vertebral body.

The anterior longitudinal ligament (ALL) and posterior longitudinal ligament (PLL) lie ventrally within the spinal segment. The ALL is the stronger of the two and extends from the occiput to the sacrum, where it merges with the SIJ capsule. The ALL has two sets of fibres. The superficial fibres span several vertebral segments, whereas the deep fibres attach loosely to the annulus of the spinal disc. The PLL exists in the cervical spine as the tectorial membrane and extends caudally to the periosteum of the sacrum. The PLL expands as it passes the intervertebral discs and narrows around the vertebral body. Because the PLL is considerably weaker than the ALL, the main ligamentous restriction to flexion is not from the PLL but from the ligamentum flavum and the facet joint capsule into which it merges. The ligamentum flavum and facet joint capsules combine to offer 52% of the passive resistance to flexion in the lumbar spine (Bogduk and Twomey 1991). The structural pairing of the PLL and the ligamentum flavum is functionally obvious as well. Load-deformation (stress–strain) curves plotted for the two ligaments are similar, suggesting in this case that the two ligaments may have a similar purpose.

The longitudinal ligaments are *viscoelastic*, meaning that they stiffen when loaded rapidly. They do not store all the energy used to stretch them because they lose some energy as heat, a feature known as *hysteresis*. When loaded repeatedly, these ligaments become even stiffer, and the hysteresis is less marked, making them more prone to fatigue failure (Hukins 1987). The supraspinous and interspinous ligaments are farther from the flexion axis and therefore need to stretch more than the PLL when they resist flexion.

Definition:

A *viscoelastic* material exhibits both viscous (flow) and elastic (spring) characteristics. *Hysteresis* is a slowing of an effect created by a force acting on a substance, causing the object to give way gradually.

With age, ligaments gradually lose their ability to absorb energy. The stiffest ligament in the spine is the PLL; the most flexible is the supraspinous (Panjabi et al. 1987). The ligamentum flavum in the lumbar spine is pretensioned (possesses tension at rest) when the spine is in its normal anatomical orientation (neutral position), a situation that compresses the spinal disc. This ligament has a high percentage of elastic fibres and contains nearly twice as much elastin as collagen. The ALL and joint capsules are among the strongest ligamentous tissues in the body, whereas the interspinous and PLLs are the weakest (Panjabi et al. 1987).

Keypoint:

The *ligamentum flavum* is the most elastic ligament in the body and the main ligament limiting flexion. It forms the anterior portion of the facet joint capsule.

Spinal discs

Twenty-four intervertebral discs lie between successive vertebrae, making the spine an alternatively rigid and then flexible column. The amount of flexibility in a particular spinal segment is determined by the size and shape of the spinal bones and disc, and by the resistance to motion of the soft tissue that supports the spinal joints. The discs increase in size as they descend the column, the lumbar discs having an average thickness of 10 mm, twice that of the cervical discs. The disc shapes are accommodated to the curvatures of the spine and to the shapes of the vertebrae. The greater anterior widths of the discs in the cervical and lumbar regions reflect the curvatures of these areas. Each disc has three closely related components—the annulus fibrosis, nucleus pulposus, and cartilage end plates (Figure 4.5).

The annulus contains layers of fibrous tissue arranged in concentric bands—about 20—like those in an onion. The fibres within each band are parallel, with the various bands angled at 45° to each other. The bands are more closely packed anteriorly and posteriorly than they are laterally, and those innermost are the thinnest. Fibre orientation, although partially determined at birth, is influenced by torsional stresses in the adult. The posterolateral regions have a more irregular makeup—possibly one reason why they become weaker with age and more predisposed to injury.

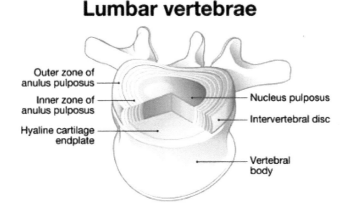

Lumbar vertebrae

Outer zone of anulus pulposus

Inner zone of anulus pulposus

Hyaline cartilage endplate

Nucleus pulposus

Intervertebral disc

Vertebral body

FIGURE 4.5 Components of the intervertebral.

Keypoint:

The spinal discs have fewer concentric bands posterolaterally than in other regions, and these are irregular—making this region of the disc more susceptible to injury.

The annular fibres pass over the edge of the cartilage end plate of the disc and are anchored to the bony rim of the vertebra and to its periosteum and body. The attaching fibres are interwoven with the fibres of the bony trabeculae of the vertebral body. The outer layer of fibres blend with the PLL but not the ALL.

Resting on the surface of the vertebra, the hyaline cartilage end plate is approximately 1 mm thick at its outer edge and becomes thinner towards its centre. The central portion of the end plate acts as a semipermeable membrane to facilitate fluid exchange into and out of the disc; it also protects the vertebral body from excessive pressure. In early life, canals from the vertebral body penetrate the end plate, but these disappear after the age of 20–30. The end plate then starts to ossify and become more brittle, whereas the central portion thins and, in some cases, is destroyed.

The nucleus pulposus is a soft hydrophilic (water-attracting) substance taking up about 25% of the total disc area. It is continuous with the annulus, but the nuclear fibres are far less dense than those of the annulus. Mucopolysaccharides called *proteoglycans* fill the spaces between the collagen fibres of the nucleus, giving the nucleus its water-retaining capacity and making it mechanically plastic. Metabolically very active, the area between the nucleus and annulus is sensitive both to physical force and to chemical and hormonal influences. Although the collagen volume of the nucleus remains unchanged, the proteoglycan content decreases with age—leading to a net reduction in water content. Early in a person's life, the water content may be as high as 80–90%, but this decreases to about 70% by middle age.

The lumbar discs are the largest avascular structures in the body. The nucleus obtains fluids by passive diffusion from the margins of the vertebral body and across the cartilage end plate—particularly across the centre of the end plate, which is more permeable than the periphery. Intense anaerobic activity within the nucleus (Holm et al. 1981) can lead to lactate build-up and low oxygen concentration, placing the nuclear cells at risk. Inadequate adenosine triphosphate (ATP) levels may lead to cell death.

Keypoint:

The lumbar spinal discs are avascular and depend on fluid exchange by passive diffusion. Regular movement and activity are vital to this process.

Some researchers hypothesise that regular exercise involving movement of the spine may improve the nutrition of the disc—and over the years might not only improve the general health of discs but even slow the loss of height attributable to water loss from discs. Experimentally, the myokine irisin which is released when muscles contract has been shown to increase nucleus pulposis cell proliferation and metabolic activity. It promotes anabolic gene expression and reduces catabolic markers suggesting a biological link (crosstalk) between muscle and intervertebral disc tissue (Vadala et al. 2022).

Definition:

A *myokine* is a protein or peptide secreted by muscle cells.

Facet joints

The facet joints are synovial joints formed between the inferior articular process of the vertebra above and the superior articular process the vertebra below. The facet joint capsule holds about 2 ml of synovial fluid. Its anterior wall is formed by the ligamentum flavum; posteriorly, the capsule is reinforced by the deep fibres of the multifidus muscle. At its superior and inferior poles, the joint leaves a small gap, creating the subscapular pockets. These are filled with fat, contained within the synovial membrane. Within the subscapular pocket lies a small foramen for passage of the fat in and out of the joint as the spine moves.

The capsule contains three structures of interest. The first is the connective tissue rim, a thickened wedge-shaped area that makes up for the curved shape of the articular cartilage in much the same way as the menisci of the knee do. The second structure is an adipose tissue pad, a 2 mm fold of synovium filled with fat and blood vessels. The third structure is the fibroadipose meniscoid, a 5 mm leaflike fold that projects from the inner surfaces of the superior and inferior capsules. The last two structures have a protective function. Flexion leaves some of the articular facets' cartilage exposed—both the adipose tissue pad and the fibroadipose meniscus cover the exposed regions (Bogduk and Engel 1984).

With ageing, cartilage of the facet joint can split parallel to the joint surface, pulling a portion of joint capsule with it. The split cartilage, with its attached piece of capsule, forms a false intra-articular meniscoid (Taylor and Twomey 1986). Flexion normally draws the fibroadipose meniscus out from the joint, and it moves back in with extension. If the meniscus fails to move back, it may buckle and remain under the capsule, possibly causing pain. A mobilisation or manipulation that combines flexion and rotation may potentially relieve pain by allowing the meniscoid to move back to its original position.

Many of the structures described here contain nociceptors and/or mechano-receptors, and so may be instigators of a nociceptive response when stressed or damaged. The nociceptive supply of spinal tissues is listed in Table 4.2.

TABLE 4.2 Nociceptive supply of spinal tissues

Structure	Nerve supply
Vertebra	No nociceptors in periosteum or blood vessels of cancellous bone
Disc	Peripheral annulus innervated. Granulation tissue may grow into degenerative disc dragging nociceptors with it
Dura & nerve root sleeve	Direct stimulation may cause pain
Facet joint capsule	Rich supply of nociceptors
Ligament & fascia	Richly innervated
Muscle	Mechanoreceptors in muscles itself, nociceptors in covering fascia

Data from Adams et al. (2002).

Effects of ageing

The length of the spinal column reduces with ageing but not generally because of reducing disc height, as is usually suggested. The reduction in general body height occurs initially through the loss of horizontal trabeculae within the vertebra itself. These horizontal fibres form ties across the vertebra a little like the rafters in a house roof. When the horizontal trabeculae degenerate, the vertical trabeculae buckle through weight bearing and, in some cases, may fracture. Eventually, the end plate becomes concave, a process that occurs earlier in females because of estrogen loss during menopause. Measurement of discal thickness shows no loss of height as part of the natural ageing process. The vertebral height changes that do occur are accompanied by horizontal expansion of the disc, causing the discal 'waist' (centre section) to thicken.

Over the years, the collagen makeup of the disc changes, and the water content of the disc decreases. Fissures occur initially in the circumference of the disc, and in time these spread into radially directed fissures. Blood vessels and even nerve fibres grow through the fissures towards the centre of the disc (Adams et al. 2002). The appearance of radial fissures may at first sight suggest an increased tendency for nuclear migration through the fissure, causing disc prolapse. However, the loss of the fluid nature of the nucleus by this time prevents significant nuclear migration.

Keypoint:

Fissures throughout the disc annulus associated with ageing do not lead to disc prolapse because there is a parallel loss of fluid within the disc nucleus.

Changes to the facet joints occur differentially between the anteromedial third and the posterior two thirds of the joint. The anteromedial aspect of the joint is stressed during lumbar flexion movements, and as a result the subchondral bone in the area hypertrophies by age 40 and begins to show vertical splitting. The posterior aspect of the joint ages more slowly because of its reduced weight-bearing function in comparison with the rest of the joint.

The proteoglycan of the disc's nucleus makes it hydrophilic, and its ability to transmit load relies on high water content, yet proteoglycan content declines from about 65% in early life to about 30% by middle age (Bogduk and Twomey 1987). When the proteoglycan content of the disc is high (up to age 30 in most subjects), the nucleus pulposus is gelatinous, producing a uniform fluid pressure. After this age, the lower water content of the disc leaves the nucleus unable to build as much fluid pressure. Less central pressure is produced, and the load is distributed more peripherally, eventually causing the annular fibres to become fibrillated and to crack. The net result is that a disc's reaction to compressive stress declines with age.

The age-related changes in discs cause greater susceptibility to injury. This fact—combined with a general reduction in fitness and changes in trunk movement patterns related to activities of daily living—can potentially increase the risk of injury in older people. Maintaining muscle strength and activity level may offset some of these effects.

Keypoint:

Maintaining muscle strength and activity level may offset some of the effects of spinal ageing.

Discal healing

The spinal disc is an avascular structure consisting of two types of cartilaginous tissue, the outer annulus fibrosis and inner nucleus pulposis. The junction between spinal bone and disc is formed by the cartilage endplate. Oxygen and glucose, both essential cell nutrients, enter the disc via blood capillaries in the disc periphery to diffuse to the disc centre. Metabolic waste products travel in the opposite direction from central disc cells to the periphery. Variation in compressive forces through movement-driven disc loading and unloading creates pumping dynamics demonstrating the importance of regular movement of the spine and the detrimental effect of prolonged inactivity.

Discal pathology such as shrinkage, thinning, Schmorl's node formation and discal migration or prolapse have traditionally been viewed as requiring surgical intervention. However, as we have seen above, many changes in the disc are age related and perfectly normal. With disc ageing water content and proteoglycan changes can be associated with fibrotic tissue formation and sclerosis of the vertebral end plates.

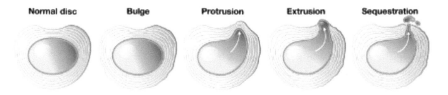

FIGURE 4.6 Disc injury stages.

> ### Definition:
>
> A *Schmorl's node* is the extrusion of disc nuclear material through the vertebral endplate into the adjacent vertebral body.

While fissure formation and osteophyte formation may exist non-symptomatically. Disc changes may indirectly lead to symptoms if they change lumbar biomechanics. Bone displacement may lead to increased forces through the facet joints leading to inflammatory changes, for example.

Disc prolapse itself may occur in several stages, with *bulging* (changed discal shape), *prolapse* (nuclear material passing into the annulus), *extrusion* (nuclear material rupturing through the annulus) and *sequestration* (nuclear material outside the disc breaking free from its central core) typically described (Figure 4.6). Such changes may or may not be symptomatic, however. Where nerve tissue is irritated mechanically or structurally, pain may occur locally or in a referral area (radicular pain). Nerve compression with altered nerve conduction (radiculopathy) may be painful or alter function. Spontaneous regression of disc prolapse is described (Kim et al. 2014, Hu et al. 2021). Nuclear material which has moved outside the annulus is likely to dehydrate and shrink, while both immune and inflammatory processes act to degrade discal material (Cunha et al. 2018). Macrophage activity and protease enzyme action may lead ultimately to symptom resolution. Sequestrated disc material has been found to contain more macrophages creating a greater inflammatory reaction than extruded disc (Virri et al. 2001), and migration of herniated material may improve its blood supply through neovascularisation facilitating reabsorption (Komori et al. 1996).

> ### Keypoint:
>
> Disc healing may occur through immune and inflammatory process which degrade the prolapsed material.

Sacroiliac joint

The sacroiliac joints (SIJ) are formed between the L-shaped surfaces of the iliac bones and those of the sacrum. The anterior one-third is said to be a true synovial joint, but the posterior two-thirds are considered as fibrous. The sacral joint surface is covered with hyaline cartilage, but the iliac surface is lined by thinner fibrocartilage. Normally the joint has minimal motion, 2–4 mm in all planes (Gartenberg et al. 2021). During the third trimester of pregnancy, release of sex hormones increases ligamentous laxity and with it pelvic joint mobility in preparation for childbirth. In contract, mobility is reduced due to ageing. From puberty the surfaces become progressively rougher and develop fibrous plaques, restricting joint motion by the age of 30 onwards. Surface fissures, chondrocyte changes, and fibrillation occur, and the capsule become collagenous by the eighth decade of life. These changes are thought to be an adaptation to shear forces associated with human bipedal stance (Kampen and Tillmann 1998).

Stability of the SIJ is provided by both *form* and *force* closure (Vleeming and Schuenke 2019). Form closure is passive and refers to the interlocking of the roughened SIJ joint surfaces. Force closure in contrast is the compression of the joint through active and passive forces generated by the ligaments, muscles, and fascia surrounding the joint.

The sacrum is inserted like the keystone of an arch, but seemingly the wrong way round, tending to be displaced rather than forced inwards with pressure. As bodyweight is taken, the tension developed in the interosseous sacroiliac ligaments pulls the two halves of the pelvic ring together producing form closure. Although no strong muscles cross the SIJ, the joint may be actively stabilised by a combination of forces acting over the joint, representing force closure. The sacrotuberous ligament (running from the sacrum to the ischial tuberosity) and the long dorsal sacroiliac ligament (sacral segments 4/5 to posterior inferior iliac spine) blend to form an expansion measuring roughly 20 mm wide by 60 mm long. This expansion attaches to the posterior layer of the TLF and to the aponeurosis of the erector spinae. A variety of trunk and lower limb muscles couple with the lumbosacral fascia and ligaments, stabilising the SIJ.

Definition:

Form closure is SIJ stability produced due to pelvic anatomy. *Force closure* is SIJ stability due to force generation of soft tissue structures (muscles, ligaments, and fascia) crossing the joint.

Several ligaments connect to structures within the region. The iliolumbar ligament attaches to the transverse process of L5, and in some subjects to those of L4 as well and passes anteromedially to the iliac crest and the surface of the ilium. The iliolumbar ligament resists movement between the sacrum and lumbar spine, particularly that of lateral flexion. When the ligament is cut, movement of the lumbar spine (L5) on the sacrum increases significantly lateral flexion by nearly 30%, and flexion, extension, and rotation by 18–23%. The superior aspect of the SIJ capsule is an extension of the iliolumbar ligament, whereas the anterior portion of the capsule merges into the sacrotuberous ligament.

The sacrotuberous ligament has a triangular shape extending between the posterior iliac spines, SIJ capsule, and coccyx (Figure 4.7). The tendon of biceps femoris (one of the hamstring muscle group) extends over the ischial tuberosity to attach to the sacrotuberous ligament; the ligament also attaches to some of the deepest fibres of the multifidus muscle (the multifidus runs vertically down the entire length of the back, on either side of the spine). Pure movement at the SIJ is described as nutation and counternutation (Table 2.3). The sacrotuberous ligament resists nutation of the sacrum, whereas the long dorsal sacroiliac ligament resists counternutation.

Greater movement ranges of the SIJ have been reported in non-weight-bearing than weight-bearing movements. Non-weight-bearing movements have exhibited as much as 12° innominate rotation during flexion, together with 8 mm of translation during extension; weight-bearing movements were reduced to 2.5° rotation and 1.6 mm maximal translation. In a study of healthy people aged 20–50 years, Jacob and Kissling (1995) found average rotational motion at the SIJ to be 2°, whereas symptomatic patients averaged 6°.

Nutation of the SIJ is an anterior tilting of the sacrum on the fixed innominate bones. The sacral base moves down and forward, whereas the sacral apex moves up, increasing the pelvic outlet. Nutation occurs in standing and increases as the lordosis deepens. By pulling the iliac bones together, nutation compresses the SIJ as well as the superior portion of the pubic symphysis. *Counternutation* is the opposite movement, with the sacral base moving up and back and the apex moving downwards. This movement occurs in non-weight-bearing situations, such as lying prone, and increases as the lordosis is reduced and the low back is flattened. During counternutation, the iliac bones move apart, the pelvic inlet increases, and the pelvic outlet reduces.

A variety of movements may occur about the SIJ during trunk actions. During forward bending of the trunk, the pelvis tilts anteriorly and the sacrum

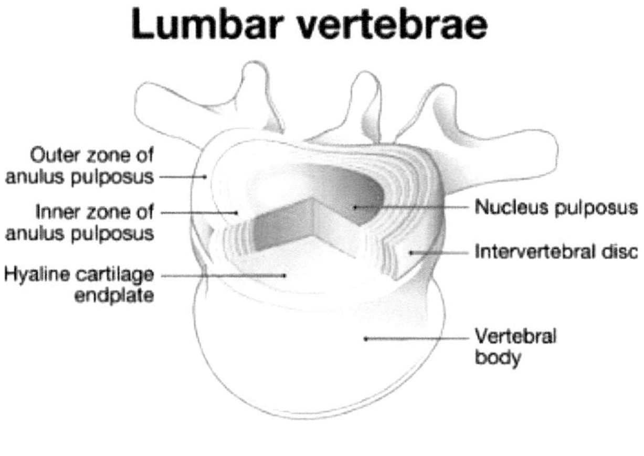

FIGURE 4.7 Components of disc.

may move into extension (coccyx moving backward; i.e., nutation around an oblique axis), causing the iliac crests and posterior superior iliac spines to approximate (i.e., press towards each other) and the ischial tuberosities and the anterior superior iliac spines to separate. During side bending, the trunk laterally flexes and the pelvis shifts to the opposite direction to maintain balance. With left lateral flexion and right pelvic shift, the right innominate bone can rotate posteriorly, and the left innominate rotates anteriorly. The sacrum rotates to the right. During trunk rotation, the pelvis rotates in the same direction; therefore, with left trunk rotation, the right innominate anteriorly rotates and the left posteriorly rotates. The sacrum is driven into left rotation. In subjects where motion cannot be detected, torsion (twisting) forces are still imposed on the joint.

Axial compression of the spine

Vertical loading of the lumbar spine (axial compression) occurs during upright (standing or sitting) postures, exacerbating certain forms of back pain. Knowledge of loading can help us to design more effective exercise programmes for people with back pain.

Compression of the vertebral bodies

Within the vertebra itself, compressive force is transmitted by both the cancellous (spongy) bone of the vertebral body and its cortical bone shell. Until about the age of 40, the cancellous bone contributes about 25–55% of the vertebra's strength. As ageing-related decreases in bone density lead to a decline in the proportion of cancellous bone, the cortical bone shell carries a greater proportion of load. As the vertebral body is compressed, early work showed a net flow of blood out of it reduces bone volume and dissipates energy (Crock and Yoshizawa 1976). Blood returns slowly as the force is reduced—leaving a latent period after the initial compression and diminishing the shock-absorbing properties of the bone. Exercises that involve prolonged periods of repeated shock to the spine (e.g., jumping on a hard surface) are therefore more likely to load the vertebrae than those that load the spine for short periods and allow recovery of the vertebral blood flow before repeating a movement.

Although this research is valuable, one limitation of this type of work is that it was normally performed using an isolated porcine (pig) spine model, or cadavers. This type of study does not necessarily correlate with healthy human tissue and would not show an offloading effect attributed to muscle. Using in vivo (within the body) approaches can account for this difference. For example, using a hybrid model of the passive lumbar spine computing disc, ligament, and facet joint stress-strain and estimated muscle forces Khoddam-Khorasani et al. (2020) found a free posture (between the extreme of kyphotic and lordotic postures) to have both active and passive systems during trunk flexion.

Compression of intervertebral discs

During standing, 12–25% of axial compression forces are transmitted between adjacent vertebrae by the facet joints; the intervertebral disc absorbs the rest of the force (Miller et al. 1983). The annulus fibrosis of a healthy disc resists buckling; even if a disc's nucleus pulposus has been removed, its annulus alone can exhibit a load-bearing capacity similar to that of the fully intact disc for a brief period. When exposed to prolonged loading, however, the collagen lamellae of the annulus eventually buckle.

Throughout the waking day, discal loading diminishes a person's height until the forces inside the disc equal the load forces (Twomey and Taylor 1994). By reducing axial loading, lying down permit's restoration of the former spinal length. Lying in a flexed position speeds the regain of lost height as the lumbar discs are distracted (unloaded) during flexion (Tyrrell et al. 1985). Application of an axial load compresses the fluid nucleus of the disc, causing it to expand laterally. This lateral expansion stretches the annular fibres, preventing them from buckling. The degree of discal compression depends on the weight imposed and the rate of loading. The stretch in the annular fibres stores energy, which is released when the compression stress is removed. The stored energy gives the disc a certain springiness, which helps to offset any deformation that occurred in the nucleus. A force applied rapidly is not lessened by this mechanism, but its rate of application is slowed, giving the spinal tissues time to adapt.

Definition:

In vivo means within a living organism, *in vitro* describes something in an experiment (from the Latin vivo 'in alive' and vitro 'in glass').

Deformation of the disc occurs more rapidly at the onset of axial load application, the majority of its deformation occurring within 10 min of onset. After this time, deformation continues but slows to a rate of about 1 mm/hr (Markolf and Morris 1974), leading to loss of height throughout the day. Under constant loading, the discs exhibit *creep* (i.e., they continue to deform even though the load is not increasing). Because compression causes an increase in fluid pressure, fluid is lost from both the nucleus and the annulus. About 10% of the water within the disc can be squeezed out by this method (Kraemer et al. 1985), the exact amount dependent on the size and duration of the applied force. When the compressive force is reduced, the fluid is absorbed back through pores in the cartilage end plates of the vertebra. Exercises that axially load the spine reduce a person's height through discal compression—squat exercises in weight training, for example, can create compression loads in the L3–L4 segment of six to ten times body weight (Cappozzo et al. 1985). Researchers have observed average height losses of 5.4 mm over a 25 min period of general weight training and 3.25 mm after a 6 km run (Leatt et al. 1986). Static axial loading of the spine with a 40 kg barbell over a 20 min period can reduce a subject's height by as much as 11.2 mm (Tyrrell et al. 1985). Exercises that involve this degree of spinal loading may be unsuitable for people with discal pathology in the acute phase of healing.

> **Keypoint:**
>
> Exercises that compress (axially load) the spine for a prolonged period result in a temporary loss of height of more than 1 cm through fluid loss from the disc nucleus.

The vertebral end plates of the discs are compressed centrally and can undergo less deformation than either the annulus or the cancellous bone. The end plates are therefore likely to fail (fracture) under high compression. Discs subjected to very high compressive loads can show permanent deformation without herniation. However, such compression forces may lead to deformation: The disc end plate (which joins the disc to the vertebral body) ruptures, and nuclear material from the disc passes through to the vertebral body itself. Bending and torsional stresses on the spine, when combined with compression, are more damaging than compression alone, and degenerated discs are particularly at risk.

Compression of facet joints

The orientations of facet joints differ among various regions of the spine, thereby altering the available motion. In the mid- and lower cervical spine, for example, rotation and lateral flexion are limited but flexion and extension are possible. In the thoracic spine, flexion and extension are limited but lateral flexion and rotation are free. At the thoracolumbar junction (T12-L1), rotation is the only movement that is limited; in the lumbar spine, both rotation and lateral flexion are limited.

The superior and inferior alignment of the facet joints in the lumbar spine means that during axial loading in the neutral position, the joint surfaces slide past each other. However, anywhere between T9 and T12, the orientation of the facet joints may change from those of the thoracic spine to those characteristic of the lumbar spine. Therefore, the level at which movements will occur can vary considerably among subjects. During lumbar movements, displacement of the facet joint surfaces causes them to impact or press together. Because the sacrum is inclined and the body and disc of L5 are wedge-shaped, during axial loading L5 is subjected to a shearing force. This force is resisted by the more anterior orientation of the L5 inferior articular processes. As the lordosis increases, the ALL and the anterior portion of the annulus fibrosis are stretched, providing tension to resist the bending force. Additional stabilisation is provided for the L5 vertebra by the iliolumbar ligament, attached to the L5 transverse process. This ligament, together with the facet joint capsules, stretches to resist the distraction force.

Once the axial compression force stops, release of the stored elastic energy in the spinal ligaments reestablishes the neutral lordosis. With compression of the lordotic lumbar spine, or in cases where gross disc narrowing has occurred, the inferior articular processes may contact the lamina of the vertebra below. In this case, the lower joints (L3-L4, L4-L5, L5-S1) may bear as much as 19% of the compression force, whereas the upper joints (L1-L2, L2-L3) bear only 11% (Adams et al. 1980).

Movements of the lumbar spine and pelvis

Flexion and extension

Both disc height and the horizontal length of the vertebral end plate affect the range of motion attainable during sagittal plane movement of the lumbar spine. Greatest range of motion occurs with a combination of maximum disc height and maximum end plate length. Because this alignment most often occurs in young females, they possess the greatest ranges of motion at the lumbar spine. With ageing, disc height and end plate length become more similar between the sexes, equalising the available range of motion for males and females in old age (Twomey and Taylor 1994).

During flexion movements, the anterior annulus of a lumbar disc is compressed, whereas the posterior fibres are stretched. Similarly, the nucleus pulposus of the disc is compressed anteriorly, whereas pressure is relieved over its posterior surface. Because the total volume of the disc remains unchanged, however, its pressure should not increase. The increases in pressure seen with posture changes are attributable not to the bending motion of the bones within the vertebral joint itself but to the soft tissue tension created to control the bending. If the pressure at the L3 disc for a 70 kg standing subject is 100%, supine lying reduces the pressure to 25%. The pressure variations increase dramatically as soon as the lumbar spine is flexed and tissue tension increases. The sitting posture increases intradiscal pressure to 140%, whereas sitting and leaning forward with a 10 kg weight in each hand increase pressure to 275% (Nachemson 1992).

The original work on discal pressure has often been misinterpreted as implying that different positions would place the disc at more risk and therefore should be avoided. However, Nachemson himself pointed out that the disc as causation for low back pain (LBP) was unproven (Danielsson et al. 2007). These pressure changes should therefore be viewed as normal variation with different body positions. Rather than displaying a constant pressure throughout a range of movements, the disc nucleus pressure varies, and the body has adapted to this. Changing intradiscal pressure would only be a significant concern where the adaptation process is impaired through injury or pathology.

> **Keypoint:**
>
> Changes in intradiscal pressure are often not directly associated with disc injury.

The posterior annulus stretches during flexion, whereas the nucleus is compressed onto the posterior wall. Because the posterior portion of the annulus is the thinnest part, the combination of stretch and pressure to this area may result in discal bulging or herniation. Since layers of annular fibres alternate in direction, rotation movements stretch only half of the fibres at any given time. The disc is more easily injured during a combination of rotation and flexion, which stretches all the fibres at the same time.

As the lumbar spine flexes, the lordosis flattens and then reverses at its upper level. Flexion of the lumbar spine involves a combination of anterior sagittal rotation and anterior translation. As sagittal rotation occurs, the articular facets move apart, permitting the translation movement to occur. Translation is limited by impaction of the inferior facet of one vertebra on the superior facet of the vertebra below. As flexion increases, or if the spine is angled forward on the hip, the surface (i.e., the top) of the vertebral body faces more vertically, increasing the shearing force attributable to gravity. The forces involved in facet impaction therefore increase to limit translation of the vertebra and stabilise the lumbar spine. Because the facet joint has a curved articular facet, the load is not concentrated evenly across the whole surface but is focussed on the anteromedial portion of the facet. Anatomical variations in vertebral structure in general and of facet joint orientation in particular (articular tropism) give rise to marked individual between subject differences with movement.

> **Keypoint:**
>
> Anatomical variations in vertebral structure can give rise to marked differences in vertebral movements between subjects practicing similar actions.

The sagittal rotation movement of the facet joint causes the joint to open and is therefore limited by the stretch of the joint capsule. The posteriorly placed spinal ligaments are also tightened. Adams and colleagues (1980) used mathematical modelling to analyse the forces that limit sagittal rotation within the lumbar spine. These investigators found that the disc contributes 29% of the limit to movement, the supraspinous and interspinous ligaments 19%, and the facet joint capsules 39%. In one experiment, the researchers cut (and thereby released) various posterior tissues in cadavers to measure the effects of those tissues on flexion range. Range of motion increased about 4° when the posterior ligaments were released and 9° when the capsule was released. Releasing the pedicles increased the flexion range by 24° in young (14–22 years) subjects. Cutting all the posterior elements increased the flexion range by 100% in the young subjects but by only 60% in the elderly (61–78 years) subjects. This type of in vitro modelling does not describe motion limitation by muscle.

During sustained flexion, tissue overstretch results in creep—gradually increasing the range of motion as tissues elongate over time. With ageing, the amount of creep is greater, but recovery takes longer (Twomey and Taylor 1994). Occupations that involve prolonged flexion with little recovery provide little chance for the overstretched tissue to recover, leading to chronic adaptation of both soft tissue and bone.

> **Keypoint:**
>
> Sustained flexion results in creep of the lumbar tissues (i.e., a gradual increase in range of motion over time). Prolonged flexion with inadequate tissue recovery can lead to chronic adaptation and consequent pain.

During extension, anterior structures are under tension, whereas posterior structures are first taken off stretch and then compressed (depending on the range of motion). Extension movements subject the vertebral bodies to posterior sagittal rotation. The inferior articular processes move downwards, causing them to press against the lamina of the vertebra below. Once the bony block has occurred, if further load is applied, the upper vertebra will axially rotate by pivoting on the impacted inferior articular process. The inferior articular process will move backward, overstretching and possibly damaging the joint capsule. Repeated movements of this type eventually can lead to erosion of the laminal periosteum. At the site of impaction, the joint capsule may catch between the opposing bones, creating another source of pain (Adams and Hutton 1983). Because structural abnormalities can alter a vertebra's axis of rotation, considerable variation exists among subjects.

Rotation and lateral flexion

During rotation, torsional stiffness is provided by the outer layers of the annulus, by the orientation of the facet joints, and by the cortical bone shell of the vertebral bodies themselves. Moreover, the annular fibres of the disc are stretched as their orientation permits; because alternating layers of fibres are angled obliquely to each other, some fibres will be stretched whereas others relax. A maximum range of approximately 3° of rotation can occur before the annular fibres will be microscopically damaged and a maximum of 12° before tissue failure. The spinous processes separate during rotation, stretching the supraspinous and interspinous ligaments. Impaction occurs between the opposing articular facets on one side, causing the articular cartilage to compress by 0.5 mm for each 1° of rotation and providing a substantial buffer mechanism (Bogduk and Twomey 1987). If rotation continues beyond this point, the vertebra pivots around the impacted facet joint, causing posterior and lateral movement. The combination of movements and forces places stress on the impacted facet joint by compression, the spinal disc by torsion and shear, and the capsule of the opposite facet joint by traction.

Keypoint:

The passive anchor to rotation comes from (a) facet joint impaction, (b) torsion and shear of the disc, and (c) stretch of both ligaments and the facet capsule.

When the lumbar spine is laterally flexed, the annular fibres towards the concavity of the curve are compressed and begin to bulge, whereas those on the convexity of the curve are stretched. The contralateral fibres of the outer annulus and the contralateral intertransverse ligaments help to resist extremes of motion. Lateral flexion and rotation occur as coupled movements. Classically, in the neutral position, rotation of the upper four lumbar segments is accompanied by lateral flexion to the opposite side; rotation of the L5–S1 joint, however, occurs with lateral flexion to the same side. The nature of the coupling varies with the degree of flexion and extension. In the neutral position, rotation and lateral flexion occur to the opposite side, called type I movement (i.e., right rotation is coupled with left lateral flexion). But when the lumbar spine is in flexion or extension, rotation and lateral flexion occur in the same direction, called type II movement (i.e., right rotation is coupled with right lateral flexion). In the concavity of lateral flexion, the inferior facet of the upper vertebra slides downwards on the superior facet of the vertebra below, reducing the area of the intervertebral foramen on that side. On the convexity of the laterally flexed spine, the inferior facet slides upwards on the superior facet of the vertebra below, increasing the diameter of the intervertebral foramen.

Between subjects variation exists depending on individual anatomical orientation. The inconsistency in patterns of coupled motions suggest that rules linking motion used for evaluation or treatment (Fryette's laws) should be used with caution (Legaspi and Edmond 2007).

Keypoint:

Inconsistency in patterns of coupled motions suggest that rules linking motion used for evaluation or treatment (Fryette's laws) should be used with caution.

Lumbar–pelvic rhythm

When people bend forward as though to touch their toes, the movement comes from both the pelvis and the lumbar spine. The pelvis anteriorly tilts on the femur, whereas the lumbar spine flexes on the pelvis. The combined movement of both lumbar and pelvic motion is called *lumbar–pelvic rhythm*. With the lumbar spine held immobile and the knees locked, the pelvis can tilt only to roughly 90° hip flexion (hamstring tightness limits further movement). To touch the floor, one must also flex the lumbar spine. Similarly, with the pelvis held immobile, lumbar flexion is limited to about 30° to 40°, with most movement occurring at the lower lumbar segments. Therefore, to achieve full forward bending, one must move both body segments. When flexing to mid-range levels during daily living, people can significantly reduce their lumbar flexion by using anterior pelvic tilt. Reduced ability to anteriorly tilt the pelvis increases the need to flex the lumbar spine, opening the possibility of postural pain through repetitive loading of the lumbar tissues.

When a person bends forward from a standing position, the pelvis and lumbar spine rotate in the same direction. Lumbar flexion accompanies anterior tilt of the pelvis. In the upright posture, the feet and shoulders are static, and the pelvis and lumbar spine move in opposite directions—lumbar extension compensates for an anteriorly tilted pelvis to maintain the head and shoulders in an upright orientation (Figure 4.8).

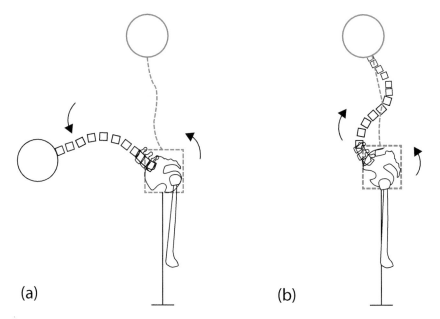

(a)   (b)

FIGURE 4.8   (a) Lumbar-pelvic rhythm in open chain formation occurs in the same direction. Anterior pelvic tilt accompanies lumbar flexion. (b) Lumbar-pelvic rhythm in closed kinetic chain formation occurs in opposite directions. Anterior pelvic tilt is compensated by lumbar extension.

Mechanics of bending and lifting

Lifting as a set of torques

Lifting an object from the ground can be viewed at a mechanical level as a set of torques involving both the body and the object to be lifted, that will produce the desired outcome Figure 4.9. The forces created during flexion by leverage, body weight, and muscle force—plus those created by the weight being lifted—must be overcome by an opposing extension force created by the hip extensor muscles as they contract on the spine.

> **Definition:**
>
> A Torque (also called a moment) is a force which causes rotation. It is measured in Newton metres (N.m.) and calculated by multiplying force and distance.

If the spine is not stable, posterior pelvic tilting brought about by the hip extensors (gluteus maximus and the hamstrings) merely increases flexion of the spine. However, where the spine is stable, the power created when the hip extensors to posteriorly tilt the pelvis is transmitted by the erector spinae along the length of the spine to the upper limb, which then delivers the force to the object being lifted.

The hip extensor muscles are better suited than the erector spinae to initiate a lift from a flexed position. Looking at a lifting scenario simplistically, A

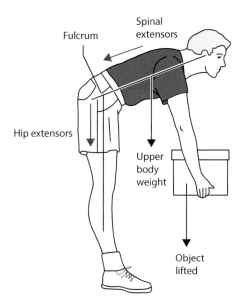

FIGURE 4.9 Mechanics of lifting.

68 kg athlete develops a torque of about 1,130 N·m in lifting a 200 kg) weight. Although the hip extensors can generate a torque of about 1,695 N·m, the erector spinae can generate only 339 N·m, or 30% of that required to perform the lift. Note that the bulk of the muscles creating the force (gluteus maximus) are some distance from the limb controlling the movement. When lifting a heavy weight emphasising use of the hip extensors working on a relatively immobile (stable) spine using a hip hinge action, rather than a spine flexion movement is usually more effective (a greater weight can be lifted).

Modelling the spine as a cantilever system according to standard mechanical principles, one can calculate the torques of various forces acting on the spine during lifting. Where the leverage is in equilibrium, the sum of the torques is zero, with flexion forces exactly balancing extension forces. It is possible to calculate both the force needed to lift an object and the resulting compression force on the lumbar spine. To lift a weight, the muscles and connective tissues in the lumbar spine must counteract the flexion caused by the weight by providing an equal amount of extension. However, because the weight is far from the fulcrum whereas the lower back muscles and tissues are very near to it, the muscles and tissues have much less leverage and must therefore exert much more force than just the weight of the object being lifted. Meanwhile, the vertebral joints experience a compression that is the sum of this force and the weight of the object. To counteract the compressive force acting on the spinal column when lifting large amounts of weight, the spine has several reinforcing mechanisms involving the soft tissues. The spine as a whole (bone and soft tissues) offers considerable resilience.

Flexion relaxation response in lifting

When bending forwards to pick something off the floor or lift, movement is occurring at the hip and spine. It would be easy to visualise the hip and spine extensors paying out (eccentric action) to lower the body towards the ground and pulling (concentric action) to lift the body back up. Looking at EMG evidence however, this is not what we see. When a subject flexes during a lift, the erector spinae are electrically silent just short of full flexion (Kippers and Parker 1984). This phenomenon, called the flexion relaxation response or critical point, is the result of elastic recoil (rebound) of the posterior elements of the spine. This point does not occur in all people (discussed later) and occurs later in the range of motion when weights are carried (Bogduk and Twomey 1991). During the final stages of flexion and from 2° to 10° extension (Sullivan 1997), movement occurs by recoil of the stretched tissues rather than by active muscle work.

Keypoint:

During bending, the erector spinae are electrically silent just short of full flexion. This phenomenon is the *flexion relaxation response*.

If the erector spinae are in protective spasm, chronic LBP often obliterates the flexion relaxation response. Failure of the muscles to relax prevents adequate perfusion with fresh blood and can lead to local ischemic muscle pain. Interestingly, during a squat lift with the back perfectly straight, the latissimus dorsi contracts powerfully at the beginning of the lift—perhaps to initiate extension by pulling on the TLF (Sullivan 1997). With extremely heavy lifts of any type, as subjects flex forward to the point of electrical silence, the positions of the vertebrae suggest that they do not reach the point at which the ligaments would be loaded (i.e., stretched or tensioned greater than at rest) (Cholewicki and McGill 1992).

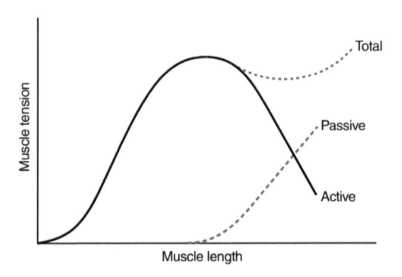

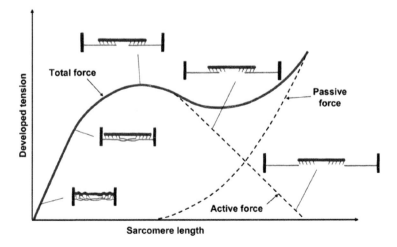

FIGURE 4.10 Length tension relationship.

The electrical silence of the muscles and the anatomical alignment of the vertebral segments suggest that the final degrees of flexion as well as the first degrees of extension occur through elastic recoil of the spinal extensor muscles. The length–tension relationship in muscles Figure 4.10 shows that a muscle loses active tension as it is stretched—but even towards the end of the range of movement, there is little decrease in total tension because an increase in passive force (recoil) largely makes up for the decrease in active contraction. As the spine returns from a fully flexed position, the ligaments may produce some 50 N·m of tension while the recoiling muscles produce 200 N·m. The combined extensor forces of the two passive systems are the major component of the posterior ligamentous system supporting the spine.

Hamstring muscle activity during bending

Bending incorporates movement at both the hip and lumbar spine. Activity of the gluteals and hamstrings controls pelvic tilt, whereas the extension force from the erector spinae muscles powers lumbar extension. Alteration in the sequencing (timing of movement of one body part relative to another) of hip and lumbar spine movement patterns during forward bending has been proposed as a risk factor for the development of LBP (Esola et al. 1996). Changes in both lumbar motion range and motion velocity have been noted in people with LBP. People with LBP demonstrate reduced hip mobility during forward bending (Porter and Wilkinson 1997), but other motions of the hip remain largely unaltered. Changes in the activity level of the hamstrings may be responsible for this movement dysfunction (Wong and Lee 2004). Interestingly, alteration in stretch tolerance rather than stiffness of the hamstrings has been shown to determine this range of motion change in people with non-specific LBP (Halbertsma et al. 2001).

Hamstring tightness is a common finding in the patient with LBP (Nourbakhsh and Arab 2002), and it has been argued that lengthening the hamstrings may allow greater motion to occur at the hips and therefore reduce stress on the lumbar spine. However, hamstring tightness is not related to pelvic tilt position during the standing static posture (Gajdosik et al. 1992) or total pelvic motion range during bending.

Investigation into the timing of the hip extensors and erector spinae muscle activity in forward bending may answer this conundrum. It has been shown that the erector spinae and hamstrings are activated before the gluteus maximus in people without LBP. In those with LBP, the muscle activation sequence is unchanged, but the duration of gluteus maximus contraction is shortened (Leinonen et al. 2000). In parallel with the flexion–relaxation phenomenon previously described for the erector spinae, activity of the hamstrings also ceases near end range (97% flexion), and the final angle of pelvic tilt is limited by elastic resistance of these muscles and tension of other posteriorly placed soft tissues.

Movement of the lumbar spine relative to that of the pelvis has been shown to change during the forward bending movement. Lumbar spine to hip flexion ratios for early (0–30°), middle (30–60°), and late (60–90°) forward bending have been given at 2:1, 1:1, and 1:2, respectively (Esola et al. 1996), showing an increase in the contribution by the pelvis as forward bending proceeds. Subjects with a history of LBP tend to have a changed pattern of forward bending compared with normal subjects, although the total range of motion for both groups is generally the same. In people with LBP, hamstring flexibility is reduced and greater electrical activity in the hamstring muscles is seen.

Keypoint:

The pattern of forward bending motion is changed in those with low back pain. Additionally, these subjects demonstrate greater electrical activity in the hamstring muscles.

Earlier lumbar motion in the activities of daily living may increase the repetitive stress imposed on the low back and could be an important factor in the recurrence of LBP, particularly because activities of daily living require only partial forward bending. Although the way in which a person bends is unlikely to be the single causal factor in the initiation of LBP, it may be important in the reactive phase following an injury if it is a driver of symptoms.

Lifting methods

There are two basic ways to lift something: in the squat lift, a person bends the knees and keeps the back relatively straight; in the stoop lift, the legs remain straight, and the back alone bends. Because the legs are apart and bent with the squat lift, an individual can generally hold the object closer to the body's line of gravity—thereby reducing the length of the lever arm from the body's line of gravity to the centre of gravity of the object. The disadvantage of the squat lift is that people are lifting more of their bodies (the legs and trunk as opposed to the trunk alone) and therefore must expend more energy than with a stoop lift. The erector spinae are more active in positions where lordosis is maintained; after people have attained a fully erect position when lifting a heavy weight, they tend to lean back to balance the weight and to use their hip flexor muscles to resist further spinal extension and to stabilise their spines.

Keypoint:

In a *squat lift*, a person can usually hold a weight closer to the body's centre of gravity, thereby reducing the torque on the spine.

In addition to differentiating between the squat lift and stoop lift, we must also examine the difference between using a squat lift with the back lordotic (lumbar spine minimally extended) and with the back flat (lumbar spine minimally flexed). Lumbar curvature is calculated as the angle formed between the surface of the vertebral body of L1 and that of the sacrum. The population mean value of this angle is 50°, although in children it is increased to 67° and in young males to as much as 74° (Bogduk and Twomey 1991) depending on posture type. The lordosis naturally results from the shapes of the vertebrae and disks of the lumbar spine. The L5-S1 vertebral disc is wedge-shaped, its posterior height typically about 7 mm less than its anterior. The L5 vertebral body also is wedge-shaped, its posterior height typically 3 mm less than its anterior. The remainder of the lordosis occurs because the discs themselves (not the vertebral bodies) are wedge-shaped. The sacrum is angled at about 30° to the horizontal, and changes to this angle affect the SIJ.

Because the orientations of the vertebrae differ between the squat and stoop lifts, the load distribution is affected. The lengths of various trunk muscles also differ between the two lifts. Because the depth of the lumbar discs (6–12 mm) is considerably smaller than the vertical height of the lumbar vertebrae (30–45 mm), even minimal changes in vertebral angles can greatly deform the discs. A flexion angle of 10° to 12°, for example, stretches the posterior annulus by more than 50% (Adams and Dolan 1997). Repeated loading in a lordotic posture can cause compressive stress within the posterior annulus of a disc and load the adjacent facet joints.

Recovery from this type of tissue stress is by no means immediate. Only 50% of intervertebral stiffness is regained after a 2 min rest period following a 20 min flexion period (McGill and Brown 1992). Minimal flexion (flat back), however, which brings the vertebral bodies into vertical alignment, equalises compressive stress across the whole disc and unloads the facets. At 60–80% of maximum flexion, the posterior tissues exert a substantial extensor torque, yet there is only a small compression effect on the lumbar discs. Moreover, tension in the TLF helps to stabilise the SIJ, and contractions of the gluteal muscles, the abdominals, and latissimus dorsi increase the TLF tension in a flat-back posture.

Looking at the resultant force taken in the lumbar spine (L1 and L3) only a marginal 4% difference has been found between the squat and stoop lifts (Dreischarf et al. 2016).

Definition:

Resultant force is the sum of that produced when two or more forces act on an object.

Comparing a squat lift to a stoop or freestyle lift (subject choice) the stoop lift was found to produce lower compressive and total load when compared to the squat or freestyle (von Arx et al. 2021). The lifting time (duration) was different between the three lift types with the freestyle being fastest, and the stoop the longest. Shear forces were generally higher in the stoop lift. Although the squat lift is often recommended, the biomechanics literature looking at spinal shrinkage, intra-discal pressure and spinal compression does not support advice to lift using a squat technique (back straight) rather than stoop technique (back bent) for the prevention of LBP (van Dieen et al. 1999).

Stabilisation mechanisms of the lumbar spine

Devoid of its musculature, the human spine is inherently unstable. The spine of a fresh cadaver stripped of muscle can sustain a load of only 4 to 5 lb (1.8–2.3 kg) before it buckles into flexion (Panjabi et al. 1989). Several tissue structures help stiffen (stabilise) the spine, including the posterior ligamentous system, the thoracolumbar fascia, direct trunk muscle action, and intra-abdominal pressure (IAP).

> **Keypoint:**
>
> The spinal column by itself is inherently unstable. Without muscle action, severe stress is imposed on the delicate joints and discs.

Posterior ligamentous system

When the muscle is stripped from a cadaveric spine, the interspinous and supraspinous ligaments, facet joint capsules, and TLF together provide passive support for the spine said to be sufficient to balance up to 55% of imposed flexion stress (Adams et al. 1980).

In the unstretched position, collagen fibres within the anterior and PLLs and the ligamentum flavum are aligned haphazardly. When the ligaments are stretched as the spine flexes or extends, however, the collagen fibres become aligned, and the ligament becomes stiffer. Pre-stressed at rest, the ligaments retract when cut. The longitudinal ligaments therefore maintain a compressive force along the axis of the spine, causing it to act somewhat like a stressed beam (Aspden 1992). The posterior ligamentous system can sustain a maximum torque of less than 25% that of the contracting erector spinae. However, two passive systems are at work here (see above). While the posterior ligamentous system is recoiling, the erector spinae muscles are also recoiling. At the point of full flexion, these muscles no longer contract (they are electrically silent), but they do exert a passive force through recoil. The force that the erector spinae create through recoil is about 200 N·m, equal to their potential contractile force. The combined posterior musculoligamentous system therefore provides a substantial stabilising mechanism in full flexion.

Many of the original studies on spinal ligaments were conducted on cadavers. When a person dies, however, the active systems of the disc stop, and because the disc material naturally absorbs water (it is hydrophilic), the disc expands slightly after death. Because the disc absorbs water in this way, the ligaments that surround the spinal segment are stretched slightly, making some of the results obtained from cadaveric tests inaccurate (McGill 2002). It has been demonstrated (Sharma et al. 1995) that of the posterior ligaments, the supraspinous ligament, rather than the PLLs or ligamentum flavum, is the passive structure that most contributes to passive spinal stability.

Thoracolumbar fascia

The TLF has three layers that cover the muscles of the back Figure 4.11 and is most developed in the lumbar region. The *anterior layer* derives from fascia covering the quadratus lumborum (QL) muscle and attaches to the transverse processes of the lumbar vertebrae. The *middle layer*, behind the quadratus lumborum, attaches both to the transverse processes and to the intertransverse ligaments. Laterally, it extends to cover transversus abdominis (TrA). The *posterior layer*, which envelops the erector spinae, attaches from the spinous processes and wraps around the back muscles to blend with the rest of the TLF laterally to the iliocostalis. The point at which the layers blend is the lateral raphe.

The superficial layer of the TLF is continuous with the latissimus dorsi and gluteus maximus. Sometimes a few fibres attach to parts of the external oblique and trapezius, and some cross the body midline (Vleeming et al. 1995). At L4–L5 level, fibres from latissimus dorsi and gluteus maximus differ in orientation, giving the superficial layer of the TLF a crosshatched appearance. This appearance may even extend down to the L5–S2 level. The fibres of the deep layer are

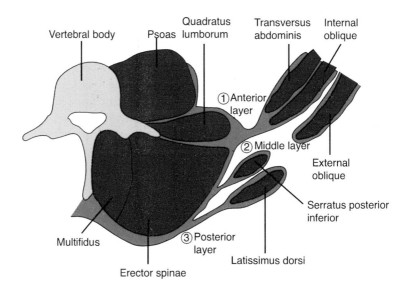

FIGURE 4.11 Cross section trunk.

continuous with the sacrotuberous ligament (and through it to the biceps femoris muscle of the upper leg), and they attach to the posterior superior iliac spines, the iliac crests, and the sacroiliac ligaments. In the thoracic region, fibres of the serratus posterior inferior are continuous with the TLF.

> ## Keypoint:
>
> The TLF is a tough fibrous sheet covering the back. It is tensioned by muscles from above, the side, and below. Through it, these muscles transmit their power across the whole spine.

The TLF contains nociceptive free nerve endings which are sensitive to chemical stimulation giving a long-term response. The nerve endings exhibit morphological changes in persons with chronic LBP. In addition, ultrasound imaging in persons with chronic LBP have demonstrated increase thickness and fat deposition (Langevin et al. 2009).

Thoracolumbar fascia action

In addition to its passive role, the TLF has two further capacities that involve muscle contraction. The TrA, through its attachment to the lateral raphe, pulls on the TLF. Although both attach to the lateral raphe, the deep laminae of the TLF angle upwards, whereas the superficial laminae angle downwards. As the TrA contracts and pulls on the lateral raphe, the deep and superficial fibres of the TLF pull laterally for the most part, although some force is transmitted along the length of the TLF. The increased force developed in this way (called the TLF gain) is small, between 3.9 and 5.9 N·m (compared with 250 Nm for the back extensor muscles) but provides some additional passive resistance to flexion by stiffening the lumbar spine.

Attachment of the TLF to the transverse processes of the lumbar vertebrae may control intervertebral motion to a certain extent (Hodges et al. 2003). Contraction force from the TrA muscle will be passed onto the TLF and indirectly affect the transverse processes. Approximation of the transverse processes (or more realistically limitation of distraction) may also occur during lateral flexion of the lumbar spine. Resistance to lateral flexion of this type has been calculated to create a force of 14.5 N (Tesh et al. 1987).

Tensioning the TLF through contraction of the TrA muscle has been shown to increase resistance to flexion loads by 9.5 N but to reduce resistance to extension loading by 6.6 N (Barker et al. 2006). Barker and colleagues showed fascial tension to affect cyclic loading during flexion by reducing vertebral displacement by 26% at the start of loading, reducing to 2% as loading continued. Fascial tension during cyclic loading in extension increased vertebral displacement by 23% at onset, reducing to 1% as loading reached 450 N.

> **Keypoint:**
>
> Tensioning of the TLF using contraction of the TrA muscle reduces vertebral displacement when the spine is loaded in flexion but increases displacement when the spine is loaded in extension.

The TLF may also act to amplify the force generated by the erector spinae muscles. The posterior layer of the TLF is retinacular tissue which envelops the erector spinae. As these muscles contract, the TLF resists the expansion of the bellies of the shortening muscles by increasing tension in the fascia. Restriction of the radial expansion of the erector spinae by the TLF has been shown to increase the stress generated by these muscles by as much as 30% (Hukins et al. 1990) and has been termed a hydraulic amplifier effect.

The TFL is likely more important as a retinaculum, spreading the forces created by muscles attaching into it across the trunk. Stiffness within the TFL may help to increase stability to the spine.

Thoracolumbar fascia coupling and the sacroiliac joint

A combination of form closure and force closure stabilises the SIJ (see above). *Form closure* is due to the shape of the pelvic bones where the sacrum forms a kind of keystone between the wings of the pelvis. *Force closure* results from muscles pulling laterally onto fascia and ligaments that pass over the joint. The combination of form and force closure creates a self-locking mechanism within the SIJ.

Nutation (see Table 4.3) tensions the SIJ ligaments, pulling the posterior parts of the iliac bones together and increasing SIJ compression. Two ligaments are of special importance to self-locking—the sacrotuberous ligament connecting the sacrum to the ischial tuberosity, and the long dorsal sacroiliac ligament from the third and fourth sacral segments to the posterior superior iliac spines. Both ligaments blend over the posterolateral aspect of the sacrum to form an expansion approximately 20 mm wide and 60 mm long. The ligaments attach to the posterior layer of the TLF and to the aponeurosis of the erector spinae. Nutation tensions the sacrotuberous ligament, whereas counternutation tensions the long dorsal sacroiliac (SI) ligament. The SI ligament is tensioned by contraction of the biceps femoris and of the gluteus maximus.

> **Keypoint:**
>
> The sacrotuberous ligament and the long dorsal sacroiliac ligament blend to form the sacroiliac expansion.

TABLE 4.3 Movements of the sacroiliac joint (SIJ)

Nutation	Counter-nutation
Anterior tilting of sacrum	Posterior tilting of sacrum
Sacral base moves down and forwards, apex moves up	Sacral base moves up and back, apex moves down
Size of pelvic outlet increases, pelvic inlet decreased	Pelvic inlet increased, outlet reduced
Occurs in standing	Occurs in non-weight bearing positions such as lying
Increased as lumbar lordosis increased	Increased as lumbar lordosis decreased
Iliac bones pulled together, SIJ impacted	Iliac bones move apart, SIJ distracted
Superior aspect of pubis compressed	Inferior aspect of pubis compressed.

Force closure of the SIJ opens the possibility of treating SIJ lesions with exercise therapy. As muscle affects the SIJ, training could improve SIJ functions. When the erector spinae contract, they pull the sacrum forward—inducing nutation of the SIJ and tensing the interosseous and sacrotuberous ligaments. The iliac portion of the muscle tends to pull the cranial aspect of the SIJ together, whereas nutation pulls the caudal aspect apart. The gluteus maximus can compress the SIJ directly and indirectly through its attachment to the sacrotuberous ligament. This occurs particularly when the gluteus maximus contracts with the contralateral latissimus dorsi and both muscles tension the TLF, whose fibres join the two muscles. Tension in the sacrotuberous ligament is increased by tensioning of the long head of the biceps femoris muscle. This occurs most noticeably in a flexed trunk or stooped position, in which the sacrotuberous ligament is also tensioned by the sacral portion of the erector spinae and the gluteus maximus.

Keypoint:

Tension generated by contraction of biceps femoris and gluteus maximus is transmitted via ligaments to the sacroiliac joint itself.

SIJ pain frequently occurs during and after pregnancy, when laxness of the SIJ ligaments reduces form closure of the joints. Female gymnasts experience similar problems: The hyperflexibility developed through gymnastics generally increases the laxity of the pelvic ligaments, reducing the form closure that they produce. The increased muscular stability resulting from the muscular demands of the sport compensates for the laxness, as long as the women continue their activity. When their muscle strength declines after they stop practicing the sport, the SIJ is left unstable and open to pathology. SIJ pain of this type is often helped by using a pelvic belt. Improving force closure of the SIJ by using stabilisation techniques for the lumbar spine and enhancing gluteal muscle strength using the hip hinge action can also reduce pain.

> **Keypoint:**
>
> Specific exercise can improve stability of the sacroiliac joint by restoring the natural mechanisms of form closure and force closure.

Stability exercise has been used successfully to treat SIJ conditions. Mooney and colleagues (2001) found changes in muscle balance tests for those suffering SIJ pain. These patients had higher levels of gluteal and latissimus dorsi muscle activity through actively 'splinting' the joint. Their core stabilising muscles were not working properly, so the gluteal and latissimus muscles had to act to compensate for this. By using rotary strengthening, these authors were able to return the patients' muscle activity to normal. Richardson and colleagues (2002) used Doppler imaging to assess SIJ laxity on patients while at the same time studying trunk muscle activity using electromyography (EMG). These authors were able to demonstrate a reduction in joint laxity (i.e., increased SIJ stability) by using TrA contraction. Reduced general back stability has also been found in people with SIJ dysfunction. Hungerford and colleagues (2003) found changes in internal oblique, multifidus, and gluteus maximus recruitment in the weight-bearing leg of those with SIJ pain. This is significant clinically, because patients with SIJ pain often present with pain that is worsened when standing in a swayback posture where they favour one leg.

Trunk muscle action

Facilitating co-contraction of the muscles surrounding the lumbar spine, can stiffen or stabilise the spine providing resistance to movement. Lumbar spine dissection (Jemmett et al. 2004) has shown individual segmental attachments to the lumbar spine for transversus, psoas, quadratus lumborum, and multifidus and these muscles are often referred to as local or primary stabilisers. The other muscles pass over the lumbar region without segmental attachment and so are considered global or secondary stabilisers. Importantly, all muscle are able to stiffen the spine and so may act to stabilise at some time during a movement.

> **Keypoint:**
>
> *Local* stabilising muscles attach directly to the lumbar vertebrae. *Global* stabilisers pass over the lumbar vertebral without segmental attachment. All muscles can stiffen or stabilise the spine.

Spinal extensor muscles

The spinal extensors may be broadly categorised as superficial muscles (the erector spinae) that travel the length of the lumbar spine and attach to the sacrum and pelvis and as deep, or intersegmental muscles (multifidi, interspinales, and intertransversarii) that span the spaces between the individual lumbar segments.

The intersegmental muscles, being more deeply placed, are closer to the centre of rotation of the spine and have a shorter lever arm than the superficial muscles. However, their closeness to the centre of rotation means that the change in length of intersegmental muscles is less for any given change in the spine's angular position, and the muscles' shorter length may give them a faster reaction time, creating a smoother and more efficient stabilising control system.

Being larger in size and farther from the centre of rotation, the superficial muscles are better placed to create gross sagittal rotation movements, whereas the intersegmental muscles may be of greater importance to spinal stability. Furthermore, because the smaller intersegmental muscles have about seven times the number of muscle spindles (Bastide et al. 1989) than the larger muscles have, the smaller muscles have a greater proprioceptive role.

Deep (Intersegmental) muscles

These muscles lie below the erector spinae, at the level of the spinous process and transverse processes of the vertebra. Of the deeply placed intersegmental muscles, the multifidus has been the focus of lumbar stability research. The fibres of the multifidus are arranged segmentally, and each fascicle of a given vertebra has a separate innervation by the medial branch of the dorsal ramus of the vertebra below (Macintosh and Bogduk 1986).

Studies have also been able to differentiate between deep and superficial portions of this muscle (Moseley et al. 2003). Using arm movements, Moseley and colleagues showed that the superficial multifidus worked with the erector spinae and varied depending on the direction of arm movement. The deep multifidus worked with the TrA, and these muscles were active to the same degree whatever the arm movement direction. In addition, it seems that the action of individual components of the multifidus is different depending on the body's preparedness for the task, that is, whether the subject is expecting the movement, as though the body was trying to fine-tune its stability response.

The primary function of each multifidus fascicle may be to control lordosis at its vertebral level and to independently counteract any imposed loading. The action of the multifidus can be resolved into a small horizontal and much larger vertical component, a configuration which enables the multifidus to produce posterior sagittal rotation (rocking) of the lumbar vertebrae (Macintosh and Bogduk 1986). This action neutralises spinal flexion caused as a secondary action when the oblique abdominals produce spinal rotation. Because the line of action of the long fascicles of the multifidus lies behind the lumbar spine, the muscle also increases lumbar lordosis. The multifidus is active through the whole range of flexion, during rotation in either direction, and during extension movements of the hip. Posterior sagittal rotation occurs during all flexion movements in order to resist the anterior sagittal rotation that naturally accompanies flexion.

Panjabi's description of instability (as a reduction in stiffness within the neutral zone of the lumbar spine) is particularly relevant to multifidus function. The multifidus is a muscle well positioned to enhance segmental stiffness in the neutral zone and contributes nearly 70% of the stiffness resulting from muscle contraction (Wilke et al. 1995).

Real-time ultrasound imaging has revealed marked asymmetry of the multifidus in patients with LBP (Hides et al. 1994). Cross-sectional area (CSA) of the multifidus was markedly reduced on the ipsilateral side to symptoms, the site of reduction corresponding to the level of lumbar lesion as assessed by manual therapy palpation. The muscle also showed a rounder shape, suggesting muscle spasm. The suggested mechanism for the CSA reduction was by inhibition through perceived pain via a long loop reflex. The level of vertebral pathology may have been targeted to protect the damaged tissues from movement. The authors suggested that the rapid muscle wasting (less than 14 days in 20 of the 26 patients studied) may have resulted from spasm-induced reduction in circulation to the muscle.

In addition to noting changes in muscle bulk, Biedermann and colleagues (1991) observed altered fibre types in the multifidus of patients with LBP; patients who tended to decrease their physical and social activities because of LBP showed a reduced ratio of slow-twitch to fast-twitch muscle fibres. This could be the muscle's adaptive response to changes in functional demand placed on it, or the injury may have caused a shift in recruitment patterns of motor units of the paraspinal muscles, with the fast-twitch motor units being recruited before the slow-twitch units. Pathologic changes in the multifidus following LBP include a moth-eaten appearance of type I fibres and an increase in fatty deposits.

In an early study comparing medical treatment alone (1–3 days of bed rest, analgesics, and anti-inflammatory medication) with medical treatment plus specific exercise therapy to the multifidus, Hides and colleagues (1996) showed that multifidus activity could be retrained. Subjects who had experienced first-episode acute LBP showed an average of 24% reduction in CSA to the multifidus on the painful side. The difference between painful and painless sides changed from nearly 17% after four weeks to 14% after ten weeks in those subjects receiving medical treatment alone. For those who received additional exercise therapy, however, the mean values were 0.7% at four weeks, decreasing to 0.24% after ten weeks.

By injecting an irritant chemical (hypertonic saline) directly into the muscle, researchers have proven that the multifidus can be a source of pain (Cornwall et al. 2006). Pain can occur in a muscle because of spasm which restricts the blood flow through a muscle producing ischemic pain. Prolonged lumbar flexion has been shown to produce spasm in the multifidus in cats used as a model for the human spine (Williams et al. 2000). However, Williams and colleagues showed that the initial multifidus spasm reduced dramatically, by more than 90% after only 3 min.

Jackson and colleagues (2001) used a cat (feline) model to subject the spine to 20 min of prolonged flexion to produce sacrospinous ligament strain and multifidus spasm. Initial decrease in Multifidus EMG activity was followed by spasm, with full recovery was not being observed after seven hours of rest.

With the plethora of research concerning the multifidus over the years, it is tempting to believe that this muscle is the key to the lumbar spine and to use it in isolation to retrain the spine. However, many of the exercises used when retraining the multifidus also target other muscles, and many subjects find isolated multifidus contractions extremely difficult.

Some interesting studies highlight the problem of muscle isolation techniques when used alone. Using computed tomography, Choi and colleagues (2005) measured the CSA of the multifidus and longissimus muscles (L4–L5 level) following a 12-week rehabilitation programme in patients who had undergone surgery for lumbar disc herniation. Resisted back extension was used rather than selective muscle isolation. Both muscles showed significant increases following the programme, the CSA of longissimus increasing by 7.2% and that of the multifidus by 29.2%. Danneels and colleagues (2003) used computed tomography to measure the CSA of the multifidus after either (a) stability training alone, (b) stability combined with dynamic resistance training, or (c) stability with static–dynamic training. Their results demonstrated significant increases in CSA only in the group using stabilisation combined with static–dynamic training.

The back extensor muscles including the multifidus have been trained in normal subjects using both resistance training alone (San Juan et al. 2005) and resistance training on unstable surfaces or a stability ball (Scott et al. 2015). Additionally, the changes seen in Multifidus because of CLBP often remain after symptom resolution (MacDonald et al. 2009), and Multifidus muscle geometry does not always predict clinical outcomes (Zielinski et al. 2013). A systematic review of motor control exercise (MCE) on morphological changes to the Multifidus (9 trials with 451 participants) found that MCE was no better than other exercise when treating people with LBP, that there was no relation between post exercise changes in Multifidus and LBP related disability and concluded that changes to the muscle are unrelated to clinical outcomes (Pinto et al. 2021).

Keypoint:

Changes to the *Multifidus* muscle may be unrelated to clinical outcomes.

Superficial muscles

These muscles lie on top of the deep muscles, above the level of the spinous process and transverse processes.

Erector spinae

The lumbar erector spinae muscle group consists of three components, iliocostalis, longissimus, and spinales (Figure 4.12). Segments of the muscles are named after the spinal regions they attach to—capitis (head), cervicis (neck), thoracis (thoracic spine), and lumborum (lumbar spine).

The force produced by the lumbar longissimus can be resolved into a large vertical vector and a smaller horizontal vector. However, the fascicle attachments are closer to the axis of sagittal rotation than those of the multifidus, so their effect on posterior sagittal rotation is less. Because the horizontal vectors of lumbar longissimus are directed backward, the muscle can draw the vertebrae backward into posterior translation and restore the anterior translation that

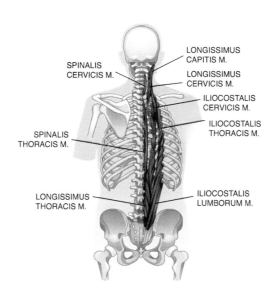

FIGURE 4.12 Components of erector spinae.

occurs with lumbar flexion. The upper lumbar fascicles are better equipped to facilitate posterior sagittal rotation, whereas the lower levels are better suited to resist anterior translation.

The lumbar iliocostalis has an action like that of the lumbar longissimus. In addition, the muscle cooperates with the multifidus to neutralise flexion caused when the abdominals rotate the trunk. The thoracic longissimus can indirectly increase lumbar lordosis via its effect on the aponeurosis of the erector spinae. It also indirectly laterally flexes the lumbar spine through its lateral flexion of the thoracic spine.

The thoracic iliocostalis attaches not to the lumbar vertebrae but to the iliac crest. On contraction, these fascicles increase lordosis; through their additional leverage from the ribs, they indirectly laterally flex the lumbar spine. During contralateral rotation, the ribs separate, stretching the thoracic iliocostalis, which can therefore limit this movement. On contraction, the thoracic iliocostalis will resist rotation of the rib cage and lumbar spine from a position of contralateral rotation.

Probably the endurance rather than the strength of the erector spinae is important to LBP rehabilitation. Endurance has been used to predict susceptibility to LBP (Biering-Sorensen 1984) and to predict chronicity following injury (Enthoven et al. 2003). The classic Biering-Sorensen test, has been shown to be a reliable measure of spinal endurance in several clinical populations, including both symptomatic and asymptomatic people (Latimer et al. 1999).

The Biering-Sorenson test measures the amount of time a person can keep their unsupported upper body horizontal with the legs fixed and arms folded. The test has been validated as a differential test for LBP, and measure hip and spinal extensor endurance. Those with LBP have a significantly lower holding time than those without. Times reported are 39.55 to 54.5 seconds for those with LBP (mixed sex) and 80–194 (male) and 146–227 seconds (female). Holding times of less than 176 seconds may be predicted of LBP occurrence and greater than 198 seconds protective (Demoulin et al. 2006).

Quadratus lumborum

The quadratus lumborum (QL) (Figure 4.13) lies deeper than the erector spinae and has medial and lateral fibres. The medial fibres connect the lumbar transverse processes to the ilium and iliolumbar ligament or the 12th rib, whereas the lateral fibres directly connect the ilium and iliolumbar ligament and 12th rib. The QL has a small extensor torque and a larger lateral flexion torque and is able to stabilise the lumbar spine via its segmental attachments. EMG with fine wire electrodes has shown the muscle to be more active during lateral bending than during extension and especially active in upright standing and unilateral carrying. Side-support actions shift some of the loading of the muscles from the discs and facet joints of the lumbar spine to the side. This role of the QL as a potential stabiliser of the lumbar spine expands the traditionally recognised role of the muscle as a prime mover of side flexion and as an auxiliary muscle of respiration.

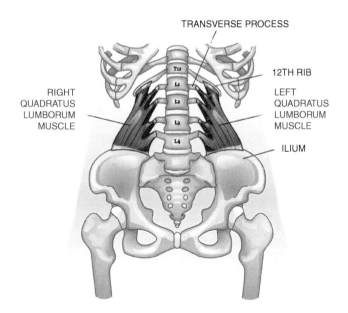

TRANSVERSE PROCESS

12TH RIB

RIGHT
QUADRATUS
LUMBORUM
MUSCLE

LEFT
QUADRATUS
LUMBORUM
MUSCLE

ILIUM

FIGURE 4.13 Quadratus lumborum.

McGill (2002) advocated retraining the QL using the horizontal side-support exercise in various guises and wrote that the normal value for an endurance hold of this action is 86 s (mean value, combined male and female scores).

Iliopsoas

The iliopsoas (Figure 4.14) consists of the separate psoas and iliacus muscles. The psoas major arises from the vertebral bodies and discs of the lumbar and 12th thoracic vertebrae and from their transverse processes. The muscle passes downwards and laterally, beneath the inguinal ligament, to blend with the fibres of iliacus and then to attach onto the posterior aspect of the lesser trochanter of the femur. The iliacus is a large triangular muscle on the anterior aspect of the pelvis. It arises primarily from the upper and posterior portions of the iliac fossa, but some fibres have been found on the sacrum and anterior sacroiliac ligament. The fibres from the iliacus pass downwards and medially to blend with those of the psoas major and attach to the lesser trochanter, with a few fibres merging with the joint capsule.

The iliopsoas flexes the hip, anteriorly tilting the pelvis and flexing the lumbar spine. Although these actions are minimal, the psoas major extends the upper lumbar spine and flexes the lower lumbar spine (Bogduk et al. 1992); far more important is the psoas major's production of compression and shear forces over the lumbar spine. The individual fascicles of psoas spiral anteromedially and are

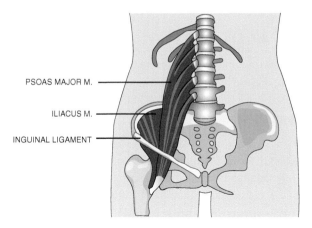

PSOAS MAJOR M.

ILIACUS M.

INGUINAL LIGAMENT

FIGURE 4.14 Iliopsoas muscle.

all of similar lengths. The lines of action of these fascicles run very close to the axis of rotation of the lumbar spine, giving the muscle fascicles very small torque arms and reducing the muscle's ability to flex the trunk on the stationary hip.

Because the two components of iliopsoas have a separate innervation (psoas from the anterior rami and L1–L3, and iliacus from the femoral nerve), they can be activated separately. In a study using fine-wire electrodes guided by high-resolution ultrasound, Andersson and colleagues (1995) showed selective recruitment of the iliacus during contralateral leg extension from single-leg standing. No postural activity was seen in either muscle during relaxed standing or with the whole trunk flexed to 30°. When the contralateral hand was loaded (34 kg weight), the psoas was active but the iliacus was electrically silent. During sitting with a straight back, the psoas was active but the iliacus relatively silent; in relaxed sitting, both muscles were inactive. Both muscles showed moderate activity when subjects sat with an anteriorly tilted pelvis and an increased lordosis. During abdominal exercise, both muscles were active during straight-leg sit-ups—with even higher activity during sit-ups with the knees and hips flexed to 90° (crunch position). However, little activity was seen when subjects performed trunk curls from the crunch position. During straight-leg raising, both muscles were active when the ipsilateral leg was lifted; both were inactive when the contralateral leg was lifted.

A stability function for the posterior fibres of the psoas has been proposed (Gibbons 2001). These smaller fibres attach from the transverse processes of the lumbar vertebrae and are located closer to the axis of spinal rotation than are the anterior fibres. They attach directly to the deep layer of the TLF and fill the inter-transverse interval. Within the 'drum' of the IAP mechanism (p. 55), the lid of the drum is the diaphragm and the base the pelvic floor. The posterior fibres of the psoas may form a link between the IAP lid and floor through the medial arcuate ligament to the diaphragm and the psoas fascia to the pelvic floor. Mathematical modelling has shown the psoas to have potential stabilising effects in upright stance (Penning 2000). We have seen that the multifidus muscle reduces in CSA as a result of back pain, and Barker and colleagues (2004) showed similar CSA changes in the psoas. Their study revealed positive correlations between the percentage decrease in CSA of the psoas on the affected side of the lumbar spine and (a) pain rating, (b) reported nerve root compression, and (c) duration of symptoms.

Abdominal muscles

The abdominal muscle group consists of four muscles, divided into two groups (Figure 4.15). The deep (anterolateral) abdominals are TrA and internal oblique; the superficial (front) abdominals are the rectus abdominis and external oblique.

Anatomy of the superficial abdominals

The rectus abdominis is positioned vertically at the front of the abdomen. It attaches from the symphysis pubis and pubic crest and runs to the xiphoid process and fifth, sixth, and seventh ribs, being broader superiorly. The lateral border (semilunaris) can be seen in lean subjects, as can the central separation between the two muscles, the linea alba. Of the three noticeable tendinous intersections of this muscle, one is level with the umbilicus, one is level with the xiphoid, and one is midway between the two. Each rectus muscle is enclosed within a fibrous sheath (the rectus sheath) formed from the aponeuroses of the internal and external oblique muscles and of the TrA. These aponeuroses join centrally to form the linea alba. The rectus sheath changes at a level midway between the pubic symphysis and the umbilicus. In the upper area of the muscle, above this point,

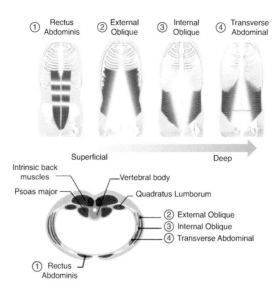

FIGURE 4.15 The abdominal muscles.

the aponeurosis of internal oblique splits into two, one part passing behind the rectus and the other in front. The aponeurosis of TrA fuses with the posterior portion of the sheath, whereas the aponeurosis of external oblique fuses with the anterior sheath. In the lower portion of the muscle (below the midpoint between the pubis and umbilicus), the oblique abdominal and TrA aponeuroses pass in front of the rectus, and as a result the rectus is less visible in this region.

The external oblique is positioned on the anterolateral aspect of the abdomen, with its fibres running downwards and medially. It attaches from the outer borders of the lower eight ribs (and their costal cartilages) and then passes towards the midline. The muscle interdigitates with the serratus anterior (above) and latissimus dorsi (below). The lateral fibres are almost vertical and attach to the iliac crest, whereas the medial fibres attach into the rectus sheath. The lower border of the muscle aponeurosis passes between the pubic tubercle and the anterior superior iliac spine to form the inguinal ligament.

> **Keypoint:**
>
> The outermost (lateral) fibres of the external oblique run vertically and work in flexion actions with the rectus abdominis.

Anatomy of the deep abdominals

The internal oblique is deep to the external oblique and attaches from the lateral two thirds of the inguinal ligament and the anterior two thirds of the iliac crest. It also takes attachment from the thoracolumbar fascia. The fibres fan outwards and upwards (the posterior fibres being almost vertical) to attach to the inferior borders of the lower four ribs. The anterior fibres pass medially to help form the rectus sheath. The portion of the muscle that attaches to the inguinal ligament joins its neighbouring fibres from TrA to form the conjoint tendon.

The TrA is the deepest of the sheetlike abdominal muscles and attaches from the lateral third of the inguinal ligament and the anterior two thirds of the inner lip of the iliac crest. In addition, it has an attachment from the TLF (where it merges with the internal oblique to form the lateral raphe) and from the lower six ribs, where it interdigitates with the diaphragm. Its fibres pass horizontally to merge into the rectus sheath, with the lower fibres attaching to the inguinal ligament and merging with the fibres of the internal oblique to form the conjoint tendon. The lower part of the TrA forms into the transversalis fascia in which lies the deep inguinal ring.

Functions of the abdominals

The rectus abdominis and lateral fibres of external oblique are the prime movers of trunk flexion; the internal oblique and TrA may be considered the major stabilisers. The rectus and external oblique are superficial muscles that often dominate trunk actions. The transversus and internal oblique are more deeply placed, and patients often are unable to contract them voluntarily.

The rectus abdominis flexes the trunk by approximating the pelvis and rib cage to which it attaches (i.e., moving them closer together). An abdominal hollowing action (pulling the umbilicus inward towards the spine) activates the internal oblique and transversus muscles, and the transversus has been said to act at the initiation of movement to stabilise the trunk in overhead and lower-limb actions (Hodges and Richardson 1996). Differentiation has been made between the various regions of the TrA (Urquhart et al. 2005). When the TrA is used for postural maintenance during limb motion, the EMG onset of the upper region of TrA is later than that of the middle and lower regions. A similar picture is said to emerge during active trunk rotation, with the recruitment patterns of the upper muscle fascicles being opposite to those of the middle and lower fascicles. During left trunk rotation, the lower and middle TrA regions of the opposite side (contralateral) muscle are more active, but in right trunk rotation the upper region of the same side (ipsilateral) muscle is more active. However, this view has been challenged by subsequent work (Morris et al. 2012) which shows TrA activity forming part of a general synergy of muscles initiating axial rotation forces which oppose arm movement. These authors argued that training pre-activation of the TrA was not justified. In addition, TrA contraction has been shown to be excessive during an active straight leg raise (ASLR) in persons with long lasting pregnancy related pelvic girdle pain (PGP). Again, the authors argued that there was no rationale for exercise prescription to enhance TrA contraction is this clinical group (Mens and Pool-Goudzwaard 2017). Looking at athletes (college golfers) with and without LBP Skibski et al. (2020) used ultrasound measures of TrA activity and observed no significant differences between painful and pain-free groups. Alteration in feed-forwards response of the TrA may represent a normal variation in motor control (Allison and Morris 2008) and may not be clinically relevant.

In resisted actions such as sport or lifting, the abdominal muscles stabilise the trunk and provide a firm base of support for the arms and legs to work against. If stability is poor (in relation to total power of the subject), some of the energy of the limb actions can displace the pelvis and trunk instead of providing the desired limb movement.

Patterns of coordination among the abdominals during spinal movement

In terms of spinal stabilisation, the contraction speed of the abdominals may be more critical than their strength when they react to a force tending to displace the lumbar spine. Moreover, the ability of a patient to dissociate deep abdominal function from that of the superficial abdominals can be important, and one of the keys to lumbar stabilisation may be the ratio rather than the intensity of muscle activity. Abdominal hollowing (rather than a sit-up movement) emphasises the TrA and internal oblique (rather than the rectus abdominis and the external oblique). O'Sullivan and colleagues (1997) found that patients with chronic low back pain (CLBP) were poorer at using the internal oblique than using the rectus abdominis and external oblique, reflecting a shift in the pattern of motor activity. As CLBP patients attempted an abdominal hollowing action, they tended to substitute the superficial muscles that override the deep abdominals. When expressed as a ratio of internal oblique over rectus abdominis, the value from the control group (non-LBP) was 8.74 whereas the CLBP group had a ratio of only 2.41—indicating a much larger proportional contribution to hollowing by the internal oblique in the control group. Pain inhibition in the subjects with CLBP may have led to altered muscle recruitment and compensatory strategies (O'Sullivan et al. 1997).

EMG measurements of trunk muscles have shown that the muscles do not simply work as prime movers of the spine but show antagonistic activity during various movements. The oblique abdominals are more active than predicted, to help stabilise the trunk. Zetterberg and colleagues (1987) reported that subjects' abdominal muscle activities during maximum trunk extension ranged from 32% to 68% of their longissimus activities. As would be expected, the ipsilateral muscles showed maximum activity in resisted lateral flexion, but the contralateral muscles were also active at about 10–20% of the maximum values.

The coordinated patterns among the abdominal muscles are task-specific. But the only muscle that is active in all patterns is the TrA. During maximum voluntary isometric trunk extension, the TrA is the only one of the abdominal muscles to show marked activity. It is also the muscle most consistently related to changes in IAP (Cresswell et al. 1992). Not only does the TrA contract whenever the trunk moves in any direction, but its activity always precedes the contraction of the other trunk muscles in the normal (non-LBP) subject (Cresswell et al. 1994). The ability of the TrA to contract before other abdominal muscles is a feature of motor control (as described subsequently).

Keypoint:

The transversus abdominis is active in trunk movements in all directions. Its activity often precedes that of the other abdominal muscles in normal subjects.

Intra-abdominal pressure

Pressure within the trunk (intratruncal pressure) includes both *intra-abdominal* and *intrathoracic* pressure. Intrathoracic pressure is created during inspiration by expanding the lungs within the rib cage to coincide with a lift or other effort. Intrabdominal pressure (IAP) involves synchronous contraction of the abdominal muscles, the diaphragm, and the muscles of the pelvic floor. The deep abdominals (TrA and internal oblique) are often considered the most important of the abdominal muscle groups in this respect because they are visceral compressors rather than flexors. Most people experience IAP in everyday life, for example, when the muscles contract reflexively to defend the abdomen from a direct blow. The theoretical basis for the IAP mechanism in lifting is that pressure within the abdomen, acting like an inflated balloon against the pelvis and diaphragm, provides additional extensor torque to the spine (Figure 4.16), providing a resistance to flexion.

Keypoint:

Intra-abdominal pressure is created by synchronous contraction of the abdominal muscles, the diaphragm, and the muscles of the pelvic floor.

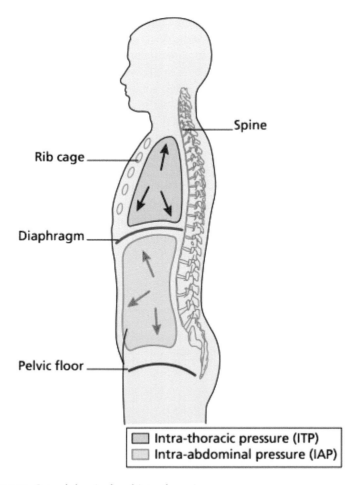

FIGURE 4.16 Intraabdominal and intrathoracic pressure.

Contraction of the TrA and the internal oblique increases IAP, providing the glottis is closed. Visualising the trunk as a cylinder, the cylinder top would be formed by the diaphragm, the bottom the pelvic floor, and the walls the deep abdominals (transversus and internal oblique). As the abdominal wall is pulled in and up, the walls of the cylinder are effectively pulled in. If a deep breath is taken, the diaphragm is lowered, compressing the cylinder from the top. If the pelvic floor (the bottom of the cylinder) is intact, the cylinder is pressurised and made more solid. In this way, it is able to better resist any bending stress applied to it.

The IAP is greater if the breath is held following a deep inspiration (Valsalva maneuver) because the diaphragm is lower and the comparative size of the abdominal cavity (the cylinder) is reduced. During lifting, the pelvic floor muscles (the floor of the cylinder) contract to maintain pelvic integrity and prevent urination. The Valsalva maneuver is therefore appropriate for normal subjects during heavy lifting as long as it occurs only briefly. However, because blood pressure changes may not be desirable in subjects with poor cardiopulmonary health, heavy lifting is not normally recommended for this group.

Making the trunk into a more solid cylinder reduces axial compression and shear loads and transmits loads over a wider area. IAP may also help to protect the spine from excessive indirect loads (those not acting directly on the spine but through limb loading), with the muscles acting to involuntarily fix the rib cage. IAP is greater when heavy lifts are performed and when the lift is rapid.

Abdominal muscle strength affects IAP—strong athletes can produce very large IAP values. Yet, strengthening the abdominal muscles with movements such as sit-ups does not permanently increase IAP because these exercises usually do not mimic the coordination among abdominal muscles that is inherent in the IAP mechanism. Investigating the effect of abdominal muscle training on IAP, Hemborg and colleagues (1985) used isometric trunk curl and twist exercises. Increased recruitment of motor units in the oblique abdominal muscles clearly demonstrated muscle strengthening, yet EMG activity of these muscles decreased during lifting, implying that the subjects did not make functional use of their increased ability to recruit more motor units. The differentiation between strength and functional ability is important: If an exercise is not specific to a task, the physiological adaptation of the musculoskeletal system may be inappropriate.

A number of important criticisms have been made against the IAP mechanism when it has been presented as an important stabilising process for the spine. First, to fully stabilise the spine during the lifting of heavy weights, the IAP would have to exceed the systolic pressure within the aorta, effectively cutting off the blood flow to the viscera and lower limbs. Competitive weightlifters have been known to black out when lifting extremely heavy weight, perhaps because of very high IAP. At the onset of a lift, there is an initial rapid increase in IAP—known as the snatch pressure—that may last for less than 0.5 s. The pressure declines during the remainder of the lift. Hemborg and colleagues (1985) calculated that a peak IAP of 250 mmHg would be required to lift a 100 kg weight. Second, the muscle force required to create a sufficiently high IAP is greater than the hoop pressure possible from the abdominal muscles (Gracovetsky et al. 1985). Third, if the rectus abdominis contracts to increase IAP, it produces a flexion torque that counteracts the anteflexion effect of IAP created as the diaphragm and pelvic floor spread apart. These criticisms of IAP have led to reexamination of its contribution to back stability. Originally, IAP was believed to reduce the compression acting on the lumbar spine by as much as 40% (Eie 1966), but more recent studies have shown this to be only 7% (McGill et al. 2002).

Keypoint:

Intra-abdominal pressure has been estimated to reduce the compression acting on the lumbar spine by only 7%.

To retrain IAP voluntarily following injury, the subject must contract the pelvic floor muscles and TrA simultaneously. Ultrasound scanning has shown the thickness of the TrA to be greater (65.8% increase) when contracted with the pelvic floor muscles than without (49.7% increase) (Critchley 2002). Breathing should also be emphasised when retraining IAP, because diaphragm action is important to this mechanism. Using direct stimulation of the phrenic nerve, Hodges and colleagues (2005) showed IAP increases of 31% without TrA contraction—the increase coming from diaphragm action alone.

Keypoint:

Both pelvic floor action and breathing control must be used alongside transversus abdominis action (abdominal hollowing) to train the IAP mechanism.

It may be tempting to see the TrA as the key to the lumbar spine, but just as with the multifidus, isolation of this muscle alone is not enough for full rehabilitation. Many of the studies quoted as targeting the TrA actually used a drawing-in action called abdominal hollowing. Using MRI scanning, Hides and colleagues (2006) showed that this action significantly increased the CSA of not just the TrA but the internal oblique as well.

Motor control strategies

The body's central nervous system (CNS) must continually monitor the forces acting on the spine and the spinal movements themselves. In so doing, the CNS must analyse the present state of stiffness (stability) in the spine and either reduce it to allow unimpeded movement or increase it to reduce unwanted motion. To do this, the CNS receives continuous signals from nerve sensors in the spinal tissues including the joints, discs, ligaments, and muscles.

When people engage in repeated movements, their bodies anticipate the predictable load and the muscles brace themselves accordingly. When back stability is controlled in advance in this way, it is known as *feedforward control*. Using fine-wire electrodes, Hodges and Richardson (1996) assessed abdominal muscle action during shoulder flexion, extension, and abduction. They found that the TrA contracted before the shoulder muscles by as much as 38.9 ms. The reaction time for the deltoid was on average 188 ms, with the abdominal muscles (except transversus) following the deltoid contraction by 9.84 ms. With subjects who had a history of LBP, however, the contraction of the transversus failed to precede that of the deltoid, indicating that the subjects had lost the anticipatory nature of stability. This finding reveals a uniform dysfunction in the motor control of the TrA in people with LBP —the problem is not simply one of muscle strength. It appears that the anticipatory nature of the transversus may be lost in those with LBP.

Keypoint:

Patients with chronic low back pain may exhibit a motor control deficit (alteration in muscle reaction timing and anticipatory bracing) in the transversus abdominis.

A number of authors have highlighted contraction of the abdominal muscles before the initiation of limb movement as an example of a feedforward postural reaction (Friedli et al. 1984, Aruin and Latash 1995). In these cases, as would be expected, the erector spinae and the external oblique contract before arm flexion, whereas the rectus abdominis contracts before arm extension. In each case, the trunk muscles limit the reactive body movement towards the moving limb. Contraction of the transversus before the other abdominal muscle was described by Cresswell and colleagues (1994) in response to trunk movements, but anticipatory contraction of this type during limb movements is a newer finding. The TrA seems to contract during posture not simply to bring the body back closer to the posture line but to increase the stiffness of the lumbar region and enhance stability.

When working in this way, the CNS is predicting the types of stresses that the spine is likely to encounter in an action. How does it know? Throughout life, as we perform actions over and over again, we build up a movement vocabulary, which we are able to use as a reference point against which to compare a new movement. In this process, when the CNS recognises a familiar movement pattern, it is able to use feedforward motion control to plan ahead and contract the stability muscles by just the right amount to optimally stabilise the spine, without stiffening the spine so much that free movement is compromised. This is a highly skilled action and occurs in many seemingly mundane actions through our daily lives.

> **Keypoint:**
>
> Feedforward motor control anticipates what stability will be required by comparing against an internal reference map of familiar actions.

When more complex actions are performed, especially those that demand a subject's close attention, the contraction latency (waiting time before contraction occurs) of muscles will change. If the brain has to throw its attention into catching a ball, for example, the muscle contraction of a moving limb seems to hesitate and so the limb contraction latency is longer. However, the latency period for the stabilising muscles of the spine has been shown not to change, suggesting that stability is an automatic action that does not require a lot of thinking—it is not under higher centre control.

When movements are not predictable, the CNS measures stress imposed on the lumbar tissues, and when it determines that this stress is excessive, the CNS invokes a protective response; this is an example of feedback motor control. This is partially attributable to rapid protective reflexes such as the stretch reflex within the muscle spindles of the spinal muscles themselves. This type of reflex is short loop (local to the spinal cord) and has also been shown to occur in spinal muscles through stimulation of the disc annulus, ligaments, and facet joint capsules. Long-loop reflexes occur more slowly, involve the spinal cord and brain, and are thought to have a greater role in postural error correction (Hodges 2004).

> **Keypoint:**
>
> Feedback motor control measures stress imposed on spinal tissues and causes muscle responses after the stress has occurred.

Criticism of the initiation of TrA activity is that there may be a disconnect between pure science on one side, and clinical practice on the other (McGill 2016). Certainly, some people seem to benefit from stability re-training, while others do not and as we have seen previously there is no difference in outcome between stability exercise and general exercise for the management of LBP in population studies (Smith et al. 2014). In addition, within a general group of mechanical low back pain persons (MLBP) those with segmental instability reacted differently to those without (Silfies et al. 2009). Both groups activated trunk extensor muscles in a feedforward manner, but the non-instability group activated earlier that the instability group. Subgrouping patients into those with too little movement likely to benefit from *mobility* and those with too much movement likely to benefit from *stability* has been shown to be effective (Fritz et al. 2005a,b). Several clinical examination tests (Table 4.4) are able to predict radiographic instability and show good reliability for predicting the presence of

TABLE 4.4 Instability evaluation

Test	Detail
Aberrant motion	Painful arc of motion, instability catch, thigh climbing, reversal of lumbopelvic rhythm. Positive if any observed.
PIT	Pt in prone position on end of couch with feet on floor. PA pressure to painful segment of lumbar spine. Test positive if pain reduced to active leg extension. Positive is pain reduced.
Passive SLR	>91° positive
Lumbar flexion ROM	Forward flexion record ROM using bubble inclinometer at Sacrum (S2) and lumbar spine (T12-L1) Subtract sacral ROM from thoracolumbar >53° positive
PLE test	Pt prone, passively raised legs to 30° and traction. Positive if pain reproduced.
PA glide test	PA glide to lumbar spine at each segment. Positive in one level not stiff (hypomobile)

ROM—range of motion, PIT—prone instability test, SLR—straight leg raise, PLE—passive lumbar extension, PA—posteroanterior.

Data from Hicks et al. (2005), Alyazedi et al. (2015).

lumbar in stability non-radiographically (Alyazedi et al. 2015). In addition to age and fear-avoidance beliefs, four main physical tests predict the potential success of a stabilisation exercise programme (Hicks et al. 2005), these are straight leg raise (SLR), prone instability test (PIT), aberrant motions, and lumbar hypermobility.

Palpation and surface marking of the low back

We have covered the anatomy of the spine above, but the only time this is freely visible is at dissection or during surgery. When examining a patient, we have to palpate through the skin, subcutaneous tissue, and muscle layers. To do this we are looking for the most easily palpable structures and these are the bony landmarks.

> **Definition:**
>
> A *bony landmark* is a location on the skin where the underlying bone is close to the surface and clearly palpable.

Working from the head down, the most prominent bone at the back of the lower skull is the external occipital protuberance (EOP). Its top is called the inion and the nuchal ligament and upper fibres of trapezius attach to it. The superior nuchal line extends either side of the EOP. Moving down from here roughly 3 cm the palpating fingertip drops into a dip, at the base of which lies the rudimentary spinous process of the first cervical vertebra (C1) also called the Atlas bone (Table 4.5). Moving towards the tail (caudally) the first spinous process we can palpate is that of the second cervical vertebra (C2) or Axis bone. Due to the inward curve of the neck (cervical lordosis) the next vertebrae (C3–5) are tightly packed and difficult to differentiate. C6 and C7 are more prominent and C7 (cervical prominens) may be distinguished from C6 by extending the neck, whereupon C6 moves deeper. Additionally, with the patient lying on their back, palpating C7 and T1 (sometimes more prominent that C7) can be differentiated by rotating the neck. As T1 is part of the thoracic spine and relatively fixed by bodyweight on the ribcage it will stay still while C7 moves with cervical rotation.

Moving downwards (caudally) along the thoracic spinous processes, T3 is roughly at the level of the root of the scapular spine and T7 level with the inferior angle of the scapula. T12 attaches to the 12th rib and so the rib attachment may be traced back to the vertebral line. The rib angles of the mid and upper thoracic region are around 3–4 cm from the tip of the transverse processes of each vertebra.

Definition:

Caudal means near the tail (inferior part of the body), *cephalic* means closer to the head (superior part of the body).

Moving from the thoracic spine to the lumbar spine (Table 4.6), the fourth lumber vertebra (L4) is roughly level with a line joining the highest point of the iliac crests (supracristal plane). The supracristal plane itself is roughly level with the umbilicus (belly button) and used to divide the upper and lower quadrants of the abdomen (the midline divides between left and right). The fifth lumbar vertebra

TABLE 4.5 Surface marking of the upper back

Level	Palpation
C1	Atlas—rudimentary spinous process 3 cms below external occipital protuberance
C2	Axis—prominent lump below C1
C7	Cervical prominens—lowest cervical vertebra. Extend neck to distinguish from C6 which disappears
T1	T1 below C7. Distinguish by rotating neck. T1 stays still, C7 moves
T3	Approximately level with the root of the scapular spine
T7	Approximately level with the inferior angle of the scapula
T12	Attached to 12th (lowest) rib. Approximately at mid-point of a line joining inferior angle of the scapula and the iliac crest.
Rib angle	3–4 cms lateral to tip of transverse process

TABLE 4.6 Surface marking of the lower back and pelvis

Level	Palpation
L4	Approximately level with top of iliac crests (supracristal plane)
L5	First dip as finger slides off sacrum in cephalic direction
Sacrum	Lateral edge defined by line between PSIS and sacral hiatus
Coccyx	Usually palpable from sacral hiatus to coccyx tip
ASIS	Anterior extremity of iliac crest
PSIS	Posterior edge of the iliac crest, at the base of the dimple of Venus
Ischial tuberosity	Approximately 5 cm from the midline, at the gluteal fold
Greater trochanter	Slide finger upwards alongside of femur to prominent lateral eminence

ASIS—anterior superior iliac spine. PSIS—posterior superior iliac spine.

(L5) has a shorter spinous process than the other lumbar vertebra and its body is more anteriorly placed, so the tip of the L5 spinous process is palpated at the base of a dip at the level of the top of the sacrum. The tips of the lumbar transverse processes lie approximately 5–6 cm lateral to the midline to the side of the erector spinae muscles.

Finding the iliac crest (best palpated using the side of the hand than the fingertips) the anterior extremity is the anterior superior iliac spine (ASIS) and the posterior extremity the posterior superior iliac spine (PSIS). The sacrum is triangular with the base uppermost and its lateral edge lies on a line from the PSIS to the sacral hiatus. The hiatus is a U-shaped space lying at the caudal part of the sacrum between the two sacral cornua. All points are fairly superficial and easily palpable.

The greater trochanter is readily palpable by sliding the palpating finger upwards from the side of the femur to the prominent lateral eminence, roughly 10 cm below the lateral aspect of the iliac crest. The ischial tuberosity (lying approximately 5 cm from the midline) lies at the gluteal fold between the lateral border of the sacrum and the greater trochanter.

References

Adams, M., Bogduk, N., Burton, K., and Dolan, P. (2002). *The biomechanics of back pain*. Edinburgh, UK: Churchill Livingstone.

Adams, M.A., and Dolan, P. (1997). The combined function of the spine, pelvis, and legs when lifting with a straight back. In Vleeming, A., Mooney, V., Dorman, T., Snijders, C., and Stoeckart, R., Eds., *Movement, stability and low back pain*. New York: Churchill Livingstone, 211–217.

Adams, M.A., and Hutton, W.C. (1983). The mechanical function of the lumbar apophyseal joints. *Spine* 8: 327–330.

Adams, M.A., Hutton, W.C., and Stott, J.R.R. (1980). The resistance to flexion of the lumbar intervertebral joint. *Spine* 5: 245–253.

Allison, G.T., and Morris, S.L. (2008). Transversus abdominis and core stability: Has the pendulum swung? *British Journal of Sports Medicine* 42(11): 930–931.

Alyazedi, F.M., Lohman, E.B., Wesley Swen, R., and Bahjri, K. (2015). The inter-rater reliability of clinical tests that best predict the subclassification of lumbar segmental instability: Structural, functional and combined instability. *The Journal of Manual & Manipulative Therapy* 23(4): 197–204.

Andersson, E., Oddsson, L., Grundstrom, H., and Thorstensson, A. (1995). The role of the psoas and iliacus muscles for stability and movement of the lumbar spine, pelvis and hip. *Scandinavian Journal of Medicine and Science in Sports* 5: 10–16.

Aruin, A.S., and Latash, M.L. (1995). Directional specificity of postural muscles in feed-forward postural reactions during fast voluntary arm movements. *Experimental Brain Research* 103: 323–332.

Aspden, R.M. (1992). Review of the functional anatomy of the spinal ligaments and the lumbar erector spinae muscles. *Clinical Anatomy* 5: 372–387.

Barker, K.L., Shamley, D.R., and Jackson, D. (2004). Changes in the cross-sectional area of multifidus and psoas in patients with unilateral back pain: The relationship to pain and disability. *Spine* 29: 515–519.

Barker, P.J., Guggenheimer, K.T., Grkovic, I., et al. (2006). Effects of tensioning the lumbar fasciae on segmental stiffness during flexion and extension. *Spine* 15(4): 397–405.

Bastide, G., Zadeh, J., and Lefebre, D. (1989). Are the little muscles what we think they are? *Surgical and Radiological Anatomy* 11: 255–256.

Biedermann, H.J., Shanks, G.L., Forrest, W.J., et al. (1991). Power spectrum analyses of electromyographic activity. *Spine* 16: 1179–1184.

Biering-Sorensen, R. (1984). Physical measurement as risk indicators for low back trouble over a one year period. *Spine* 9: 106–119.

Bogduk, N., and Engel, R. (1984). The menisci of the lumbar zygapophyseal joints. A review of their anatomy and clinical significance. *Spine* 9: 454–460.

Bogduk, N., and Twomey, L.T. (1987). *Clinical anatomy of the lumbar spine*. Edinburgh, UK: Churchill Livingstone.

Bogduk, N., and Twomey, L.T. (1991). *Clinical anatomy of the lumbar spine* (2nd ed). Edinburgh, UK: Churchill Livingstone.

Bogduk, N., Pearcy, M., and Hadfield, G. (1992). Anatomy and biomechanics of psoas major. *Clinical Biomechanics* 7: 109–119.

Cappozzo, A., Felici, F., Figura, F., and Gazzani, F. (1985). Lumbar spine loading during half-squat exercises. *Medicine and Science in Sports and Exercise* 17(5): 613–620.

Chiu, C.C., Chuang, T.Y., Chang, K.H., Wu, C.H., Lin, P.W., & Hsu, W.Y. (2015). The probability of spontaneous regression of lumbar herniated disc: a systematic review. *Clinical Rehabilitation* 29(2): 184–195.

Cholewicki, J., and McGill, S.M. (1992). Lumbar posterior ligament involvement during extremely heavy lifts estimated from fluoroscopic measurements. *Journal of Biomechanics* 25: 17–28.

Cornwall, J., John-Harris, A., and Mercer, S.R. (2006). The lumbar multifidus muscle and patterns of pain. *Manual Therapy* 11: 40–45.

Cresswell, A.G., Grundstrom, H., and Thorstensson, A. (1992). Observations on intra-abdominal pressure and patterns of abdominal intra-muscular activity in man. *Acta Physiologica Scandinavica* 144: 409–418.

Cresswell, A.G., Oddsson, L., and Thorstensson, A. (1994). The influence of sudden perturbations on trunk muscle activity and intra-abdominal pressure while standing. *Experimental Brain Research* 98: 336–341.

Critchley, D. (2002). Instructing pelvic floor contraction facilitates transversus abdominis thickness increase during low-abdominal hollowing. *Physiotherapy Research International* 7: 65–75.

Crock, H.V., and Yoshizawa, H. (1976). The blood supply of the lumbar vertebral column. *Clinical Orthopaedics* 115: 6–21.

Cunha, Silva, A. J., Pereira, P., Vaz, R., Gonçalves, R. M., & Barbosa, M. A. (2018). The inflammatory response in the regression of lumbar disc herniation. *Arthritis Research & Therapy* 20(1): 251. https://doi.org/10.1186/s13075-018-1743-4

Danielsson A., Brisby, H., Hansson, T.H. et al. (2007). A Tribute to Alf Nachemson: The Spine Interview. *The back letter* 22(2): 13, 18–21, February 2007.

Demoulin, C., Vanderthommen, M., Duysens, C., et al. (2006). Spinal muscle evaluation using the Sorensen test: A critical appraisal of the literature. *Joint Bone Spine* 73(1): 43–50.

Dreischarf, M., Rohlmann, A., Graichen, F., et al. (2016). In vivo loads on a vertebral body replacement during different lifting techniques. *Journal of Biomechanics* 49(6): 890–895.

Dumas, G.A., Beudoin, L., and Drouin, G. (1987). In situ mechanical behavior of posterior spinal ligaments in the lumbar region. *Journal of Biomechanics* 20: 301–310.

Eie, N. (1966). Load capacity of the low back. *Journal of Oslo City Hospitals* 16: 73–98.

Enthoven, P., Skargren, E., and Kjellman, G. (2003). Course of back pain in primary care: A prospective study of physical measures. *Journal of Rehabilitation Medicine* 35: 168–173.

Esola, M.A., McClure, P.W., Fitzgerald, G.K., et al. (1996). Analysis of lumbar spine and hip motion during forward bending in subjects with and without a history of low back pain. *Spine* 21: 71–78.

Farfan, H.F., Osteria, V., and Lamy, C. (1976). The mechanical etiology of spondylolysis and spondylolisthesis. *Clinical Orthopedics and Related Research* 117: 40–55.

Friedli, W.G., Hallet, M., and Simon, S.R. (1984). Postural adjustments associated with rapid voluntary arm movements. Electromyographic data. *Journal of Neurology, Neurosurgery and Psychiatry* 47: 611–622.

Fritz, J.M., Piva, S.R., and Childs, J.D. (2005a). Accuracy of the clinical examination to predict radiographic instability of the lumbar spine. *European Spine Journal* 14(8): 743–750.

Fritz, J.M., Whitman, J.M., and Childs, J.D. (2005b). Lumbar spine segmental mobility assessment: An examination of validity for determining intervention strategies in patients with low back pain. *Archives of Physical Medicine and Rehabilitation* 86(9): 1745–1752.

Gajdosik, R.L., Hatcher, C.K., and Whitsell, S. (1992). Influence of short hamstring muscles on the pelvis and lumbar spine in standing and during the toe touch test. *Clinical Biomechanics* 7: 38–42.

Gartenberg, A., Nessim, A., and Cho, W. (2021). Sacroiliac joint dysfunction: Pathophysiology, diagnosis, and treatment. *European Spine Journal* 30(10): 2936–2943.

Gibbons, S. (2001). Biomechanics and stability mechanisms of psoas major. In *The 4th Interdisciplinary World Congress on Low Back Pain*. Montreal. Canada: European Conference Organizers, 17–19.

Gracovetsky, S., Farfan, H.F., and Helleur, C. (1985). The abdominal mechanism. *Spine* 10: 317–324.

Gruss, L.T., Gruss, R., and Schmitt, D. (2017). Pelvic breadth and locomotor kinematics in human evolution. *Anatomical Record* 300: 739–751.

Halbertsma, J.P., Goeken, L.N., Hof, A.L., Groothoff, J.W., and Eisma W.H. (2001). Extensibility and stiffness of the hamstrings in patients with non-specific low back pain. *Archives of Physical Medicine and Rehabilitation* 82: 232–238.

Hemborg, B., Moritz, U., Hamberg, J., et al. (1985). Intra-abdominal pressure and trunk muscle activity during lifting. III. Effects of abdominal muscle training in chronic low-back patients. *Scandinavian Journal of Rehabilitation Medicine* 17: 15–24.

Hicks, G.E., Fritz, J.M., Delitto, A., et al. (2005). Preliminary development of a clinical prediction rule for determining which patients with low back pain will respond to a stabilization exercise program. *Archives of Physical Medicine and Rehabilitation* 86(9): 1753–1762.

Hides, J.A., Stokes, M.J., Saide, M., et al. (1994). Evidence of lumbar multifidus muscle wasting ipsilateral to symptoms in patients with acute/subacute low back pain. *Spine* 19(2): 165–172.

Hides, J., Wilson, S., and Stanton, W. (2006). An MRI investigation into the function of the transversus abdominis muscle during drawing in of the abdominal wall. *Spine* 31: 175–178.

Hides, J.A., Richardson, C.A., and Jull, G.A. (1996). Multifidus muscle recovery is not automatic after resolution of acute, first-episode low back pain. *Spine* 21: 2763–2769.

Hodges, P. (2004). Lumbopelvic stability: A functional mode of the biomechanics and motor control. In Richardson, C., Hodgesand, P., Hides, J., Eds., *Therapeutic exercise for lumbopelvic stabilization*. Edinburgh, UK: Churchill Livingstone, 42–47.

Hodges, P., Kaigle Holm, A., Holm, S., and Ekstrom, L. (2003). Intervertebral stiffness of the spine is increased by evoked contraction of the transversus abdominis and the diaphragm. *Spine* 28: 2594–2601.

Hodges, P.W., and Richardson, C.A. (1996). Contraction of transversus abdominis invariably precedes movement of the upper and lower limb. In *Proceedings of the 6th International Conference of the International Federation of Orthopaedic Manipulative Therapists*, Lillehammer, Norway, 71–76.

Hodges, P.W., Eriksson, A.E., Shirley, D., and Gandevia, S.C. (2005). Intra-abdominal pressure increases stiffness of the lumbar spine. *Journal of Biomechanics* 38: 1873–1880.

Holm, S., Maroudas, A., Urban, J.P.G., Selstam, G., et al. (1981). Nutrition of the intervertebral disc: Solute transport and metabolism. *Connective Tissue Research* 8: 101–119.

Hu, C., Lin, B., Li, Z., et al. (2021). Spontaneous regression of a large sequestered lumbar disc herniation: A case report and literature review. *Journal of International Medical Research* 49(11): 1–9.

Hukins, D.W.L. (1987). Properties of spinal materials. In Jayson, M.I.V., Ed., *The lumbar spine and back pain*. Edinburgh, UK: Churchill Livingstone, 84–89.

Hukins, D.W.L., Aspden, R.M., and Hickey, D.S. (1990). Thoracolumbar fascia can increase the efficiency of the erector spinae muscles. *Clinical Biomechanics* 5: 30–34.

Hungerford, B., Gilleard, W., and Hodges, P. (2003). Evidence of altered lumbopelvic muscle recruitment in the presence of sacroiliac joint pain. *Spine* 28: 1593–1600.

Jackson, M., Solomonow, M., and Zhou, B. (2001). Multifidus EMG and tension-relaxation recovery after prolonged static lumbar flexion. *Spine* 26: 715–723.

Jacob, H.A.C., and Kissling, R.O. (1995). The mobility of the sacroiliac joints in healthy volunteers between 20 and 50 years of age. *Clinical Biomechanics* 10: 352–361.

Jemmett, R. S., Macdonald, D. A., Agur, A. M. (2004). Anatomical relationships between selected segmental muscles of the lumbar spine in the context of multi-planar segmental motion: A preliminary investigation. *Manual Therapy* 4: 203–210.

Kampen, W. U., and Tillmann, B. (1998). Age-related changes in the articular cartilage of human sacroiliac joint. *Anatomy and Embryology* 198(6): 505–513.

Khoddam-Khorasani, P., Arjmand, N., and Shirazi-Adl, A. (2020). Effect of changes in the lumbar posture in lifting on trunk muscle and spinal loads: A combined in vivo, musculoskeletal, and finite element model study. *Journal of Biomechanics* 104: 109728.

Kim, E.S., Oladunjoye, A.O., Li, J.A., et al. (2014) Spontaneous regression of herniated lumbar discs. *Journal of Clinical Neuroscience* 21: 909–913.

Kippers, V., and Parker, A.W. (1984). Posture related to myoelectric silence of erectores spinae during trunk flexion. *Spine* 9: 740–745.

Komori, H., Shinomiya, K., Nakai, O., et al. (1996). The natural history of herniated nucleus pulposus with radiculopathy. *Spine* 21: 225–229.

Kraemer, J., Kolditz, D., and Gowin, R. (1985). Water and electrolyte content of human intervertebral discs under variable load. *Spine* 10: 69–71.

Langevin, H.M., Stevens-Tuttle, D., Fox, J.R., et al. (2009a). Ultrasound evidence of altered lumbar connective tissue structure in human subjects with chronic low back pain. *BMC Musculoskeletal Disorders* 10, 151.

Langevin, H.M., Stevens-Tuttle, D., Fox, J.R., et al. (2009b). Ultrasound evidence of altered lumbar connective tissue structure in human subjects with chronic low back pain. *BMC Musculoskeletal Disorders* 10: 151.

Latimer, J., Maher, C.G., and Refshauge, S. (1999). The reliability and validity of the Biering-Sorensen test in asymptomatic subjects reporting current or previous non-specific low back pain. *Spine* 24: 2085–2090.

Leatt, P., Reilly, T., and Troup, J.G.D. (1986). Spinal loading during circuit weight-training and running. *British Journal of Sports Medicine* 20(3): 119–124.

Legaspi, O., and Edmond, S.L. (2007). Does the evidence support the existence of lumbar spine coupled motion? A critical review of the literature. *Journal of Orthopaedic & Sports Physical* 37(4): 169–78.

Leinonen, V., Kankaanpaa, M., Airaksinen, O., et al. (2000). Back and hip extensor activities during trunk flexion/extension: Effects of low back pain and rehabilitation. *Archives of Physical Medicine and Rehabilitation* 81: 32–37.

MacDonald, D., Moseley, G.L., Hodges, P.W. (2009). Why do some patients keep hurting their back? Evidence of ongoing back muscle dysfunction during remission from recurrent back pain. *Pain* 142(3): 183–188.

Macintosh, J.E., and Bogduk, N. (1986). The biomechanics of the lumbar multifidus. *Clinical Biomechanics* 1: 205–213.

Markolf, K.L., and Morris, J.M. (1974). The structural components of the intervertebral disc. *Journal of Bone and Joint Surgery* 56A: 675–687.

McGill, S. (2002). *Low back disorders*. Champaign, IL: Human Kinetics.

McGill, S. (2016). *Low back disorders* (3rd ed). Champaign, IL: Human Kinetics.

McGill, S.M., and Brown, S. (1992). Creep response of the lumbar spine to prolonged lumbar flexion. *Clinical Biomechanics* 7: 43.

Mens, J., and Pool-Goudzwaard, A. (2017). The transverse abdominal muscle is excessively active during active straight leg raising in pregnancy-related posterior pelvic girdle pain: An observational study. *BMC Musculoskeletal Disorders* 18(1): 372.

Miller, J.A.A., Haderspeck, K.A., and Schultz, A.B. (1983). Posterior element loads in lumbar motion segments. *Spine* 8: 331–337.

Mooney, V., Pozos, R., and Vleeming, A. (2001). Exercise treatment for sacroiliac pain. *Orthopedics* 24: 29–32.

Morris, S.L., Lay, B., & Allison, G.T. (2012). Corset hypothesis rebutted—transversus abdominis does not co-contract in unison prior to rapid arm movements. *Clinical Biomechanics (Bristol, Avon)* 27(3): 249–254.

Moseley, G.L., Hodges, P.W., and Gandevia, S.C. (2003). External perturbation of the trunk in standing humans differentially activates components of the medial back muscles. *Journal of Physiology* 547: 581–587.

Nachemson, A.L. (1992). Newest knowledge of low back pain. *Clinical Orthopaedics* 279: 8.

Nourbakhsh, M.R., and Arab, A.M. (2002). Relationship between mechanical factors and incidence of low back pain. *Journal of Orthopaedic and Sports Physical Therapy* 32: 447–460.

O'Sullivan, P.B., Twomey, L.T., and Allison, G.T. (1997). Evaluation of specific stabilizing exercise in the treatment of chronic low back pain with radiologic diagnosis of spondylolysis or spondylolisthesis. *Spine* 22: 2959–2967.

Panjabi, M.M., Abumi, K., Duranceau, J., and Oxland, T. (1989). Spinal stability and intersegmental muscle forces. A biomechanical model. *Spine* 14: 194–200.

Panjabi, M.M., Hult, J.E., and White, A.A. (1987). Biomechanics studies in cadaveric spines. In Jayson, M.I.V., Ed., *The lumbar spine and back pain*. Edinburgh, UK: Churchill Livingstone, 34–38.

Penning, L. (2000). Psoas muscle and lumbar spine stability: A concept uniting existing controversies. Critical review and hypothesis. *European Spine Journal* 9(6): 577–585.

Pinto, S.M., Boghra, S.B., Macedo, et al. (2021). Does motor control exercise restore normal morphology of lumbar multifidus muscle in people with low back pain? – A systematic review. *Journal of Pain Research* 14: 2543–2562.

Porter, J.L., and Wilkinson, A. (1997). Lumbar-hip flexion motion. A comparative study between asymptomatic and chronic low back pain in 18 to 36 year old men. *Spine* 22(13): 1508–1513.

Richardson, C.A., Snijders, C.J., and Hides, J.A. (2002). The relation between the transversus abdominis muscles, sacroliliac joint mechanics, and low back pain. *Spine* 27: 399–405.

San Juan, J.G., Yaggie, J.A., Levy, S.S., et al. (2005). Effects of pelvic stabilization on lumbar muscle activity during dynamic exercise. *Journal of Strength and Conditioning Research* 19(4): 903–907.

Scott, I.R., Vaughan, A., and Hall, J. (2015). Swiss ball enhances lumbar multifidus activity in chronic low back pain. *Physical Therapy in Sport* 16(3): 40–44.

Sharma, M., Langrama, N.A., and Rodriguez, J. (1995). Role of ligaments and facets in lumbar spine stability. *Spine* 20: 887.

Silfies, S.P., Mehta, R., Smith, S.S., et al. (2009). Differences in feed forward trunk muscle activity in subgroups of patients with mechanical low back pain. *Archives of Physical Medicine and Rehabilitation* 90(7): 1159–1169.

Skibski, A., Burkholder, E., and Goetschius, J. (2020). Transverse abdominis activity and ultrasound biofeedback in college golfers with and without low back pain. *Physical Therapy in Sport* 46: 249–253.

Smith, B.E., Littlewood, C., and May, S. (2014). An update of stabilisation exercises for low back pain: a systematic review with meta-analysis. *BMC Musculoskelet Disorders* 15: 416.

Sullivan, M.S. (1997). Lifting and back pain. In Twomey, L.T. and Taylor, J.R., Eds., *Physical therapy of the low back*. Edinburgh, UK: Churchill Livingstone, 92–97.

Taylor, J.R., and Twomey, L.T. (1986). Age changes in lumbar zygapophyseal joints. *Spine* 11: 739–745.

Tesh, K.M., Shaw-Dunn, J., and Evans, J.H. (1987). The abdominal muscles and vertebral stability. *Spine* 12: 501–508.

Twomey, L.T., and Taylor, J.R. (1994). Factors influencing ranges of movement in the spine. In Twomey, L.T. and Taylor, J.R., Eds., *Physical therapy of the low back* (2nd ed). Edinburgh, UK: Churchill Livingstone, 56–62.

Tyrrell, A.R., Reilly, T., and Troup, J.D.G. (1985). Circadian variation in stature and the effects of spinal loading. *Spine* 10: 161–164.

Urquhart, D.M., Hodges, P.W., and Story, I.H. (2005). Postural activity of the abdominal muscles varies between regions of these muscles and between body positions. *Gait Posture* 22: 295–301.

Vadalà, G., Di Giacomo, G., Ambrosio, L., et al. (2022). The effect of Irisin on human nucleus pulposus cells: New insights into the biological crosstalk between the muscle and intervertebral disc. *Spine*, Advance online publication.

van Dieën, J.H., Hoozemans, M.J., and Toussaint, H.M. (1999). Stoop or squat: A review of biomechanical studies on lifting technique. *Clinical Biomechanics (Bristol, Avon)* 14(10): 685–696.

Virri, J., Gronblad, M., Seitsalo, S., et al. (2001). Comparison of the prevalence of inflammatory cells in subtypes of disc herniations and associations with straight leg raising. *Spine* 26: 2311–2315.

Vleeming, A., and Schuenke, M. (2019). Form and force closure of the sacroiliac joints. *Physical Medicine & Rehabilitaiton* 11(Suppl 1): S24–S31.

Vleeming, A., Pool-Goudzwaard, A.L., Stoeckart, R., Wingerden, J.P., and Snijders, C.J. (1995). The posterior layer of the thoracolumbar fascia: Its function in load transfer from spine to legs. *Spine* 20: 753–758.

von Arx, M., Liechti, M., Connolly, L., Bangerter, C., et al. (2021). From stoop to squat: A comprehensive analysis of lumbar loading among different lifting styles. *Frontiers in Bioengineering and Biotechnology* 9: 769117.

Wilke, H.J., Wolf, S., Claes, L.E., Arand, M., and Weisend, A. (1995). Stability increase of the lumbar spine with different muscle groups: A biomechanical in vitro study. *Spine* 20: 192–198.

Willard, F.H. (1997). The muscular, ligamentous and neural structure of the low back and its relation to back pain. In Vleeming, A., Mooney, V., Dorman, T., Snijders, C., and Stoeckart, R., Eds., *Movement stability and low back pain*. Edinburgh, UK: Churchill Livingstone, 43–51.

Williams, M., Solomonow, M., Zhou, B.H., et al. (2000). Multifidus spasms elicited by prolonged lumbar flexion. *Spine* 25(22): 2916–2924.

Wong, T.K., and Lee, R.Y. (2004). Effects of low back pain on the relationship between the movements of the lumbar spine and hip. *Human Movement Science* 23(1): 21–34.

Zetterberg, C., Andersson, G.B.J., and Schultz, A.B. (1987). The activity of individual trunk muscles during heavy physical loading. *Spine* 12: 1035–1040.

Zielinski, K.A., Henry, S.M., Ouellette-Morton, R.H., and DeSarno, M.J. (2013). Lumbar multifidus muscle thickness does not predict patients with low back pain who improve with trunk stabilization exercises. *Archives of Physical Medicine and Rehabilitation* 94(6): 1132–1138.

5

ASSESSMENT—PATHOLOGY AND PERFORMANCE

Basic musculoskeletal assessment

Let's begin this chapter with an overview of basic musculoskeletal (MSK) assessment. For more detailed information on this subject, see Norris (2019). A simple pneumonic to use as a guide to the assessment process and its documentation is SOAP, standing for *Subjective, Objective, Assessment and Plan*. The SOAP format records evidence of patient interaction and clinical reasoning (CR) in a systematic and concise way. It is part of a wider approach originated in problem-orientated medical records (POMR) and is often found in electronic medical records.

Subjective assessment

The subjective assessment means questioning a person, or taking a history, and getting a description of a person's problems in their own words. Clinical conditions often have a definite pattern, for example, an acute injury (one which happens suddenly) would normally have a history of injury, a twist or strain, for example, while a chronic injury (one developing slowly) will usually have resulted from overuse of a bodypart during a regular activity such as sport. Now, by extending our subjective assessment we aim to identify these patterns. To do this we can ask questions in a variety of categories expanded below, from the approach originally pioneered by James Cyriax, an orthopaedic medicine consultant from St Thomas's hospital in London (Table 5.1). Although his approach was very much structurally based, and things have moved on since then, the simplicity of the basic format is a useful starting point. Bear in mind however, that a vital part of the subjective examination is to hear the person's story. By this, I mean what the person has been through, and how it has affected them. For example, a person may have picked something up in the garden and felt their back suddenly 'go'. It is tempting to immediately ask

DOI: 10.4324/9781003366188-5

TABLE 5.1 Subjective assessment guide

Category	Meaning
Age & occupation	How old is the client and what job/sports/activity do they do
Site & spread	Where do they feel their symptom(s) and does this travel or vary
Onset & duration	When did their symptoms begin and have they changed since that time
Symptoms & behaviour	What are their symptoms and how to they vary throughout the day
Medical considerations	Are there other consideration/co-morbidities

where the pain is, what level of pain they have, and how it affects them through the day. All of these points are relevant, but by sitting back and allowing a person to talk rather than reading a list of questions, we are more likely to discover the psychosocial effects of their back condition, rather than just identifying a site of potential pain generation (nociception).

Age and occupation is important, because certain conditions such are osteoarthritis (OA) are more common in older clients. Low back pain (LBP) can occur in anyone, but manual workers have very different stresses imposed on the spine than desk bound individuals, for example. In addition, the advice for aftercare will obviously vary, so knowledge of the typical activities which a client is returning to is important. Within this category we should note what the person does for a job or their occupational history (OccH) and what sports or activities they engage in, their social history (SocH).

Site and spread of symptoms (something a client complains of) can give clues to pain referral. For example, a disc injury in the low back may trap the sciatic nerve giving pain into the leg (sciatica). Sometimes a client may complain of leg pain and be unaware that they have a back condition. Equally, pain can be referred from a condition even when a nerve is not trapped. For example, a hip condition can often give leg pain which appears to come from the back and vice versa.

Onset and duration of symptoms clarifies the difference between a sudden onset (acute) condition and that which develops slowly overtime (overuse) and helps us to identify the stage of healing and the likely condition of the injured tissues. Also, the 24-hour pattern of the symptoms should be noted. For example, does the person have pain at night (does it wake them up) or only when they wake up in the morning. Throughout the day do symptoms build up (related to *activity*) or does the person wake with the symptom which then gradually wears off (normally associated with *stiffness*).

Symptoms and behaviour of these symptoms gives us information about things which make the clients' condition better (easing factor) or worse (aggravating factors). For example, as noted above a chronic stiff joint is typically better for gentle mobilising exercise, while an acute joint normally reacts to exercise with increasing pain as the condition is stirred up. Behaviour of symptoms also gives us information about activities which may be driving a person's symptoms and so an indication about social factors and how we can help manage these. For example, does someone's back pain get worse when they push a young child in a buggy (pushchair) when taking an older sibling to school.

> **Keypoint:**
>
> Establish *aggravating* (aggs) and *easing* (ease) factors. What makes the person's symptoms worse or better?

Medical considerations are important, and a medical history should be taken. It is important to know if a person has medical conditions other than the injury they are presenting with, and if they are taking any tablets or drugs (medications) which may affect or be affected by rehabilitation. A simple medical questionnaire should be filled in prior to treatment, and you should question a person more closely on areas which are likely to be affected by rehab. Past medical history (PMH) and past surgical history (PSH) may be relevant and should be noted, as should family history (FH) and any medications a person is taking, called the drug history (DH). Often an older person may present with back pain but also several other clinical conditions which affect their lifestyle. The factors (called co-morbidities) may have to be considered when prescribing exercise and may require exercise adaptation. For example, high blood pressure (hypertension) or arthritis in a peripheral joint may preclude strenuous or prolonged weight bearing actions, or require additional recovery time.

> **Definition:**
>
> A *co-morbidity* is the simultaneous presence of two or more medical conditions in a patient.

It is also important to establish what a person wants to achieve from treatment or rehabilitation—what are their goals and expectations? This can be crucial, first because their expectations should be realistic. If a person presents with a swollen joint after a traumatic injury, it is not realistic to expect to play competitive sports pain free the next day. Establishing what is realistic from the start prepares an individual for the timescale of healing and expected length of treatment.

SIN factors

One of the things we are interested in, especially when prescribing a rehab programme is how easily a condition is stirred up. We call this establishing the 'SIN'

TABLE 5.2 Establishing the SIN factors of a condition

Factor	Meaning	How described
Severity	Intensity of symptoms and how they restrict a person's movement or activity	Mild, moderate, severe NRS (1–10) or VAS (marked on a line)
Irritability	Degree to which a symptom increases or decreases.	Low, medium, high
Nature	Related to the pattern of a pathology	Pathological description (e.g., inflammatory, neurogenic, mechanical)

NRS—numerical rating scale. VAS—visual analogue scale.

of a condition, standing for Severity, Irritability, and Nature (Table 5.2). Originally used mainly in the manual therapy domain, SIN has become equally important with exercise prescription. The *severity* of a condition relates to the intensity of symptoms and how they restrict a person's movement or activity. Typically, we can grade this as mild, moderate, or severe and score it using a numerical rating scale (1–10 with 10 being most severe). *Irritability* refers to the degree to which a symptom increases or decreases. A highly irritable symptoms increases easily and with little provocation—in common parlance it is easily stirred up. *Nature* of a condition is related to the pattern of a pathology. For example, an inflamed joint can be expected to feel tight to movement, whereas a neurogenic (nerve) condition will typically give altered sensations such as burning or tingling.

Where a condition has high severity and irritability, the person will not be able to tolerate extensive physical testing or exercise and will usually require more time to recover between exercise/activity bouts. Those with low severity and irritability will be able to tolerate more tissue stress (exercise or testing), but this can make it more difficult to reproduce symptoms during the objective examination (below).

Definition:

A *sign* is something which is measurable (objective) a *symptom* is something which is described (subjective).

Objective assessment

Objective assessment is the physical evaluation of the person, and for the lumbar spine region we can structure the process into a broad *screening evaluation* and more specific *special tests*, the latter being more relevant to the clinic rather than the gym. Physical evaluation uses a mixture of *active*, *passive*, and *resisted* movements. Active movements are those which the client performs themselves, passive movements are those performed by the therapist upon the client, and resisted movements involve no joint action but use an isometric muscle contraction instead.

Keypoint:

Active movements are performed by the client themselves; *passive* movements are performed by the therapist on the client, and *resisted* movements use isometric muscle contraction with the client's joints not moving.

Active movements show the quality of movement and the willingness to move. Movement quality can be changed by pain, tissue, and joint changes, and learnt responses. Willingness to move again reflects pain but also psychosocial factors. Performing a passive movement allows the client's muscles to relax, while the joint and other tissues are moved normally. For this reason, passive movements more accurately reflect potential injury to the joint structures rather than contracting muscles. Emphasis is placed on muscles by using a resisted movement. For this we choose an isometric contraction where the muscle is contracting against the resistance supplied by the therapist, but the client's joint does not move appreciably. In this way there is little displacement of the joint and its surrounding tissues, but stress is placed upon the contracting muscle as it works isometrically.

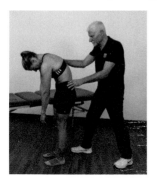 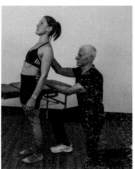 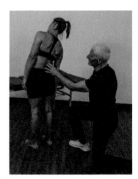

| PHOTO 5.1 | PHOTO 5.2 | PHOTO 5.3 |

Assessing active movements Photo 5.1 spinal flexion. Photo 5.2 spinal extension. Photo 5.3 spinal lateral flexion

For *active* movements of the lumbar spine, the client begins in a normal standing position with the feet, either together or hip width apart to assist their balance. Forward bending (flexion), backward bending (extension), and side bending (lateral flexion) are performed to full comfortable end range (Photos 5.1–5.3). Although the same movements can be performed to resistance, only lateral flexion is performed in standing. For this action, stand to the side of your client and hold their right hand with your left as they attempt to sideband to the left. To give yourself a mechanical advantage it is best to ask the client to separate their feet further, and place one of your feet between theirs whilst at the same time placing your left hand against their shoulder to provide further resistance (Photo 5.4). The same side bending action is performed to the right with you reversing your grip. *Resisted* flexion and extension movements are best carried out with your client lying on an examination couch or gym mat. For resisted flexion, they perform a trunk curl action whilst you resist the spinal flexion by placing resistance using the flat of your hand on their breastbone (sternum) (Photo 5.5). For resisted extension. They lie on the front with their hands by their sides. From this position, they attempt to lift their chest off the couch as you provide pressure between their shoulder blades (scapulae) (Photo 5.6). Lateral flexion and rotation are coupled movements in the lumbar spine, meaning that they occur together. For this reason, both actions do not need to be examined clinically. However, where you decide that rotation should be examined, it is easier to do so with your client sitting on an examination couch or high stool (Photo 5.7). The sitting position fixes their pelvis so that the rotation movement is limited to the spine. Stand behind your client and place resistance on their shoulders using your hands.

Evaluation of the hips and pelvis should also be carried out where a client has a lumbar condition because movement of these three areas (lumbar spine, hips, and pelvis) are so closely related. Again, active, passive, and resisted movements are used for all the anatomical movements of the hip (flexion/extension, abduction/adduction, medial rotation/lateral rotation) (see Table 5.3). Typically, these will be performed either on a treatment couch (plinth) or gym mat on the floor. In addition, nerve stretch, and conductivity can be examined using a straight leg raise (SLR) test and PKB (see below).

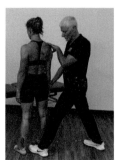
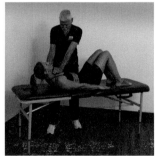

PHOTO 5.4   PHOTO 5.5

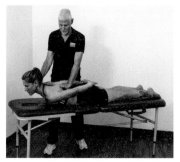
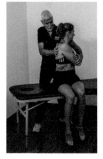

PHOTO 5.6   PHOTO 5.7

Assessing resisted motion Photo 5.4 side flexion. Photo 5.5 flexion Photo 5.6 extension photo 5.7 rotation.

TABLE 5.3 Active, passive, and resisted movement of the hip joint

Movement	Active	Passive	Resisted
Flexion	Knee to chest in supine	Knee to chest in supine	Stand at pts shoulders, place hand on femur above knee
Extension	Prone hip extension (leg lift)	Prone hip extension	Hand on posterior thigh above knee
Abduction	Standing scissor action	Supine supported scissor action	Side lying, target leg uppermost. Hand on thigh above knee as leg is lifted
Adduction	Standing scissor action	Supine supported scissor action	Supine lying, leg abducted (legs open). Hand on inside of thigh above knee to resist adduction (leg closing)
Lateral rotation	Prone lying knee flexed—shin moves inwards	Prone lying knee flexed. Shin moving inwards (legs crossing)	Either *prone lying* knee flexed (hip joint in neural) or *supine lying* hip and knee flexed (hip at 90°). Monitor skin movement from bodyline.
Medial rotation	Prone lying knee flexed—shin moves outwards	Prone lying knee flexed. Shin moving outwards (legs moving apart)	

Neurodynamic testing

The neurological system with reference to the lumbar spine is examined using either assessment of *neural integrity* (the ability of nerves to conduct impulses) and/ or tests of *neural sensitivity* (movement of nerves and nerve palpation). Sensory (feeling) and motor (movement) tests and reflex testing are used to assess nerve conduction while *neurodynamic testing* assesses movement of nerves. Only neuro-dynamics will be described as it is the most relevant to rehabilitation and train-ing. Where reflex testing or sensory testing is needed, the person should be referred to a physiotherapist or medical practitioner.

A note on dermatomes

Sensation (typically increased or decreased) relates to the nerve supplying the skin in the region being tested and this area is referred to as a *dermatome*. Dermatome maps are commonly used in assessment to help define if a spinal nerve is affected. The maps were first described in the early 1930s and formalised by Keegan and Garrett (1948). The spinal nerves run in 31 pairs from the dorsal and ventral horns of the spinal cord to exit through the intervertebral foramina. Within the low back region there are five lumbar, five sacral, and one coccygeal pair. Although dermatome maps are widely used, there is much overlap between dermatomes

Anatomical location	Classical map
C6 - Thumb	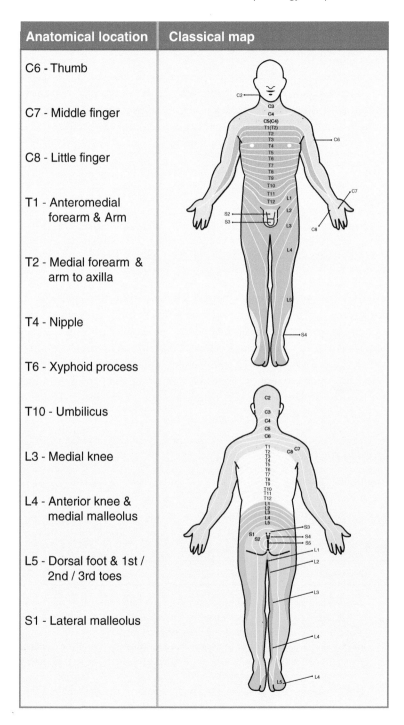
C7 - Middle finger	
C8 - Little finger	
T1 - Anteromedial forearm & Arm	
T2 - Medial forearm & arm to axilla	
T4 - Nipple	
T6 - Xyphoid process	
T10 - Umbilicus	
L3 - Medial knee	
L4 - Anterior knee & medial malleolus	
L5 - Dorsal foot & 1st / 2nd / 3rd toes	
S1 - Lateral malleolus	

FIGURE 5.1 Dermatomes.

and inconsistency between individuals. Anatomical landmarks related to the dermatomal levels are often more useful clinically to give an approximate regional location (Figure 5.1)

Reflex testing relevant to the lumbar spine is to the *knee jerk* (L3-L4) and *ankle jerk* (S1-S2), the figure in brackets representing the nerve root responsible for controlling the region. Where a reflex produces an exaggerated muscle reaction, this (along with other signs) may suggest an upper motor neuron (UMN) lesion. Where reflexes are reduced or non-existent, lower motor neuron (LMN) lesions are more likely.

> **Definition:**
>
> An *upper motor neuron* (UMN) originates in the cerebral cortex and travels down to the brain stem or spinal cord. A *lower motor neuron* (LMN) begins in the spinal cord and travels to a muscle or gland.

Motor tests assess muscle strength with reference to the spinal nerve supplying a muscle group (myotome). The traditional tests are listed in Table 5.4 and performed by comparing one side of the body to the other. Whilst not being 100% accurate, weakness in a myotome in association with other clinical findings can indicate the likely level of a nerve compression (radiculopathy).

Three neurodynamic tests are most relevant to the lumbar spine and may be used for both assessment and as part of rehabilitation or training. These are the SLR, slump test, and the PKB.

Straight leg raise test

The straight leg raise test (SLR) or Lasegue's sign is used to assess the sciatic nerve in cases of back pain. In addition to its effect on the sciatic nerve, the SLR also stretches the hamstrings and buttock tissues, and places stress over the sacroiliac

TABLE 5.4 Myotome testing for the lumbar spine

Level	Movement	Resisted test
S1	Ankle plantar flexion	In standing ask pt to raise onto the ball of their foot. Resisted ankle plantar flexion and eversion in lying.
S2	Knee flexion	Supine lying resisted knee flexion
L5	Big toe extension	Resist the big toe as pt pulls it up towards their face
L4	Ankle dorsiflexion	Stabilise the lower shin and ask the pt to pull their foot upwards
L3	Knee extension	Place on hand under the knee and the other on the lower leg to provide resistance
L1/2	Hip flexion	In supine lying resist SLR or bent knee hip flexion

Pt—patient. SLR—straight leg raise.

joint, posterior lumbar ligaments, and facet joints as well as lengthening the spinal canal. Confirmation that the nerve root is the source of pain rather than the other tissues may be improved by raising the leg to the point of pain and then lowering it a few degrees. The nerve and its sheath are then further stretched either from below by dorsiflexing the foot or applying firm pressure to the popliteal fossa over the posterior tibial nerve. Pressure from above is produced by flexing the cervical spine. When performing the SLR, as the leg is raised the knee should not be allowed to bend and the pelvis should stay on the couch.

Keypoint:

The *straight leg raise* (SLR) test places the sciatic nerve on stretch and may be refined by lowering the leg until pain is eased and either dorsiflexing the ankle or flexing the neck.

Testing the unaffected leg (crossed SLR or 'well leg' test) may also give symptoms. This manoeuvre pulls the nerve root and associated tissue distally and medially but increases the pressure on the nerve complex by less than half that of the standard SLR test. When the SLR is performed on the affected leg, the tissues connected to the nerve pathway are sensitised. Because the crossed SLR stretches the neural structures less, the resting tension of these tissues must be higher to cause pain. The crossed SLR may therefore be a more reliable predictor of lumbar disc conditions than the standard SLR (Photo 5.8).

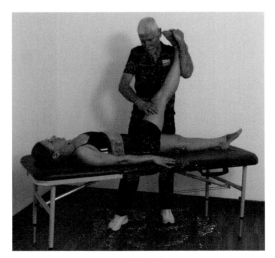

PHOTO 5.8

Slump test

The slump is a neurodynamic test used to assess tension in the pain-sensitive structures around the vertebral canal or intervertebral foramen, and to ensure that these structures can stretch properly. It is also used to differentiate the hamstrings from the sciatic nerve in cases of posterior thigh pain.

To perform the manoeuvre, the person being tested sits unsupported over the couch side or sideways on a chair with the knees together and flexed to 90°. The posterior thigh is in contact with the couch/chair. The person is then instructed to relax the spine completely and 'slump' forward, keeping the cervical spine in its neutral position ('look forwards, not down'). The therapist (standing to the side) places overpressure onto the person's shoulders to increase the movement, attempting to bow the spine rather than increase hip flexion (Photo 5.8A).

From this position, the person is asked to flex their neck ('chin to chest') and then straighten the leg on the unaffected (non-painful) side first. In each case, the examiner places mild overpressure on the area and assesses the result. The tested person is then asked to dorsiflex the ankle ('pull your toes up'). Neck flexion is slowly released, and the response monitored. The opposite leg is then tested. A normal test result is one where there is a pain free lack of knee extension by about 30° and slight central pain over T9/10.

> **CASE NOTE**
>
> A 25-year-old male presented for treatment with posterior thigh pain, which had been present for 2 months. He was a regular runner, training 3–5 times per week up to 6 miles per run. His work was office based and he drove as part of this work, often between 80–100 miles per day. He stated that this thigh pain came on at the start of a run and would ease and sometimes disappear altogether only to return when sitting watching TV in the evening. His pain was worse with driving and eased within 5 minutes when getting out of the car and walking. On examination resisted knee flexion was painless, but straight leg raise gave mild posterior thigh symptoms. Sensation to the shin, foot, and ankle was normal and resisted foot and toe extension demonstrated full power.
>
> When performing the slump test, his posterior thigh pain brought on in the full slump position (trunk flexed, hands behind back and leg straight with ankle dorsiflexed). His symptoms were eased by releasing neck flexion to look at the ceiling or releasing ankle dorsiflexion by pointing the toes.
>
> Treatment was directed at managing radicular pain using the slump as a stretching position and reducing lumbar flexion when sitting. Pain began to ease within 3 days and the patient was pain free within 10 days.

Prone knee bend test

The prone knee bend (PKB) test, also called the Femoral Nerve Tension Test (FNTT) or reversed Lasegue examines the femoral nerve travelling in the anterior aspect of the thigh. The person lies on their front and the knee is flexed initially to 90°. Where pain in the anterior thigh occurs, we must differentiate between the femoral nerve and rectus femoris muscle. Stabilising the pelvis with

TABLE 5.5 Nerve palpation in the lower limb

Nerve	Palpation location
Sciatic	Midpoint of a line joining the ischial tuberosity and greater trochanter
Common peroneal	(i) Medial to the tendon of Biceps femoris
	(ii) Posterior to the head of the fibula
Tibial	(i) Centrally over the posterior knee crease, medial to the popliteal artery
	(ii) Behind the medial malleolus with the ankle dorsiflexed
Superficial peroneal	On the dorsum of the foot on an imaginary line along the 4th metatarsal with the foot plantarflexed and inverted
Deep peroneal	Between the 1st and 2nd metatarsals lateral to the extensor hallucis tendon
Sural	Behind the lateral malleolus, between the malleolus and Achilles tendon.

Source: Data from Worsfold (2018).

one hand (hand on sacrum) maximally flex the knee to place a focus on the muscle and compare the sensation to that occurring when the hip is extended passively, and knee flexed to 90° where stretch is taken from the muscle and placed on the nerve. Hold each position for 45–60 seconds to bring symptoms on from L2 to L4 impingement. Performing the test (hip extension and knee flexion) and adding hip adduction places stress onto the Cutaneous nerve while abduction the hip stresses the Saphenous nerve.

Where neurodynamic tests are positive, nerve palpation may be useful to determine the precise nerve likely giving rise to symptoms. Table 5.5 shows nerve palpation locations for the lower limb.

Passive movements

Passive movements are those performed by a therapist or trainer on the person being tested. Passive movements look at both the amount of movement which occurs (movement range) and how that movement occurs (movement quality). We say that passive movements test the *inert* structures of the joint. These are the tissues other than muscle (which is defined by contrast as *contractile*), such as the ligaments, fascia, cartilage, and nerve. Bear in mind also that this distinction between tissues is not precise. Although isometric contraction (resisted) tests the muscles, a relaxed muscle or tendon acts as an inert structure when placed on stretch, so it is impossible to accurately differentiate a single tissue without surgically removing it!

The information gained from passive movements looks at pain, movement range, and end feel. This latter feature deals with the sensation that the therapist feels through their hands when the movement of the joint stops. A *hard* end feel indicates that bone is limiting movement, and a typical example would be elbow extension where motion range is normal. A hard end feel where motion range is limited compared to the unaffected side may be accompanied by grating (crepitus) and is abnormal. A *soft* end feel indicates that soft tissues are pressing against each other to limit movement, the typical example being elbow flexion. Finally, an *elastic* end feel occurs when tissues are stretched, and a typical example would be a SLR where the hamstrings limited the movement range. These three types of end feel can all be viewed as normal. Abnormal end feels include a *springy* sensation where something is trapped within a joint and an *empty* end feel where muscles go into spasm to block the final degrees of movement and protect the joint. End feel examples are shown in (Table 5.6).

Movements of individual spinal segments or individual joints have been described using the mobilisation techniques of Maitland, a pioneering Australian physiotherapist. Passive physiological intervertebral movements (PPIVM) are used to assess intervertebral movement at a single joint. Passive accessory intervertebral movement (PAIVM) is a mobilisation technique aiming at producing movement of a mobile vertebral segment without significant participation of muscles related to the body segment. Although these classical techniques have been widely used, their reliability and validity in their original form is questionable. Pain provocation, motion, and landmark location tests have only acceptable reliability, with regional motion range measurement more reliable than segmental (Seffinger et al. 2004).

Two types of passive movement are described in the mobilisation and manipulation literature, physiological and accessory. *Physiological movements* are those which can be performed by a person actively and these may be assessed for quality (stiffness, end feel) and quantity (motion range) and for their connection to symptom reproduction. *Accessory movements* (also called joint play) are those which a joint can perform, but over which a person has no active control. Accessory movements include roll, spin, and slide where roll is a rotary motion with one

TABLE 5.6 End feel during passive joint examination

Movement range	End feel and example
NORMAL (full ROM)	• Bone close contact (e.g. elbow extension)
• **Hard**	• Soft tissue compression (e.g. elbow flexion)
• **Soft**	• Tissues on stretch (e.g. straight leg raise)
• **Elastic**	
ABNORMAL (ROM limited)	• Complete block often accompanied by joint grating (crepitus)
• **Hard**	• Movement stops prematurely as though something
• **Springy**	is trapped
• **Empty**	• Movement halted prematurely by client's action alone

ROM–range of motion.

bone rolling over another as a car tyre rolling over the road. Spin is again a rotary movement, but this time one component is spinning on the other as with a car type moving without the car travelling forwards. Slide is a translatory motion with one joint surface sliding over the other as with a car tyre skidding.

> **Definition:**
>
> A *physiological* joint movement is one which can be performed by a person themselves. An *accessory* joint movement is one which can occur at a joint, but over which a person has no voluntary control.

Analysis

Once the therapist has all of the subjective and objective information in front of them, they summarise to form an analysis (SOAP assessment) of the client's problems. In this section, the therapist synthesises the findings of the subjective and objective assessment and uses a process of CR (below) to move on to the treatment plan. Importantly the analysis stage is when treatment decisions are justified.

Analysis may be of a simple alteration in movement, for example, limited lumbar flexion, or a clinical impression such as altered feeling from a nerve suggesting radiculopathy. Scope of practice is important within the sphere of analysis. As detailed above, *medical diagnosis* focusses on finding a single structure or system responsible for a person's signs and symptoms and is typically made by a medical practitioner or allied health professionals to identify a structural target for treatment. A *functional assessment* is normally made by an allied health professional or exercise professional and typically identifies alteration in movement (dynamic) or alignment (static) and forms the basis of a rehabilitation plan.

> **Keypoint:**
>
> *Scope of practice* must be remembered when analysing a person's signs and symptoms, and test findings. Contrast a medical diagnosis with a functional assessment.

Plan

Having obtained information from the subjective and objective phases of an evaluation and formed an assessment of the clinical condition, the therapist or exercise professional must now plan a rehabilitation programme. The process of decision-making to obtain the plan is clinical reasoning, described below. The management programme must be suitable for the condition and should be monitored continually and changed as the condition varies. For example, the evaluation may have revealed less movement of the spine to right lateral flexion compared to left, and muscle weakness on one side of the body compared to the other. The assessment is of movement limitation and muscle weakness, and the plan may be of mobility exercises to increase range of motion and strength exercises to rebuild muscle. Each plan should have clear aims and objectives to both guide treatment and give an understanding of the timescales involved in the overall programme.

Definition:

Aims are what the therapist hopes to achieve, the goal of treatment (e.g., restore full lumbar flexion) while *objectives* are the steps taken to achieve this, which are measurable (e.g., perform lumbar flexion exercises for 3 sets of 10 reps). A goal is therefore the outcome of a series of completed objectives.

Red flags and contraindications to rehabilitation

During client assessment, a lot of information is available to us. We talk to our clients during our consultation, taking a history of their condition, ask questions and listen to the clients' replies (subjective assessment). We examine our clients' testing movements, tissues, and function (objective assessment). We then use this information to make an assessment of the client's condition and plan a rehabilitation programme. Through our evaluation, we have access to a variety of findings and must determine how important each of these is. To make this task easier, we can highlight certain findings, which are more important than others. We use a process of flags which highlight findings, which may require referral for further investigation or close monitoring. Red flags are physical in nature and refer to findings that may indicate a more serious medical problem (pathology). Items such as infection, fracture, or presence of a tumour would fall into this category. Yellow flags are psychosocial and indicate a psychological (mind) or social (environmental issue) factor which may be influencing the condition and have a bearing on the progress of rehabilitation (see Chapter 4).

Keypoint:

(i) *Red flags* are physical findings which may suggest a more serious condition underlying a clients' back pain, (ii) *Yellow flags* are psychosocial factors which may influence a client's recovery.

The first process we need to go through when examining the client with LBP is diagnostic triage. This process can categorise LBP into one of three types, simple back pain, nerve root pain, and possible serious pathology. The primary aim of diagnostic triage is to exclude serious pathology. Simple LBP, which occurs within the age group 20–55, shows pain which is mechanical in nature (meaning it is affected by a client's movements) and restricted to the lumbosacral or buttock area. It is categorised as low risk where the patient is generally medically well. Nerve root pain presents as unilateral symptoms, with pain intensity in the leg generally being greater than that in the lower back. Pain can radiate to the foot, giving altered sensation (paraesthesia), numbness, and localised neurological deficit, such as reduction in reflexes or skin sensation, or muscle weakness, for example.

Definition:

A *neurological deficit* is an abnormality of a body part due to altered function of the brain, spinal cord, or nerves. Examples in the low back include decreased sensation, weakness, altered walking pattern, balance problems, abnormal reflexes (increased or decreased), and loss of bladder/bowel control.

SLR testing generally reproduces pain, as this position stretches the sciatic nerve travelling along the back of the thigh from the lower back (see above). If something compresses this nerve or alters its conduction of electrical impulses, stretching the nerve using the SLR test reproduces the client's symptoms.

Possible serious spinal pathology can exist where there is evidence of red flags, especially in clients younger than 20 years or older than 55. Pain is non-mechanical in nature (not influence by movement) and there may be a history of previous cancers, prolonged steroid drug use, or HIV (aids virus present). Marked structural deformity may also be present and the patient can be generally unwell showing weight loss. Severe early-morning stiffness and thoracic pain should also be of note. Table 5.7 illustrates red flags in low back examination. Where red flags are present, clients should be referred to a medical practitioner for further investigation.

We have seen earlier that back pain may be affected by psychosocial factors indicated by the presence of yellow flags. These are potential psychosocial barriers to recovery, such as the belief that pain is harmful (correlation between hurt and harm), fear avoidance behaviour (avoiding a movement because you think it will hurt even when you have not tried it), and depression or low mood state. The belief that passive treatments such as medication, rather than active treatment such as rehabilitation is the only possible course of intervention is also classified as a yellow flag, as is the presence of a compensation claim. Table 5.8 indicates yellow flags in low back examination.

CASE NOTE

A 72-year-old male presented with low back pain of 4 months duration. He had pain at night, often forcing him to get out of bed and walk around the house. This eased his pain but sometimes it would occur again and

TABLE 5.7 Red flags in the examination of Low Back Pain

- Cauda equina syndrome.
    - Bilateral sciatica
    - Severe or progressive bilateral neurological deficit of the legs, such as major motor weakness with knee extension, ankle eversion, or foot dorsiflexion.
    - Difficulty initiating micturition or impaired sensation of urinary flow
        - Urinary retention with overflow urinary incontinence
    - Loss of sensation of rectal fullness
        - Faecal incontinence
    - Saddle anaesthesia or paraesthesia).
    - Laxity of the anal sphincter.
- Spinal fracture.
    - Sudden onset of severe central spinal pain which is relieved by lying down.
    - History of major trauma (such as a road traffic collision or fall from a height), minor trauma, or even just strenuous lifting in people with osteoporosis or those taking corticosteroids.
    - Structural deformity of the spine (step) with possible point tenderness
- Cancer.
    - Patient aged > 50 years of age
    - Gradual onset of symptoms.
    - Severe unremitting pain that remains when patient is supine
    - Aching night pain which disturbs sleep
    - Pain aggravated by straining at stool, or coughing/sneezing)
    - Localised spinal tenderness.
    - No symptomatic improvement after 4–6 weeks of conservative management
    - Unexplained weight loss.
    - Past history of cancer
- Infection
    - Fever
    - Tuberculosis, or recent urinary tract infection.
    - Diabetes.
    - History of intravenous drug use.
    - Patient immunocompromised

Source: Data from: Nice clinical knowledge summary—Sciatica (lumbar radiculopathy) https://cks.nice.org.uk/sciatica-lumbar-radiculopathy#!diagnosisSub:1 accessed 19/09/2019.

sometimes not. He was a regular gardener and golfer and put his back pain down to doing too much. He had moderately high cholesterol levels and was on statins. He had a history of prostate cancer ten years ago treated with radiotherapy. The patient had seen his GP and was told that he had sciatica and been given a course of pain killers. On examination he had pain to end range flexion and end range extension in standing and his side flexion gave him a feeling of tightness, but the range was unlimited. Straight leg raise gave low back pain but no pain in the leg. Sensation and power in the lower limb was normal, and there was generalised low back pain (5–6 on a 10-point NRS) to palpation. Examination of the pelvis was unremarkable.

TABLE 5.8 Yellow flags in low back pain

Attitudes	*Pt willing or unwilling to engage in self-management.*
Beliefs	Pt feels they have something serious causing their problem leading to *catastrophising*.
Compensation	Pt waiting for legal proceedings or payment.
Diagnosis	Inappropriate communication and misunderstanding may lead to *iatrogenesis*.
Emotions	Emotional traits such as anxiety and/or depression at high risk of developing chronic pain.
Family	Overbearing or under supportive
Work	Pressure or responsibility from work situation

Source: After www.sheffieldachesandpains.com accessed 16/08/2022.

The patient was treated with manual therapy to target local pain and muscle tightness and begun on a general lumbar exercise program beginning with lumbar mobility (sitting rotation) and strength (kneeling leg extension with trunk supported on a chair seat). Following two treatment sessions the patient said that his back felt better in the daytime, but he still had night pain and occasional severe stabbing pain. Moving onto the treatment couch and turning gave severe pain. The patient was referred back to his GP requesting a scan as the following red flags were demonstrated: age, history of cancer, night pain, symptoms worsening. MRI scan revealed lumbar metastases secondary to a return of prostate cancer which were both treatable.

Clinical reasoning

Clinical reasoning (CR) is a systematic approach used by clinicians to decide which treatments or interventions are appropriate, when they should be used, and why. Rather than applying standard treatment programmes and using the same techniques with each person, we should assess to determine individual needs, and tailor a programme accordingly, an example of person-centred care. CR is really the thinking process that we go through during the evaluation and application of back rehabilitation. Through interaction with a person, we gather information and use this to develop an idea (called a hypothesis) about what could be wrong and what we should do to help.

Keypoint:

In clinical reasoning, a *hypothesis* is a theory which could explain a person's symptom.

Within a BPS model, our reasoning must go beyond a simple structural diagnosis (pathology focus) to touch on how a condition is affecting the patient as an individual (patient focus). Table 5.9 lists some categories of hypothesis which have been proposed within physiotherapy (Jones 1987, Jones and Rivett 2019).

The process of CR involves interaction with the person being treated, in other words, it is a two-way process. When we do this, we are really looking at the person through a lens made up from our past knowledge and beliefs. Clearly,

TABLE 5.9 Hypothesis categories in clinical reasoning

Category	Example
Activity restriction	Patients' functional abilities and restrictions (e.g., walking, STS, lifting)
Psychosocial status	Beliefs, expectations, emotions, social circumstances, coping strategies, peer perception.
Pain type	Nociceptive (protective), Neuropathic (related to nervous system), Nociplastic (central sensitisation).
Symptom source	Secondary to primary complaint (e.g., weakness, giving way, incontinence)
Pathology	Tissue disease or trauma—does this relate to pain or activity change
Body impairment	Whole person BPS effect. Maladaptive effect (yellow flag)
Contributing factors	Associated factor implicated in development or maintenance of condition (e.g., stiff hip altering gait and placing stress on knee).
Contraindications & cautions	Is immediate referral required or are further tests needed prior to therapy commencement.
Treatment selection & progression	Is patient advocacy required (e.g., insurers, employers, coaches). Consideration of dosage in relation to co-morbidities or BPS factors.
Prognosis	Estimate of treatment intervention, effect, and natural course of MSK recovery, influential BPS factors.

STS—sit to stand. BPS—Biopsychosocial. MSK—musculoskeletal. After Jones and Rivett (2019).

TABLE 5.10 Components of clinical reasoning

Beliefs	**Hypothesis**
What are the therapist beliefs about injury and healing and how does this influence treatment selection	What condition does the therapist thin could explain the patients' signs and symptoms
Assessment	**Expertise**
What information has been gained from the client prior to, during, and after treatment	What clinical experience does the therapist have of this particular condition

Source: After Norris (2012).

the way that we look at a person as a qualified therapist or trainer will be very different to the way we would have looked before we entered these professions. CR involves four basic components (Table 5.10). It entails collecting data (subjective and objective examination), analysing this data (making decisions) and then developing a treatment plan, as used in the SOAP format described above.

As soon as a person walks into the room, the professional is *assessing* them. How they walk, talk, and move will all give clues, however subtle. For example, contrast the view of someone who bounces into the room, bends over effortlessly to kick off their shoes and tells us they have just come back from a five-mile run, with someone who walks in slowly with a pained expression on their face, unable to bend or reach forwards. The former person is less likely to have chronic low back pain (CLBP) than the latter. We have no proof of this at this stage, but our hypothesis is that because one person has unlimited movement and the other reacts in a way that we have seen in those with back pain, that this particular person may also have back pain. The essential feature here is that the professional has received information and compared it to their previous experience. Clearly, the experienced practitioner will be able to do this far better than a student, so the level of expertise that we have in relation to a clinical condition will influence your choice of treatment.

Keypoint:

Expertise in relation to a clinical condition will influence the choice of treatment.

First impressions count

When we see anyone for the first time, we get a first impression of them. It is the same with a patient. As soon as we meet them, we get an impression of what may be wrong with them. This process is *intuitive* and is often referred to as fast thinking or system 1 processing. We are comparing them to our previous experiences and trying to recognise patterns. We do this throughout life. If you see a four-legged furry animal with paws and a wet nose, you may recognise it as a dog even if you have never seen it before. This is because we compare it to an internal image, we have of what it means to be a dog, and if it compares favourably to our pattern, we categorise it. However, sometimes this can go wrong. The same four-legged animal may be a cow, a different category to the dog. Equally a Chikwawa looks very different to a German Shepherd, but it is still a dog because both are within the same category. How do we know? Because whilst there are similarities, we can be *analytical*. This is known as slow thinking or system 2 processing. We know that both animals are dogs but the cow is not because the cow does not have claws, but hoofs. Dogs are carnivores with sharp teeth and cows are herbivores with flatter teeth and a very different digestive tract with a four chambered stomach.

> **Keypoint:**
> ___
> *Fast thinking* (system 1 processing) is intuitive and creates a first impression. *Slow thinking* (system 2 processing) is analytical and can be used to refine our initial impression.

To recognise patterns, we need experience—we must have seen several examples of the pattern to be reliable. This is why a student therapist may spend more time methodically analysing a patient's signs and symptoms whereas an experienced clinician can recognise a condition in a shorter time. Importantly, accuracy depends on the number of times we have seen a pattern (experience) rather than the amount of factual information we may have built up (academic knowledge).

Both fast and slow thinking is important in CR, but novice and experienced clinicians will clinically reason differently.

Make a plan

At the end of an assessment, a decision has been made about the source of a person's symptoms (e.g., their back) and as the professional goes through the assessment and gains further information, they will support or disprove this hypothesis.

By continuing to gather information and compare it to what they think is wrong, a professional is using a process of *reviewing* the hypothesis. Sometimes the information may support the hypothesis. If we think a person has back pain when they come into the room, the fact that they appear to experience pain when they bend to untie their shoes supports this. If they can bend freely and are able to get onto the couch easily, the original hypothesis of severe back pain may be incorrect.

> **Keypoint:**
> ___
> As treatment progresses, a professional gains further information from a person and applies the process of reflection to support, modify, or refute the initial hypothesis.

Contributing factors are those associated with a person's condition. These can sometimes be more important that the source of the problem itself. For example, the source of the problem may be a person's back muscles (erector spinae) and the contributing factor repeated bending at work. Clearly unless you give a person advice about good back care and avoiding bending, when their pain is acute, their condition will not improve.

Cautions to evaluation and/or treatment are things which keep a person's condition there (repeated bending in the above example) or make it worse. These are important as you would need to identify anything which stirs a person's condition up to avoid making them worse. If, for example, a person has an inflamed joint in their back which is made worse by mild movement, it would be unwise to use a vigorous treatment technique or exercise. The fact that mild movement has made it worse would suggest that movement if applied excessively may make their condition worse (*symptom exacerbation*).

The choice of management must consider if exercise therapy is appropriate. It is easy to assume that because a person has come to see you, they need treatment. It is important, however, to be able to say that a particular treatment technique is inappropriate at this stage and to refer on to another healthcare provider or medical practitioner. If you consider that strength training is appropriate, for example, you must now decide which techniques should be used and why (*justification of technique*). As you treat, you will continually gain feedback from a person—what they feel, how their body reacts to treatment, and how they felt after treatment. These factors will give you an idea about the likely outcome following treatment (*prognosis*) and enable you to prepare a person for this. For example, is it likely that a person who has suffered from LBP for six months will be pain free after a single intervention? They may expect to be, but a professional's clinical experience with other people and the nature of the healing process would suggest that several sessions will be required to allow adaptation.

Keypoint:

Be realistic about the likely outcome of treatment (prognosis).

Common errors

We can make errors with both fast (intuitive) and slow (analytical) thinking (Table 5.11). Although we are getting a first impression when we meet a patient, this may be skewed (biased) from information we already have. For example, a referral letter stating a diagnosis, or the results of scan findings can stop us being totally objective, an error called *priming*. If we have often seen a pattern, we may jump to a conclusion that the patient in front of us fits that pattern (confirmation bias), or we may be swayed by the memory of a very good result we once had and want to repeat (memory bias). This can be extended when we convince ourselves

TABLE 5.11 Deduction errors in clinical reasoning

Type	
Priming	Influenced through prior information (e.g., imaging findings)
Confirmation bias	Focus on data confirming existing hypothesis
Memory bias	Data similar to case with very successful outcome
Representativeness heuristic	Comparing to concept we already have in mind
Stickiness	Hypothesis not revised in the face of subsequent information

Source: Data from Jones and Rivett (2019).

TABLE 5.12 Clinical reasoning strategies

Type	Emphasis
Diagnostic	Functional limitations associated with physical or movement impairment
Narrative	Understand the patient's illness or disability
Procedure	Application of clinical guidelines with progress compared to outcome measure
Interactive	Aiming to build/maintain clinician-patient rapport
Collaborative	Shared decision making throughout treatment course
Teaching	Facilitation of change such as beliefs, coping, capabilities
Predictive	Effect/timing of selected intervention on overall prognosis
Ethical	Where ethics impinge of patient's ability to make decisions regarding their health and/or treatment

Source: Data from Edwards et al. (2004), Jones and Rivett (2019).

that the patient's signs and symptoms fit in with a pattern category (representative heuristic). Finally, slow analytical thinking is only useful if it is used to modify our first impression. If we fail to do this and are blind to the results, we see before us an error called *stickiness* is being made.

Strategies

How we conduct CR can vary on the aim. Most commonly a reductionist medical model is used, and a structural diagnosis made. This in turn leads to physical alterations such as muscle weakness or joint tightness which then reflect on functional limitations noticeable to the patient. CR based on this type of pathway is termed diagnostic CR, but as we have seen within a biopsychosocial (BPS) model of healthcare, the *biological* features (pathology, disorder) are only one aspect of patient-centred care. Internal personal influences such as beliefs, culture, self-efficacy, for example, represent *psychological* influences. External environmental influences such as family, work, sport, culture exemplify the *social* effects. Other models of CR must also be considered (Table 5.12) as they extend our reasoning and can offer a far better treatment result.

Prioritising treatment

Often, several people with LBP will appear to have similar needs, while another looks very different. This is because most clinical conditions have patterns which can be identified, and it is often helpful to sort through these patterns to determine more accurately who is likely to benefit from which treatment type. This approach is termed *subgrouping* and seeks to identify members of a larger general group who have similar needs. Putting similar subgroups together for treatment is the aim of stratified care.

TABLE 5.13 Examples of subgroups within low back pain management

Approach	Features
Posture classification (Kendall)	Posture plumbline & posture types.
Movement system impairment (Sahrmann)	Symptom provocation, muscle stiffness and bodypart dissociation.
System classification (O'Sullivan)	Direction of symptom provocation control of spine regions. Fear avoidance behaviour
Cross syndrome (Janda)	Posture & muscle imbalance around pelvic and shoulder girdle.
Pain provoking motion (McGill)	Pain provoking postures & load tolerance direct corrective exercise. Segmental stiffness & compliance.
Mechanical diagnosis (McKenzie)	Response to repeated loading with aim to centralise and abolish symptoms.
Cognitive functional therapy	Movement pattern identification. Focus on behavioural psychology
Motor Control Training	Focus on movement quality. Individualisation based on features identified in assessment.
Pain mechanism	Identify predominant pain mechanism—nociceptive, neuropathic, or central inputs.

Source: Data from Hodges et al. (2013) and Hodges (2019).

Definition:

Stratified care involves matching subgroups of people to specific treatment approaches with the aim of improving outcomes.

In the past within the therapy world, people have attempted to subgroup patient by various means with a view to directing treatment (Table 5.13). Treatments are largely either classified according to structural features such as a pathology or mechanical diagnosis (e.g., lumbar disc lesion, OA, inflammation) or from by the response to treatment (e.g., manual therapy, stabilisation, directional exercise).

Subgrouping, according to patient prognosis, has been successfully practised using the Startback screening tool (Hill et al. 2008), readily downloadable at this link, https://startback.hfac.keele.ac.uk/ The start back screening tool (SBST) aims to match patients to treatments which are most appropriate to them. It is available both as a questionnaire and an online calculator, and involves nine questions to categorise people into low, medium, or high risk of having psycho-social factors which may influence their treatment outcome (yellow flags). Of the nine questions (referred leg pain, co-morbid pain, disability (two items), bother-someness, catastrophising, fear, anxiety, and depression), the latter five have been identified as a psychosocial subscale. Those at low risk require a brief assessment and mainly advice with a focus on staying active, while those at medium risk are similarly managed but may require therapy intervention depending on findings at assessment. High risk individuals may require an additional behavioural focus to care.

Assessing movement quality

Control of movement within the lumbar spine has been proposed as an important factor in both the development of LBP and its treatment (Panjabi 1992, Hodges et al. 2013). Assessing movement can be useful to assist programme design and to identify therapy direction. However, it is often unclear if movement changes are a cause or a consequence of LBP, and whether changing movement is possible or desirable (see Chapter 1). Previously motor control changes have been seen as essentially mechanical faults using a classical medical model but using the BPS model, they are considered more multifactorial. Rather than tight or lax tissues altering movement patterns, willingness to move and fear of pain (kinesiophobia) are now considered more important factors driving movement changes (O'Sullivan et al. 2016). It has been suggested that rather than a description of poor motor control, a change in *motor control strategy* may be more valuable (Low 2018).

Certainly, in population studies movement quality is rarely related to treatment outcomes but changing movement can often be a factor in symptom modification. A variety of motion tests have been used for the lumbo-pelvic region (Norris 2008), and a test battery of the most useful tests has been proposed (Adelt et al. 2021) using 277 participants with non-specific low back pain (NSLBP) patients assessed by 21 physiotherapists. In this study, 80% of participants were found to have at least one direction specific lumbar movement control (LMC) change which was below average. Three directions were used to determine LMC, flexion, extension, and rotation/lateral flexion and loss of control was observed when a minimum of two tests were positive in one direction. The tests were rated for difficulty enabling the starting test to be selected for the person's expected ability. The study authors recommended the most difficult of each directional test if screening is to be performed, with four-point kneeling rocking backwards (flexion), supine leg lift and hold (extension), and prone single hip rotation (rotation/lateral flexion) being used. Table 5.14 illustrates the tests and LMC directions, grading them from A (easy), B (intermediate), and C (hard).

Assessing posture

The way a person positions their body is termed posture, and assessment of this position may be either static (at rest) or dynamic (when moving). Historically, posture assessment has changed. In the 18th century, posture was linked to military training to mould an individual into a soldier, with upright standing considered desirable. At the same time, posture entered the public gaze with the health

TABLE 5.14 Lumbar movement control (LMC) test battery

Test position	Grade	Movement	Loss of control on visual inspection
Forward bend (Flexion)	A	Bend forwards towards the floor and allow the arms to hang loosely	• Lumbar spine initiates movement and contributes more (>25°) than hip and thoracic spine. • On return LS unrolls later
Backward bend (extension)	A	Fold the arms across the chest and keep knees locked. Lean backwards.	• Initiates movement with excessive forward sway (>10 cms). • Hip and TS contribute less. • Return to neural LS occurs later
Chest drop (flexion)	B	Sit upright with hands on thighs. Bend the neck and look towards the floor. Stop the movement as soon as the LS begins to move	• LS starts to flex before full TS flexion is achieved. • LS not dissociated from TS flexion.
Tripod test (flexion or rotation/ lateral flexion)	A	Sit upright and straighten your right/ left knee. Perform the action only so far that the LS remains upright.	• LS flexes too early in ROM of knee extension (early/ mid-range). • Excessive LS flexion or rotation/lateral flexion)

(Continued)

TABLE 5.14 (Continued)

Test position	Grade	Movement	Loss of control on visual inspection
 Kneeling rockback/forwards (flexion or extension)	C	Begin in 4-point kneeling and rock the buttocks towards the feet, stop at mid-calf level. Return to the start and then rock forwards towards the hands, stopping with the waist moves beyond the knee. Aim to keep the back the same as the starting position throughout.	• LS flexion occurs in first half of movement when buttocks move back. • LS extension occurs in first half of movement when buttocks move forwards. • Subject is not aware of their LS movement.
 Prone single leg lift (extension or rotation)	B	Lift the right/left leg keeping the knee straight. Try to avoid moving the LS.	Before the hip reaches 10° extension: • Lumbar spine extends • LS rotation/lateral flexion occurs • Anterior pelvic tilt
 Lying bent leg lift (extension or flexion)	C	Begin with knees bent and feet flat. Lift both legs together and stop when the knees are above the hips. Where this is painful, perform a single leg action	• LS moves (flexion or extension) before knees are above hips. • Subject is unable to dissociate movement of LS from pelvis. • Bulging abdominal wall • LMC loss may be in assent or descent.

Test position	Grade	Movement	Loss of control on visual inspection
 Bent knee fall out (extension, flexion, rotation)	C	Begin with the knee bent and feet flat. Lower the right/left leg to the side. Stop at 45° and then return. Throughout the movement keep the LS in the same position as the start.	Before 45° hip rotation: • Pelvis begins to rotate • Subject unable to dissociate movement of hip from that of LS or pelvis. • LMC loss may be unilateral.
 Clamshell (extension, flexion, rotation)	B	Lie on your side with your knees and hips bent. Raise your knee towards the ceiling and stop at 15° hip abduction	Before 15° hip abduction: • LS movement into flexion or extension • LS movement into rotation • May be unilateral.
 Prone hip rotation (rotation/ lateral flexion).	C	Begin lying prone with the knee flexed to 90°. Lower the foot outwards and then inwards. Keep the pelvis in the start position.	• LS rotation occurs before the hip reaches 30° medial or lateral rotation. Subject cannot dissociate hip rotation from lumbopelvic movement. • May be unilateral.

Grade: A—easy. B—intermediate. C—hard.

LS—lumbar spine. TS—thoracic spine. ROM—range of motion. LMC—lumbar movement control.

Source: Data after Adelt et al. (2021).

and wellness movement linked to Swedish gymnastics and an upright posture became linked to morality, and something to aspire to (Gilman 2014). As an upright military posture was seen as desirable, so a relaxed (flexed) posture was seen as undesirable. Going further, this relaxed posture was viewed as uncivilised or even 'ape like' (Thompson, 1922). By the 20th century, posture had become medicalised (Jesson 2016) with its assessment taking a mechanical viewpoint directed to alignment of body segments and changes in muscle activity and joint loading.

After the Second World War, posture was described by the Posture Committee of the American Academy of Orthopaedic Surgeons in 1947 as the arrangement of body parts in a state of balance that protects the supporting structures of the body against injury or progressive deformity (Cailliet 1983). A good posture was therefore said to be effortless, non-fatiguing, and painless when the person maintains it over a long period. In the late 1980s, posture became intertwined as part of a muscle balance approach used in physiotherapy and it was said that muscles function most efficiently when postural alignment was optimal, and the joints are positioned and loaded evenly (Bullock-Saxton 1988). Optimal posture was said to combine both minimal muscle work and minimal joint loading (Norris 1995). The combination of these two factors was said to be important, and where optimal posture is lost (e.g., in slouched standing), the muscle activity would reduce, and joint loading increase, potentially increasing the risk of pain and injury.

It was argued that joint loading should be minimised over time, with an even distribution of force being preferable to point pressure. From a mechanical perspective, contact pressure is directly proportional to the transmitted force but inversely proportional to area. Distributing force over a larger area by optimising segmental alignment, was said to reduce joint surface compression and lessen the risk of degenerative changes to a joint.

Change in the alignment of one body segment usually causes neighbouring segments to move to maintain equilibrium. If one body segment moves forward, for example, another must move backward to keep the body's line of gravity (LOG) within the base of support. Over time, changes in force per unit area may cause tissue adaptation, such as selective atrophy or shortening.

Static posture (when the body is stationary) reflects the alignment of body segments and is often used as an initial examination of the body (observation) in both therapy and the exercise professions. Static posture examples include standing, sitting, and lying. Dynamic posture (body position during movement) can give information about body segment alignment, muscle actions, and motor skill. Typical dynamic postures are walking, running, jumping, and lifting. Excessive changes in posture from a presumed optimal position can give rise to asymmetrical tissue tension. Ultimately, tissue failure can result from repeated passive tissue strain if the tissue does not have time to adapt. Avoidance of end-range postures that load the soft tissues excessively may reduce short-term pain as well as long-term pain caused by overuse. Alteration in lumbar spine stiffness has been demonstrated through prolonged sitting (two hours) in normal healthy subjects with the authors suggesting these changes may contribute to LBP and may increase the risk of injury (Beach et al. 2005). Interestingly Scannell and McGill (2003) studied subjects who had either increased lordosis (hyperlordosis) or reduced lordosis (hypolordosis). The investigators modified subjects' posture using a 12-week exercise programme and demonstrated a change in posture towards a mid-range (neutral) lordosis, suggesting that exercise may influence posture.

Keypoint:

Static posture reflects body segment alignment at one moment in time only. *Dynamic posture* involves alignment during movement.

Postural stability and body sway

Although static posture assessment observes the body when stationary, in normal unsupported standing constant movement occurs. When standing erect, the human body has a small base of support attributable to its bipedal stance and comparatively high centre of gravity (approximately at the second sacral segment S2). Humans are therefore relatively unstable compared with quadrupeds (four-legged animals), which have a larger base of support and lower centre of gravity. Maintaining an erect posture takes surprisingly little energy, however, because of constant motion brought about by postural control. This motion (postural sway) depends on kinesthesis, or motion sense, which enables us to detect the position of our body parts through organs of proprioception, vision, the vestibular apparatus in the inner ear, and skin receptors. Normal postural sway consists of a small continuous motion in the sagittal plane. This oscillation of the centre of gravity results from alternating muscle activity—possibly a relief mechanism to reduce lower-limb fatigue and to aid blood flow (Bullock-Saxton et al. 1991).

Excessive postural sway generally reveals poor balance and stability, a situation commonly seen in elderly and inactive people. Levels of postural sway can predict risk of recurrent falls among frail nursing home residents. Comparing average speed of body sway between fallers and non-fallers greater speed is seen in those with a history of falls (Fernie et al. 1982). Generally, no significant difference is found with feet wide apart, but changes are seen with a narrow stance in a mediolateral or anteroposterior direction. Research on body sway is typically carried out by measuring displacement of the centre of pressure measured on a force platform in the laboratory or using inertial measurement units (IMU) during functional tasks (Ghahramani et al. 2019). In the clinic, body sway is often determined using the Berg Balance Scale (BBS) protocol (Berg and Normal 1993).

> **Definition:**
>
> The *Berg Balance Scale* (BBS) is a 14-item test with each test scored from 0 (low level function) to 4 (highest level function). Actions include common daily tasks such as sit to stand, standing unsupported, with feet together or eyes closed, reaching forwards, picking something up from the floor, turning, placing one foot on a stool.

Heavy people also may exhibit greater body sway (Sugano and Takeya 1970), as may tall people (Murray et al. 1975). Training usually can reduce postural sway. In elderly people, strength training may improve stability and limit postural sway (Hughes et al. 1996). Following ankle injury, postural sway increases, but balance and coordination training can return body sway to normal values (Bernier and Perrin 1998). Lord and colleagues (1996) reduced fracture risk in women (ages 60–85) using a general aerobic exercise programme whose effect was to improve postural sway rather than to change bone density, and Pilates exercise has been shown to have a favourable effect on postural balance in a systematic review and meta-analysis (Casonatto and Yamacita 2020).

> **Keypoint:**
>
> *Postural body sway* is greater when balance and stability are poor. Exercise that includes balance and coordination training can restore body sway to normal values.

Basic postural assessment

Observation is part of client assessment in both therapy and exercise situations, and basic postural assessment is useful to give an overview of a client's general body alignment. It enables the therapist or exercise professional to focus more closely on areas of interest with more specific tests. By its nature, postural assessment compares a person's posture to a theoretical ideal or optimal posture. Deviation from this imaginary ideal can lead the person being assessed to presume their posture is the cause of their condition (guilt) or that something is wrong with them (catastrophising)—both negative views which should be avoided.

Line of gravity

Static posture classically compares the body to a standard reference line (Kendall et al. 1993) that represents the LOG. The laws of physics dictate that the LOG must pass within the body's base of support to maintain stability. The closer the body segments are to the LOG, the less torque there is around a joint. Where the LOG passes through the joint axis, no torque is created around that joint at all. If the LOG passes some distance from the joint axis, gravitational torque will tend to move the body segment towards the LOG where the segment not counter-balanced by elastic recoil of soft tissue and muscle action (Norkin and Levangie 1992). With the LOG anterior to the joint axis, the proximal segment of the body connected to the joint tends to move anteriorly; posterior motion tends to occur when the LOG is posterior to the joint axis.

In the standard posture viewed from the side, the subject is positioned with a plumb line representing the LOG, passing just in front of the lateral malleolus. In an ideal posture, this line should pass just anterior to the midline of the knee and then through the greater trochanter, bodies of the lumbar vertebrae, shoulder joint, bodies of the cervical vertebrae, and lobe of the ear. Because the LOG is anterior to the ankle joint, gravity is continuously pulling the tibia anteriorly. This would result in enough dorsiflexion to un-balance the body were it not for constant opposing resistance provided by muscle action from the soleus (Norkin and Levangie 1992). The LOG passes in front of the knee joint axis (but behind the patella), forcing the femur anteriorly and creating an extension torque resisted by the posterior knee structures.

When viewed from the front, with the feet 3–4 in. (7–10 cm) apart, the LOG should bisect the body into two equal halves. The anterior superior iliac spines (ASIS) should be approximately in the same horizontal plane, and the pubis and ASIS should be in the same vertical plane (Kendall et al. 1993). This alignment defines the neutral lumbar–pelvic alignment, which typically is about 5° to the horizontal. The joint axes of the hips, knees, and ankles should be equidistant from the LOG, and the LOG should transect the vertebral bodies. The gravitational torque imposed on one side of the body should equal that of the other side.

Anatomical landmarks that provide comparisons for horizontal level on the right and left sides of the body include the knee creases, buttock creases, pelvic rim, inferior angle of the scapulae, acromion processes, ears, and external occipital protuberances. You also can observe alignment of the spinous processes and rib angles; minor scoliosis becomes more evident when assessed in Adam's position (forward flexion in standing). Unequal distances between arms and trunk (referred to as the keyhole), various skin creases, or unequal muscle bulk should prompt closer examination. Foot and ankle alignment should also be assessed (Figure 5.2).

Both plumbline measures (single line) and posture grid measures (standing behind a Perspex screen marked with lines) can be useful more as outcome measures to demonstrate ongoing change within therapy or exercise. When used diagnostically to suggest that a postural type or alignment is linked to a clinical condition they are off less value, as a causal factor or even when correlated.

Keypoint:

Posture assessment provides one baseline measure which may be used to plan a rehab programme. It does not indicate abnormality.

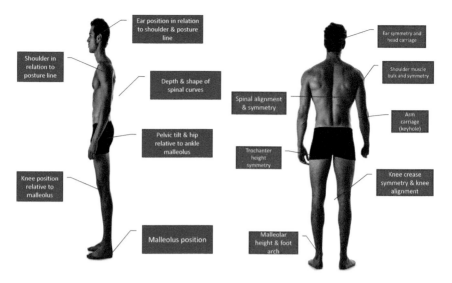

FIGURE 5.2 Posture assessment.

Posture types

There are several classic posture types described in the literature, with subdivisions and overlap between them (Figure 5.3). In the lordotic posture, the main feature is an increased anterior pelvic tilt. Anterior displacement of the pelvis characterises the swayback, whereas the flat-back posture has slight posterior pelvic tilting and reduction of the lumbar lordosis. In the kyphotic posture, the thoracic curve is increased, and this is typically associated with a forward head posture. The lordotic and kyphotic postures can co-exist, a position termed kypho-lordotic. Importantly, these traditional descriptions are all normal postures in that they are normal to the individual who possesses them.

In the classic lordotic or hollow-back posture, the greater trochanter remains on the LOG, but the pelvis tilts anteriorly, moving the anterior superior iliac spine (ASIS) forward and downward in relation to the pubic bone, something which is often visible in a lean person especially. This posture type is common in dancers and in young gymnasts, and can be noticeable in women after childbirth, especially with multiple births.

In the swayback (slouched or slumped) posture, the pelvis remains level but the hip joint is pushed forward, the greater trochanter lying anterior to the LOG. Whereas in classically described standard posture the sternum is the most anterior structure, now the pelvis has shifted and becomes the more anterior body segment, with the LOG moving from the ankle to the midfoot and toes. The hip is effectively extended increasing forces active on the anterior hip structures (Lewis and Sahrmann 2015). The lumbar lordosis now often changes shape from an even curve to a deeper, shorter curve with a prominent crease normally at mid

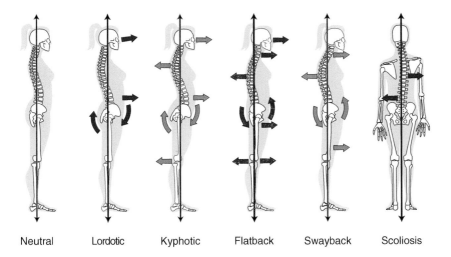

| Neutral | Lordotic | Kyphotic | Flatback | Swayback | Scoliosis |

FIGURE 5.3 Classic posture types.

lumbar level. The kyphosis can be longer and may extend into the lumbar spine. The lower lumbar region is typically flatter, and the pelvis may be minimally posteriorly tilted. The swayback posture may be combined with dominance of one leg in standing (hanging on the hip) and can be associated with lateral hip pain where the posture is maintained.

> **Keypoint:**
>
> In the swayback posture, the pelvis is placed forward of the chest.

The flat-back posture is typically correlated with lack of mobility in the lumbar spine and a flattening of the lordosis (lumbar flexion). This posture reflects the extension dysfunction originally described by McKenzie (1981) and is common in CLBP after extended periods of inactivity and rest in a sitting or lying position. The pelvis may be posteriorly tilted compared with the reference line, and the lumbar tissues are often thickened and immobile. The flat-back posture can also be seen in subjects who practise a high number of sit-up type exercises (repeated lumbar flexion). In this case, the lumbar spine may be mobile, but the repeated flexion movements may lead to habitual postural changes with or without tissue adaptation. In most cases, this will be painless and tissue adaptation will have occurred over time. Where CLBP is suffered, temporarily changing the posture by increasing the lordosis either with a spinal extension exercise or a lumbar support may alleviate symptoms and allow tissue irritability to settle.

The kyphotic posture is often referred to colloquially as a "round shouldered" carriage in youth or a "dowager's hump" in seniors. The shoulder joint may be held anterior to the posture line, increasing the thoracic kyphosis. In classical posture assessment, upper limb alignment is often said to be optimal when the scapulae are approximately the width of three fingers from the spine, and the medial borders of the scapulae are vertical. Scapular abduction can lead over time to a protracted shoulder position, in turn increasing thoracic flexion. Equally, osteoporosis can lead to vertebral wedging changing the kyphosis. In each case, further examination is required to establish a person's rehabilitation needs.

Scoliotic posture is a lateral curvature of the spine, usually associated with a twisted (rotation) appearance and rib flaring on forward bend. Where there is a specific bone change giving rise to scoliosis, it is often termed *structural*, but frequently no obvious cause is found, and the scoliosis is classified as idiopathic or *functional*. A structural scoliosis would include change in bone shape during growth or ageing, while the functional condition can be due to changes in tissue (ligament or fascia length) or muscle tone and strength. Often both types of scoliosis have elements of changes in lifestyle (sitting posture, for example) and psychological traits (anxiety and depression, for instance).

Any posture type (classically optimal or sub-optimal) can give symptoms if tissues are overloaded, and recovery is not sufficient. In addition, a posture type may not be permanent in that a person may stand in a particular posture temporarily and alter their posture when they move. In Figure 5.4, the subject is standing with their pelvic pressed forwards (sway), their thoracic spine flexed (increased kyphosis) and shoulders drawn forwards (protracted). This is clearly a temporary posture for her, and she can correct it at will. The subject's posture is entirely normal for her and would only present as clinically relevant if either

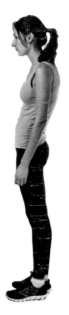 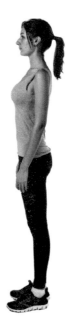

FIGURE 5.4 Temporary posture change.

posture was held for a prolonged period in which case tissue tension changes may become painful.

Posture and pain

Each person has a different posture and rarely are postural changes related to pain or performance over the long term. The shape of the curve in the upper spine (thoracic kyphosis) has been shown not to be related to shoulder pain in a systematic review which examined ten leading studies (Barrett et al. 2016). Neck posture assessment carried out using 2-dimensional photographic analysis of a group of over 1,000 adolescents has shown no association between neck pain and headaches and posture category such as upright, intermediate, slumped, and forward head postures (Richards et al. 2016). However, the same study did demonstrate a relationship between slumped and forward head position and depression (see below). Reviewing 54 studies looking at spinal curves, no association was found between curve shape and spinal pain (Christensen & Hartviqsen 2008). Looking at standing posture both overall (global alignment) and locally (spinopelvic characteristics) in over 1,000 adolescents, only a minimal relationship between posture and pain was found with global measures and none with local parameters (Dolphens et al. 2012). The amount of time spent in a sub-optimal posture would also seem to be unrelated to pain. Looking at a group of blue-collar workers, the time spent in a forward bent position was not associated with LBP intensity. In fact, in this study those who bent forward for longer periods had lower intensity LBP (Villumsen et al. 2015). Similarly, fashionable terms related to posture such as 'text neck' have been investigated as part of postural assessment and found wanting. In a study of 150 young adults (18–21) no association was found between neck posture and neck pain (Damasceno et al. 2018).

So, posture does not usually cause pain, but it can be associated with it. In other words, someone with pain may take up a different posture, and remaining in a particular posture for a long period may be painful. In a study producing pain by injecting saline into the leg muscles, researchers were able to show that posture factors altered. Body sway and EMG activity were shown to increase as a result of the experimentally induced pain. Interestingly, several studies have looked at the effect of posture on psychological (behavioural) changes. In one study, adopting a more 'powerful' posture (one which is more open and expansive) was shown to increase testosterone levels, lower cortisol, and lead to increased feelings of power and tolerance to risk. When individuals are subjected to a stressful stimulus (Trier social stress test), upright posture has been shown to improve a number of psychological states (arousal level and feelings of power) and physiological effects (systolic blood pressure, galvanic skin response, and skin temperature) compared to a slumped posture (Hackford et al. 2019). This may be important as thoughts and emotions can often be associated with facial expressions or posture. A seated upright posture (compared to slumped) has been shown to reduce sleepiness and increase feelings of power when subjected to stress. Those sitting upright had higher self-esteem, more arousal, better mood, and lower fear, compared to slumped subjects (Nair et al. 2015). Both muscular and autonomic states may be influenced by emotion an observation referred to embodied cognition theory in psychological fields.

A slumped posture is associated with depression, and although the above research show changes in mood state in healthy subjects, it was not conducted on depressed individuals. In a preliminary study by Wilkes et al. (2017) 61 individuals with mild to moderate depression received postural taping in sitting. Those with taping significantly improved sitting posture demonstrated lower negative affect and lower anxiety measured on the Trier Social Stress Test (TSST).

Definition:

The TSST is a 15-minute laboratory procedure which induces stress in three 5-minute sections (tasks). It is conducted as an interview with three trained assessors, with the subject preparing (task 1) and then presenting (task 2), a presentation followed by a mental arithmetic task (task 3). During the test, saliva and blood samples are taken and heart rate monitored.

Biopsychosocial approach to posture

So, are we looking at things the wrong way? Within the field of persistent pain, especially CLBP, we have seen a gradual shift away from a traditional biomedical mechanistic thinking towards a BPS view. The traditional mechanistic view is that pain is directly related to tissue damage— nervous impulses travel from the tissue to a 'pain centre' in the brain, for example. If something hurts more, there is greater damage and as pain lessens tissues are healing. The BPS model views pain as an indicator of perceived threat. Nervous impulses travel to the brain where different areas of the brain interpret this information. By comparing the signal to things such as past experience, beliefs, social pressure, or expected behaviours, for example, the signal may or may not be judged as threatening to an individual and therefore interpreted as pain. The key difference here is that in the biomedical model (BM) biological effects predominate, while with the BPS model biological effects occur in parallel with psychological effects and social influences. Perhaps posture should be viewed in the same way.

Keypoint:

The major difference between the *biomedical* model (BM) and the *biopsychosocial* model (BPSM) is that, in the BM biological effects predominate, while with the BPSM biological effects occur in parallel with psychological effects and social influences.

Traditionally posture has been viewed mechanistically. Altered joint angles and bodypart alignment produces stress on soft tissue, influences muscle work, and alters joint loading. However, if we view posture from a BPS perspective psychological and social influences are also important. As we have seen posture does not have a significant causal effect on pain but can influence psychological states and have social interactions—so to simply say it is unimportant can be an error. Posture may still be important to some people at different stages of an injury or condition. Posture still warrants consideration in many conditions, just perhaps not for the reasons previously proposed.

When might posture be important?

Although posture is rarely a direct cause of injury, there are occasions when its correlation with injury risk or impaired performance is important (Table 5.15). Where tissues are sensitive, maintenance of an alignment which overloads the tissue may cause tissue irritation or inflammation giving pain. In the short-term, tissue may be unloaded by modifying the posture (taping or bracing) or using a mirror image exercise which places the body in the opposite alignment. Once irritability has ceased, if the person reverts to the previous posture, they may be pain free. Where loading is low, but tissue irritability high, temporary postural modification may still be required. This may stop as irritability eases, and/or tissue adaptation occurs. The keypoint here is that it is the time spent in a posture rather than the posture itself which is the significant factor.

Keypoint:

Time spent in a posture rather than the posture itself is often the more significant factor.

Where tissues are placed under higher loads, the margin of error between tissue tolerance and injury becomes smaller. Postural alignment therefore becomes

TABLE 5.15 When might posture be important?

Tissue sensitivity	High load action	Low load action	Psychosocial factors
• If postural change alters symptoms • Take stress off stretched tissues • Allow irritable tissue to recover (offload)	• Margin of error very small • Single actions where no time to adapt	• Where tissue adaptation is not complete • Allow time for adaptation	• Depression • Self efficacy • Chronic fatigue

more important as loads increase. However, even with high loads injury may not occur providing tissue adaptation has occurred. Many elite athletes have postures which may have been considered suboptimal in the past, but the athlete has avoided injury because their tissues have adapted over many years of use.

Finally, we have seen that posture may be associated with psychological factors such as depression, body Image and self-efficacy. Psychological factors have been shown to be one of several factors which can interact in CLBP, so alterations in posture may be appropriate at least temporarily in the management of this condition.

Needs analysis

Just as a therapist would always assess a patient prior to selecting and applying treatment, before an exercise programme can be prescribed, a *needs analysis* should be performed (Table 5.16). The needs analysis looks at both the subject and the task or sport to be performed. Information gained about these two areas serves as a foundation for designing an individualised programme. Exercise history and current fitness level give a starting point in terms of skills which the subject possesses, and within these areas we should consider injury history and any exercise adaptations required because of injury. Tests of neuromuscular skill level may be relevant and can form part of a functional screen targeting the skill base of the task or sport to be performed. For example, a manual worker with a history of LBP may require screening for lifting and bending actions which mimic their working environment (height/weight/complexity), while a trail runner may need screening of lower limb alignment in a single leg squat to reflect hill descent on uneven ground. Movement analysis forms an essential part of the preparation and gives information on joint movements and muscle work especially. From this, the physiological requirements of the task/sport can be implied, and a programme planned accordingly, with specific aims and objectives (see definition box above).

Movement screening

Clinical examination uses a reductionist approach, often aiming to identify a single structure which may be responsible for a patient's symptoms. Assessment for sports performance or exercise can follow a similar pattern, trying to identify weak muscles

TABLE 5.16 Needs analysis components

Subject/athlete	Task/sport
Exercise history	Movement analysis
Current fitness level	Physiological requirements
Neuromuscular skill level	Injury risk

Source: Data from Baechle and Earle (2015).

or tight tissues, for example. Focussing on one body region or structure within that region is only one approach, and one which parallels the BM of healthcare. As we have seen the adoption of the biopsychosocial model (BPSM) is a broader more holistic approach, and in exercise programming this can be reflected by assessing whole body movement using movement screening. Classically in medicine, screening is used within a population to detect disease or to identify individuals currently without signs or symptoms who may have a pathology (Bahr 2016). Within the exercise domain, movement screening has often been aimed at injury prevention or performance enhancement. The use of movements which match those used in sport or everyday function has been popular with functional movement screening (FMS) becoming a commercial product. Although widely popular, this type of screening has been shown to have only moderate inter-rater and intra-rater reliability (Moran et al. 2016). In addition, a systematic review and meta-analysis (24 studies using the Quality of Cohort Studies assessment tool) has shown the FMS composite score not to support its use as an injury prediction tool (Moran et al. 2017).

Although movement screening cannot accurately predict injury risk, it can form the basis of exercise programme development, acting as part of a needs analysis. In some cases, it may identify individuals at risk who are just starting a fitness programme, and it can provide a tool to monitor progress and enhance motivation. Screening tests typically reflect activities which a person will likely be exposed to and may be chosen on a basis of a particular sport or occupation. For example, a

TABLE 5.17 Examples of movement screen actions (a) Functional movement screen (FMS)

Action	Description	Scoring
Overhead squat	Hold pole overhead with arms wide apart	Timing and body/limb alignment assessed.
Hurdle step	Pole across shoulders, place foot above knee high hurdle	Each exercise scored from 0 (unable to perform) to 3 (ideal) giving a potential maximum score of 21.
In-line lunge	Pole held along spine, step forwards and lower back knee to ground	
Shoulder mobility	Combine hand behind back and hand behind head—measure distance between fingers of each hand	
Rotary stability	4-point kneeling alternate arm and leg raise (Birddog exercise). Assess spinal alignment	
Active SLR	Keep non-moving leg straight on floor. Measure ROM at high flexion of moving musculoskeletal.	
Trunk stability push up	Press-up position held and shoulders and spine alignment assessed	

SLR—straight leg raise. ROM—range of motion.

Source: Data after Cook et al. (2014).

TABLE 5.17 (B) Athletic ability assessment (AAA)

Action	Description	Scoring
Prone hold	Press-up position	Timing and body/
Side hold	Side plank position	limb alignment
Overhead squat	Hold pole overhead with arms apart	assessed.
Single leg squat	Performed on a knee-high bench	3 (max) to 1 (min)
Walking lunge	Performed with a pole across the shoulders	giving a potential
Single leg hop	Performed in a forward direction	maximum of 18.

Source: Data after McKeown et al. (2014).

screen for an individual returning to work following injury may include very different actions to those chosen for someone returning to sport. An individual whose job involves lifting, carrying, and ladder climbing would require actions similar to these tasks, while an athlete whose sport involves sprinting, change of direction, acceleration/deceleration and jumping would require actions to mimic these.

Table 5.17 features exercises from the functional movement screen (FMS) and the athletic ability assessment (AAA) to demonstrate the types of actions commonly used. Movement screens may be designed to mimic the tasks which a person is to undergo either during rehabilitation or as part of general training. Forward bend and squat actions are useful for those involved in lifting, while overhead reach at a wall (wall angel) or overhead squat are informative of thoracic spine mobility in relation to shoulder movement. Sit-to-stand, balance actions, and single leg standing are useful for seniors (see Berg balance score above), while jump down (bilateral or unilateral) and hop-and-hold movements are informative of lower limb alignment following knee injury.

References

Adelt, E., Schoettker-Koeniger, T., Luedtke, K., et al. (2021). Lumbar movement control in non-specific chronic low back pain: Evaluation of a direction-specific battery of tests using item response theory. *Musculoskeletal Science & Practice* 55: 102406.

Baechle T.R., and Earle, R.W (2015) *Essential and strength and conditioning (3rd ed)*. Illinois: Human Kinetics. Champaign.

Bahr, R. (2016). Why screening tests to predict injury do not work—And probably never will. A critical review. *British Journal of Sports Medicine* 50: 776–780.

Barrett, E., O'Keeffe, M., O'Sullivan, K., et al. (2016). Is thoracic spine posture associated with shoulder pain, range of motion and function? A systematic review. *Manual Therapy* 26: 38–46.

Beach, T.A., Parkinson, R.J., Stothart, J.P., et al. (2005). Effects of prolonged sitting on the passive flexion stiffness of the in vivo lumbar spine. *The Spine Journal* 5(2): 145–154.

Berg, K., and Norman, K. (1993). Functional assessment of balance and gait. *Gait Balance Disorders* 12(4): 705–723.

Bernier, J.N., and Perrin, D.H. (1998). Effect of coordination training on proprioception of the functionally unstable ankle. *Journal of Orthopedic and Sports Physical Therapy* 27: 264–275.

Bullock-Saxton, J.E., Bullock, M.I., Tod, C., et al. (1991). Postural stability in young adult men and women. *New Zealand Journal of Physiotherapy* 3: 7–10.

Cailliet, R. (1983). *Soft tissue pain and disability.* Philadelphia, PA: Davis.

Casonatto, J., and Yamacia, C.M. (2020). Pilates exercise and postural balance in older adults: A systematic review and meta-analysis of randomized controlled trials. *Complementary Therapies in Medicine* 48: 1–7.

Christensen, S.T., and Hartvigsen, J. (2008). Spinal curves and health: A systematic critical review of the epidemiological literature dealing with associations between sagittal spinal curves and health. *Journal of Manipulative and Physiological Therapeutics* 31(9): 690–714.

Cook, G., Burton, L., et al. (2014). Functional movement screening: the use of fundamental movements as an assessment of function – Part 1. *International Journal of Sports Physical Therapy* 9(3): 396–409.

Damasceno, G.M., Ferreira, A.S., Nogueira, L.A.C., et al. (2018). Text neck and neck pain in 18–21-year-old young adults. *European Spine Journal* 27(6): 1249–1254.

Dolphens, M., Cagnie, B., Coorevits, P., et al. (2012). Sagittal standing posture and its association with spinal pain: A school-based epidemiological study of 1196 Flemish adolescents before age at peak height velocity. *Spine* 37(19): 1657–1666.

Edwards, I., Jones, M., Carr, J., et al., 2004a. *Clinical reasoning strategies in physical therapy. Phys. Ther.* 84, 312–335

Fernie, G.R., Gryfe, C.I., Holliday, P.J., et al. (1982). The relationship of postural sway in standing to the incidence of falls in geriatric subjects. *Age Ageing* 11(1): 11–16.

Ghahramani, M., Stirling, D., Naghdy, F., et al. (2019). Body postural sway analysis in older people with different fall histories. *Medical & Biological Engineering & Computing* 57: 533–542.

Hackford, J., Mackey, A., and Broadbent, E. (2019). The effects of walking posture on affective and physiological states during stress. *Journal of Behavior Therapy and Experimental Psychiatry* 62: 80–87.

Hill, J.C., Dunn, K.M., Lewis, C.L., et al. (2008). A primary care back pain screening tool: Identifying patient subgroups for initial treatment. *Arthritis & Rheumatism* 59: 632–641.

Hodges, P.W., Cholewicki, J., Dieen, J., et al. (2013). *Spinal control: The rehabilitation of back pain.* London: Churchill Livingstone.

Hodges, P.W. (2019). Hybrid approach to treatment tailoring for low back pain: A proposed model of care. *The Journal of Orthopaedic and Sports Physical Therapy* 49(6): 453–463.

Hodges, P.W., Cholewicki, J., van Dieen, J., Eds. (2013). *Spinal control: The rehabilitation of back pain.* Edinburgh: Elsevier.

Hughes, M.A., Duncan, P.W., Rose, D.K., et al. (1996). The relationship of postural sway to sensorimotor function, functional performance, and disability in the elderly. *Archives of Physical Medicine and Rehabilitation* 77: 567–572.

Jesson, T. (2016). Upright and uptight. The invention of posture. *Medium.com.* Accessed July 2016.

Jones, M.A. (1987). The clinical reasoning process in manipulative therapy. In Dalziel, B.A. and Snowsill, J.C., Eds., *Proceedings of the Fifth Biennial Conference of the Manipulative Therapists Association of Australia.* Melbourne, VIC, Australia, 62–69.

Jones, M.A., and Rivett, D.A (2019). *Clinical reasoning in musculoskeletal practice* (2nd ed). Elsevier. London.

Keegan, J.J., and Garrett, F.D. (1948). The segmental distribution of the cutaneous nerves in the limbs of man. *The Anatomical Record* 102(4): 409–437.

Kendall, F.P., McCreary, E.K., and Provance, P.G. (1993). *Muscles. Testing and function* (4th ed). Baltimore, MD: Williams & Wilkins.

Lewis, C.L., and Sahrmann, S.A. (2015). Effect of posture on hip angles and moments during gait. *Manual Therapy* 20(1): 176–182.

Low, M. (2018). A time to reflect on motor control in musculoskeletal physical therapy. *The Journal of Orthopaedic and Sports Physical Therapy* 48(11): 833–836.

McKenzie, R.A. (1981). *The lumbar spine. Mechanical diagnosis and therapy.* Lower Hutt, New Zealand: Spinal Publications.

McKeown, I., Taylor-McKeown, K., et al. (2014). Athletic ability assessment: A movement assessment protocol for athletes. *International Journal of Sports Physical Therapy* 9(7): 862–873.

Moran, R.W., Schneiders, A.G., Major, K.M., et al. (2016). How reliable are functional movement screening scores? A systematic review of rater reliability. *British Journal of Sports Medicine* 50: 527–536.

Moran, R.W., Schneiders, A.G., Mason, J., et al. (2017). Do functional movement screen (FMS) composite scores predict subsequent injury? A systematic review with meta-analysis. *British Journal of Sports Medicine* 51: 1661–1669.

Murray, M.P., Seireg, A., and Sepic, S.B. (1975). Normal postural stability and steadiness: Quantitative assessment. *Journal of Bone and Joint Surgery* 57A: 510–516.

Nair, S., Sagar, M., Sollers, J., et al. (2015). Do slumped and upright postures affect stress responses? A randomized trial. *Health Psychology: Official Journal of the Division of Health Psychology, American Psychological Association* 34(6): 632–641.

Norkin, C.C., and Levangie, P.K. (1992). *Joint structure and function. A comprehensive analysis* (2nd ed). Philadelphia, PA: Davis.

Norris, C.M. (1995). Spinal stabilisation: 5. An exercise programme to enhance lumbar stabilization. *Physiotherapy* 81(3): 138–146.

Norris, C.M. (2008). *Back stability – integrating science and therapy* (2nd ed). Champaign. IL: Human Kinetics.

Norris, C.M. (2012) *Complete guide to clinical massage.* London: Bloomsbury.

Norris, C.M. (2019). *Sports and soft tissue injuries: A guide for students and therapists.* London: Routledge.

O'Sullivan, P., Caneiro, J. P., O'Keeffe, M., et al. (2016). Unraveling the complexity of low back pain. *The Journal of Orthopaedic and Sports Physical Therapy* 46(11): 932–937.

Panjabi, M.M. (1992). The stabilizing system of the spine. Part I. Function, dysfunction, adaptation, and enhancement. *Journal of Spinal Disorders* 5(4): 383–397.

Richards, K.V., Beales, D.J., Smith, A.J., et al. (2016). Neck posture clusters and their association with biopsychosocial factors and neck pain in Australian adolescents. *Physical Therapy* 96(10): 1576–1587.

Scannell, J.P., and McGill, S.M. (2003). Lumbar posture: Should it and can it be modified? *Physical Therapy* 83: 907–917.

Seffinger, M.A., Najm, W.I., Mishra, S.I., Adams, A., Dickerson, V.M., Murphy, L.S., and Reinsch, S. (2004). Reliability of spinal palpation for diagnosis of back and neck pain: A systematic review of the literature. *Spine* 29(19): E413–E425.

Sugano, H., and Takeya, T. (1970). Measurement of body movement and its clinical application. *Japanese Journal of Physiology* 20: 296–308.

Thompson, J.E. (1922). The erect posture. *Lancet* 199(5133): 107–110.

Villumsen, M., Samani, A., Jørgensen, M.B., et al. (2015) Are forward bending of the trunk and low back pain associated among Danish blue-collar workers? A cross-sectional field study based on objective measures. *Ergonomics* 58(2): 246–258.

Wilkes, C., Kydd, R., Sagar, M., et al. (2017). Upright posture improves affect and fatigue in people with depressive symptoms. *Journal of Behavior Therapy and Experimental Psychiatry* 54: 143–149.

Worsfold, C. (2018). Examination of the Lumbar region. In Petty, N.J. and Ryder, D., Eds., *Musculoskeletal examination and assessment.* Oxford: Elsevier.

6

THE 3RS APPROACH—A CLINICAL FRAMEWORK

As we have seen in Chapter 1, the 3Rs approach is a clinical framework for practitioners and exercise teachers to prescribe exercise to those recovering from low back pain (LBP). The approach can be used at any stage of the condition, and incorporates aspects of pain management, patient education, and physical conditioning. It aims to present patient-centred therapeutic management within a biopsychosocial framework. As such the emphasis is on whole person management rather than tissue specific treatment alone. The three phases of the 3R's approach represent a progression over time (temporal) and of activity grade (functional), and broadly adhere to the healing timescale of a pathology. As normal healing progresses, pain and inflammation typically subside and recovery ensues, with patients returning to some level of function without rehabilitation. However, the nature of LBP is such that function is often reduced and recurrence of symptoms is typical. The 3Rs approach aims to increase a patient's capacity by improving function and lessen the likelihood of injury recurrence.

The 3Rs approach divides the rehabilitation process into three interrelated phases aligned with the healing timescale but representing the patient experience of injury and recovery (Norris 2020). The three phases are termed Reactive (R1), Recovery (R2), and Resilience (R3).

> **Keypoint:**
> The three phases of the 3Rs approach to back training and rehabilitation are called *Reactive* (R1), *Recovery* (R2), and *Resilience* (R3).

DOI: 10.4324/9781003366188-6

Tissue capacity

We have seen in Chapter 2 that tissue is adaptive, and loading may cause positive adaptation (training) but also negative (overtraining) if sufficient recovery is not allowed. Back pain is a condition which affects the whole person rather than an isolated tissue, a premise which underlies the biopsychosocial model (BPSM) used in its management (Chapter 1). However, the concept of tissue overload typically used in the management of peripheral soft tissue injury, can also provide a useful initial guideline to structuring a back-rehabilitation programme. Tissue overload occurs when the load imposed on a tissue exceeds its capacity; the capacity in this case being how much the tissue can be loaded or stressed without breaking down.

Definition:

Tissue capacity is how much a tissue can be loaded or stressed before it causes a negative reaction or breaks down.

Tissue capacity will differ between individuals depending on the requirements of their work or sport, the condition of their tissues, and age amongst other things. To maintain tissue capacity there is a continuous process of physiological maintenance via adaptations in the body metabolism, a process which represents *tissue homeostasis*. Injury or overuse can disrupt homeostasis leading to a cascade of biochemical changes. Excessive (supra-physiological) loading on tissue will cause adaptation providing there is sufficient time for recovery, a fact that underlies the general adaptation syndrome (GAS) seen in Chapter 2. A sudden imposition of extreme force, however, may exceed the load capacity of tissue, leading to maladaptation (trauma). Similarly, repetitive small forces which occur too frequently may not allow enough time for the tissue to adapt to the new loading level (overuse). At the other extreme, too little (sub-physiological) loading, such as would occur with prolonged rest, also disrupts homeostasis leading to changes such as

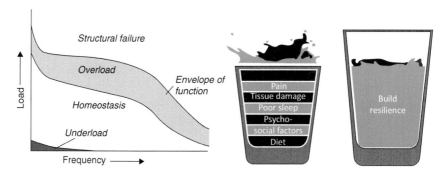

FIGURE 6.1 Models of tissue capacity.

muscle atrophy and bone mineral loss, reflecting deconditioning and reduced tissue capacity (Norris 2017).

Keypoint:

Excessive loading of a tissue may occur all at once (trauma) or build over a period of time (overuse).

The region of loading between under and over usage has been described as an 'envelope of function' and represents the area of load acceptance (Dye 2005) in day-to-day life (Figure 6.1a). Where loading exceeds the capacity of a bodypart, the action can be envisaged as occurring outside the envelope of function, and the tissues may enter the reactive phase of a musculoskeletal (MSK) condition (Cook and Docking 2015). At this stage reducing or changing loading may restore homeostasis, with a view to later increasing tissue capacity with progressive exercise and elevating the upper limit of the functional envelope.

Clearly, tissue capacity is a biological feature and within the BPSM (Chapter 1) we need to also address the psychosocial features of an individual's capacity. A useful analogy here is the overflowing cup used in psychology with reference to stressors, where the model is known as the stress cup or emotional bucket (Brabban and Turkington 2002). This has been adapted within the physiotherapy world to cover BPS factors (Lehman 2017) (Figure 6.1b). In this analogy, the cup is filled with physical factors which would make pain or injury more likely such as muscle weakness, or joint stiffness as well as psychological factors such as stress and anxiety and social factors such as life or work events. Reducing the number of these factors makes pain less likely (emptying the cup), but another method of achieving this aim would be to make the cup bigger. BPS factors which may achieve this might include muscle strength (bio), mindfulness (psycho), or support from family and friends (social). Within the 3Rs approach making the cup larger would represent building resilience. The balance between reducing the contents and the cup and increasing the cup size is usefully summed up as "calm things down, build things up", the "things" being the BPS factors.

Poor load management can have effects both on the body as a whole, and at a local tissue level. Repetitive loading without sufficient recovery can cause cumulative tissue fatigue and increase susceptibility to injury. At whole body level, inappropriate loading can prejudice a patient both psychologically and physiologically. Joint kinematics and neural feedback can be compromised with possible ongoing detriment to joint stability. Locally, excessive micro-damage may occur if the magnitude of loading is beyond the individual tissue's load-bearing capacity. Initially when loaded, tissue changes are short-term and reflect temporary *reaction*. These include changes such as increased blood flow through muscle and increased metabolic activity. When loading stops, these changes are reversed, homeostasis restored, and the tissue resumes its resting state. Repeated loading causes the tissue to change more permanently, and adaptation occurs with the tissue progressing to a *recovery* stage. Adaptation (for example, increased muscle strength) allows the body to tolerate higher loads. Training loads which are too low may not stimulate adequate adaptation and can therefore impair the tissue's ability to cope with higher loads in the future. Effective training stimulates biological adaptation to increase the patient's capacity to accept and withstand load, building *resilience*. The concept of resilience has both physical and psychological features. Physically, changes in the 'S' factors of fitness (see Chapter 2) must occur whilst psychologically factors such as fear of movement (kinesiophobia) and movement confidence are important to build self-efficacy.

CASE NOTE

A 35-year-old patient presented with left sided low back pain from performing deadlifts in his local gym. He used deadlifts regularly and his typical weight was 80–100 kg at a bodyweight of 75 kg. He generally performed his first set at a lower weight and typically used a pyramid of 12/10/8 reps. On this occasion he was challenged to lift 120 kg and because he was rushed, although warmed up from performing other exercises he performed the lift without a build-up. He performed 3 reps without a problem but on his 5th rep he felt a sudden flash of pain on the right side of his back causing him to drop (bounce) the weight. He stated afterwards that while his first 2 reps had felt strong, his 3rd rep felt weaker, and he experienced pain on his 4th rep but continued to the 5th. On examination his low back muscles were tight and painful and he described them as being "in spasm" and his back felt "locked". He had intense local low back pain to flexion, tightness only to extension and lateral flexion. His straight leg raise (SLR) was full and painless, and his hip movements were unremarkable. The night of his injury onset he was unable to sleep through the night due to pain and got up and walked for a short while which eased the pain slightly (NRS 8/10 down to NRS 6/10). Throughout the next day his pain eased gradually and by the evening he was able to sit relatively comfortably. He slept through the night. His back pain gradually eased over a period of 1 week and he returned to light training. It was hypothesised that he had exceeded the capacity of his back musculature resulting in local inflammation and pain with protective muscle spasm. The rapid recovery implied no traumatic injury to joint or neural based tissues.

Definition:

When measuring pain intensity, two scales are commonly used. A *numerical rating scale* (NRS) asks the person to rate their pain on a scale of 1 to 10. A *visual analogue scale* (VAS) rates pain on a visual scale from nil pain through mild pain to intense pain. The user is asked to mark a point on the line which is later converted by the tester to a number.

Healing timescale

After injury, tissue heals following a loosely defined timescale of interacting phases (Norris 2019). *Injury* (tissue disruption) usually instigates *inflammation*, the two phases representing the reactive period of recovery when a patient's tissues are irritable, and symptoms easily exacerbated. This aspect of tissue behaviour was encompassed in the pneumonic SIN standing for severity, irritability, and nature described in Chapter 5. This phase typically lasts no longer than 3–4 days post-injury, although tissue may be repeatedly re-irritated and re-enter the reactive phase. The reactive phase, traditionally called the acute phase of recovery, is followed by a sub-acute phase (which may last up to 14–21 days post-injury) where inflammation leads to tissue regeneration. As irritability dies down and tissue can be loaded without increasing symptoms, the patient enters the recovery period.

> **Keypoint:**
>
> Tissue may remain reactive to some degree in the acute (up to 3–5 days post-injury) and sub-acute (up to 14–21 days post-injury) phases of healing.

At the completion of this sub-acute phase (typically, a maximum of 3–6 weeks) tissue healing is complete, but the patient remains deconditioned (often termed the chronic phase of an injury). Rehabilitation now aims to build resilience to increase the body's capacity to withstand loading, enhancing performance, and reducing the likelihood of reinjury. The terms reactive (R1), recovery (R2), and resilience (R3) are used as nomenclature within the 3Rs approach.

One aim of 3Rs rehabilitation is to increase the capacity of the injured tissue, and to offload it by enhancing the strength of surrounding muscle. Tissue capacity may be built with progressive overload, involving exercise which is either simple or complex. Simple loading targets the specific tissue (for example, the medial collateral ligament of the knee), while complex loading targets the tissue within the context of the whole limb or body region (for example, a squat action). The load chosen for 3Rs' back rehabilitation must accurately reflect the type of load the tissue may be placed under during any functional action in daily living or sport. Training specificity (see Chapter 2) of this kind is vital to increase tissue capacity relevant to the patient's actions (patient-centred) rather than increasing capacity to fulfil pre-determined goals (therapist-centred).

> **Definition:**
>
> *Simple* (isolation) exercise targets a single structure while *complex* (compound) exercise targets the tissue within a body region or the whole body.

Reactive phase

The reactive phase (R1) of the 3Rs approach represents the stage in which the patient and therapist form an alliance. The patient is often fearful and in pain, so assessment, clinical reasoning, and education form a major part of patient management at this stage. The reactive phase is the time when a treatment hypothesis is formed, and treatment plan outlined. Typical treatment aims in the reactive phase are highlighted in Table 6.1, but this can only be a general guide as they are dependent on assessment findings.

Assessment of the patient with a low back injury may begin using a diagnostic triage process by the first contact practitioner (see Chapter 5). Absence of red flags helps to rule out serious spinal pathology and identify those patients with non-specific LBP. A risk stratification such as the STarT back risk assessment tool (Hill et al. 2011, Sowden et al. 2018) can be useful to identify those at high risk of a poor treatment outcome. Additionally, patient prognosis, responsiveness to treatment, and possible underlying mechanisms may form part of a stratified care process to match patients to treatment subgroups (Foster et al. 2015). Identifying those patients at low risk of a poor outcome ensures that patients are not overtreated or overmedicalised, and imaging is not routinely used (NICE 2016). Equally, identifying those at high risk ensures that yellow or red flags are not missed, and more intensive support is given where required, such as psychological intervention or onward referral.

Once treatment begins, patient education and maintenance of normal activity should form the primary part of care for those at low risk of a poor outcome, with self-management emphasised. The reactive phase of 3Rs' back rehabilitation represents the period where the patient's tissues may be irritable, and/or the patient fearful. Local inflammation with or without tissue damage may occur. Unloading the reactive or damaged tissue by avoiding tissue stressing actions or protecting the area by using a support may allow the irritable tissues to settle, and anxiety to reduce. LBP is a multifactorial condition, which may occur without tissue damage. Where tissue damage is present, temporary reduction of activities

TABLE 6.1 Reactive phase—treatment aims

- Triage for red and yellow flags to determine direction of care
- Consider therapy to target pain (e.g., manual therapies/medication) and protect region to limit irritability (e.g., rest, activity modification, taping)
- Assess for increased levels of co-contraction (splinting) & hypervigilance.
- Encourage relaxed movement for short term benefit
- Begin pain education to challenge maladaptive beliefs
- Consider introducing relaxation training/mindful movement/breathing/ mindfulness
- Aerobic exercise integrated into current lifestyle (exercise versus 'function-cise')
- Use appropriate exercise depending on contraindications (isolation/protected progressing to compound)

may be required to allow symptoms to settle, with general (non-spinal specific) activity re-starting as soon as possible to avoid kinesiophobia.

Short-term pain relief (hours, days) is often not considered significant in LBP trials which measure efficacy over long-term outcomes (months, years). However, this type of relief is considered important by individuals suffering from the condition itself (Setchell et al. 2019). Within the reactive phase of 3Rs back rehabilitation short-term pain relief is appropriate providing it is given alongside patient education which aims to first differentiate pain from tissue damage (hurt from harm), and second to reassure the patient that some pain is normal. The use of manual therapy (joint or soft tissue-based), needling (acupuncture and dry needling), and supports (taping and braces) may all have their place with certain patients to enable them to get over a barrier to progress within 3Rs back rehabilitation. No technique is superior to another, and none should be used long term or where patients become dependent upon them. Where possible, self-management should be encouraged with patients applying cold or hot packs, supports, or using resting positions to make them more comfortable as healing progresses. These aids should be used for pre-arranged time periods only, and in conjunction with clear aims and outcomes. Active strategies can be taught to find different ways to move in the reactive phase to ease pain and improve sleep patterns, and relaxation techniques may be used to reduce fear and anxiety, and muscle bracing.

Patient education forms a large part of the management of LBP, and in the reactive phase (R1) this begins with validation of the person's pain experience through active listening. Using principles of motivational interviewing (MI) such as reflective listening, affirmation and summarising can be helpful to direct the patient towards active management choices. In addition, the essentials of pain neuroscience education (PNE) can begin at this stage (see Chapter 1).

Definition:

Motivational interviewing (MI) is a person-centred communication style which focusses on the language of change. It aims to uncover a person's own reasons for change and to strengthen that motivation.

Establishing that flare-ups and setbacks are common elements of LBP is important at this stage. A flare-up is a sudden increase in symptoms, while a setback is a reduction in progress. Whilst traditionally back pain has been seen as either acute or chronic, it is probably more accurately described as fluctuating (episodic) with symptoms varying both in duration and intensity. Most patients can be expected to experience at least one flare-up; however, these can mean different things to different people. Looking at 130 individuals with LBP, Setchell et al. (2017) identified several aspects to be important (Table 6.2), including pain, symptom location, reduction in functioning, and negative psychological effects.

TABLE 6.2 Aspects of flare-up in low back pain

An increase in pain, paraesthesia, muscle tension or other uncomfortable sensation.
An increase in the area, quality and/or duration of symptoms
A reduction in physical, cognitive and/or social functioning
Negative psychological and/or emotional factors

Source: Data from Setchell et al. (2017).

During a flare-up, it is common for patients to experience a sense of disablement, mood changes, lack of understanding from others and to need to use coping strategies (Tan et al. 2019), with flare-ups having a negative effect on many life areas. Preparing patients for this and giving coping strategies such as resting positions, pacing, activity instruction, and self-applied pain reduction methods is important.

During both flare-ups and setbacks, it is important to give a person tools to cope. First, they must realise that both are normal, and they should not feel guilty when they occur. They should be conscious not to jump to the conclusion that something has gone wrong, or their injury has become worse (catastrophising). Emphasise that flare-ups and setbacks are typically time limited and that there is normally a trigger which they may be able to identify to prevent future episodes. Encourage them to take time, breath and aim to relax as best they can when a flare-up happens. Teach rest and recovery positions and plan to gradually build back up as symptoms ease.

Definition:

A *flare-up* is a sudden increase is symptoms while a *setback* is a reduction in progress.

Recovery phase

Treatment aims in the recovery phase (R2) of the 3Rs approach are shown in Table 6.3. In any soft tissue injury, as the regeneration phase of healing begins, mechanical loading of the injured tissue will upregulate gene expression of proteins and mechanotransduction resulting from movement may enhance the healing process (Khan and Scott 2009). The key question is often how much loading should be given, and when it should occur. Optimal tissue loading has been defined as "the load applied to structures that maximises physiological adaptation" (Glasgow et al. 2015). In the case of peripheral soft tissue injuries, optimal loading must address both the mechanical properties of the affected tissues and the central nervous system (CNS), to challenge the complete neuromusculoskeletal system (Norris 2017). Rather than simply increasing load on tissues, we are aiming to increase variation in movement to encourage tissue adaptation in

TABLE 6.3 Recovery phase—treatment aims

- Progress from phase 1 when pain and/or fear no longer limits (able to walk 10 mins and sit to stand 3–5 reps)
- Teach that movement and loading are good for the spine
- Progressive exercise (simple to compound increasing in complexity)
- Coaching to give feedback (tactile, auditory, visual)
- Decrease fear of movement—introduce variety and challenge beliefs (e.g. bending/lifting)
- Build patients' confidence with static hold of heavy loads—Isometrics if positive effect on pain (self efficacy).
- Build 'S' factors related to patient requirements

parallel with changes to motor control. Three categories of load variation may be used with soft tissue injuries, and this may be adapted for back rehabilitation. First, to reduce repetitive loading, magnitude, direction, and rate of loading should be varied. Second stimulation of the mechanotransduction effect may be enhanced by varying loading to prevent accommodation to stimuli (the body getting used to a stimulus so that it no longer has a substantial effect). Finally, variable tensile, compressive, and torsional forces may build a stronger biological scaffold which creates tissue resilience equipped to withstand a wider range of loading (Glasgow et al. 2015).

> **Keypoint:**
>
> Using variation in movements can encourage both *tissue adaptation* and changes in *motor control*.

The use of activity in the recovery phase of back rehabilitation may either emphasise common actions built into a patient's lifestyle or be formed from individual exercises. Where exercise is used, it is commonly either general (whole body) or specific (spine related), and various components of fitness may be targeted to structure a programme as detailed in Chapter 2. Several fitness components ('S' factors) may be emphasised depending on requirements and increased or reduced in demand (exercise progression and regression). Demand is typically measured as exercise volume or dosage using the F.I.T.T mnemonic.

Precision of movement can be important to avoid actions which exacerbate a patient's symptoms. Cueing is used to give feedback and enhance learning, and this may be visual (demonstration, mirror, video feedback), verbal (instructions, metaphor, tone of voice), tac-tile (touching, adjustment, mobilisation with movement), or cognitive (implicit meaning, visualisation). Close coaching places some of the responsibility for the movement outcome on the instructor, which is reassuring to the person exercising in phase 1 (R1) of the 3Rs approach. Later in the programme (R2) coaching is gradually de-emphasised and then withdrawn

(R3), to transfer responsibility for decision-making onto the person performing the exercise. Similarly, exercise tasks become less targeted, changing from explicit instruction (aim clearly stated, e.g., dumbbell shoulder press 2 sets of 10 reps with 10 kg weight) to implicit meaning (aim not clearly stated, e.g., place that weight on a high shelf). By reducing the focus of an exercise, variability is increased and decision-making enhanced.

Definition:

An instruction is *explicit* when something is expressed directly. *Implicit* meaning is implied by an action or outcome.

In many cases tissue damage may be minimal in LBP, and less emphasis should be placed on the bio aspect of the BPS model and more on the psychosocial aspects. Exercise or activity is used earlier in these cases (sometimes from day one) partly for its analgesic effect, and to prevent kinesiophobia. Use of graded activity (progressive exercise) is commonplace in both wellness programmes and rehabilitation to produce overload and instigate tissue adaptation. However, if pain onset is used as an end point (stopping point) rather than rating of perceived exertion (RPE) it may reinforce the perception that 'hurt equals harm' and encourage a belief that painful activity may result in damage to the back with a resultant exacerbation of suffering (Bunzli et al. 2015, Lagerman 2018). Using a time contingent approach rather than symptom continent de-emphasises the focus on tissue and pain (Nijs et al. 2014). Use of training volume with the FITT mnemonic gives the opportunity to change several variables in addition to time to suit patient requirements. Use of exercise dosage in this way may be used to influence threat perception (Lagerman 2018).

Keypoint:

Using a *time contingent* approach (stopping after a certain time or number of reps) rather than *symptom continent* approach (stopping when soreness occurs) de-emphasises the mental link between tissue and pain.

Resilience phase

Treatment aims for the resilience phase (R3) of the 3Rs approach are shown in Table 6.4 Resilience—sometimes referred to colloquially as 'toughness' is the capacity to recover quickly from difficulties which may be physical or mental in nature. Resilience is an individual's ability to return to a natural state of balance (homeostasis) outlined above. It can be viewed as the capacity to 'get back up when you are knocked down'. As with all phases of the 3Rs approach, it can be viewed from a biopsychosocial (BPS) viewpoint. Mental or emotional resilience

TABLE 6.4 Resilience phase—treatment aims

- Progress from phase 2 when pain free and/or returned to typical daily function
- Improve exercise variability while increasing movement confidence, and reducing coaching
- Increase physical capacity and enhance function further using greater variety of 'S' factors
- Improve full body conditioning—lifting, pushing, pulling, jumping, COD drills
- Exercises specific to functional requirements of patient—lifestyle/work/sport.
- Challenge subject by introducing variation of environment, movement complexity, apparatus, and decision making

COD—change of direction.

TABLE 6.5 Aspects of mental resilience

Positive attitude
Optimism
Ability to regulate emotions
Seeing failure as helpful feedback
Building social support & developing relationships

Source: Data from Psychologytoday.com, 2019, APA (2022).

is a process of adapting to challenging life experiences, and how well a person adapts depends on how they engage with the world, what coping strategies they have, and their social support (APA 2022). Mental resilience has been said to have several factors; a positive attitude, optimism, the ability to regulate emotions, the ability to see failure as helpful feedback. Social resilience reflects lifestyle factors such as a supportive network of family and friends (Table 6.5).

Physical resilience is the body's capacity to adapt to challenges or demands and to recover effectively and will rely heavily on the 'S' factors of fitness. In addition, a good diet with adequate relaxation and sleep all support recovery and help avoid burnout having effects via all three of the BPS components.

Resilience is an important concept, because LBP is a condition which has been described as be overtreated (Deyo et al. 2009). Pain is part of everyday life and does not necessarily indicate harm and should not automatically lead to suffering. Whilst an individual may seek treatment for pain in the low back after gardening, viewing the pain as negative (potential harm) they probably would not seek treatment for muscle pain following a gym workout, viewing this incident of pain as positive (sign of a good workout).

Within the 3Rs back rehabilitation approach, the resilience phase is the final stage of a progression of graded activity and graded exposure. Throughout the recovery phase, physical capacity has been redeveloped and should, by now exceed pre-injury levels, and the individual will have built confidence and optimism in movement. These abilities are now increased with whole body challenging tasks.

All through the 3Rs progression, movement (motor) and knowledge of this movement (sensory) are combined leading to sensorimotor training. In the early stages there is less emphasis on this combination, and in the later stages more. Sensorimotor training combines general control of the whole body with specific control of individual bodyparts. Actions fuse aspects of free movement (mobility) and stiffness (stability), and considerable variation will occur between patients. Initially, variation may be reduced where the style of performing an action drives symptoms. As we progress to the resilience phase of the 3Rs approach, movement variability is emphasised as it gives patients a greater number of movements to select from, increasing the likelihood of optimising the action for each individual.

Definition:

Sensorimotor training aims to enhance control of movement by maximising sensory input from several parts of the body simultaneously.

In the resilience phase (R3) of the 3Rs approach, the complex actions used can mimic requirements of a task which the person is hesitant to perform as a result of their injury. In so doing they may be termed functional or task specific. In addition, phase 3 (R3) exercises may simply increase overload to take selected fitness 'S' factors to a higher level. Strength should be increased with a variety of exercises to load a bodypart in different ways to increase movement variability. For example, a barbell shoulder press action (resisted overhead reach) used in the R2 (recovery) may be performed with a light weight to limited range and in a seated position to reduce coordination demands and decrease body sway. The same action type in R3 (resilience) would be performed with a higher resistance, in standing to increase demands of both strength and coordination. Variation would be added by using unilateral (dumbbell) rather than bilateral (barbell) actions, both behind the neck (press behind neck) and in front of the head (military press). Strength can be progressed to speed (rate of movement) and power (rate of doing work). Overhead ball throwing (single or double handed) can be progressed to a medicine ball throw against a wall (predictable environment) and then into the air (less predictable environment), and finally with the action performed on an unstable base.

Predictability of the environment is an important consideration in motor skill training (Table 6.6), with a closed skill performed in a predictable environment and an open skill performed in an unpredictable environment. Skill training may also be varied by altering movement organisation. A single standalone action (isolated) requires close focus and so aids learning. Performing multiple repetitions of the action (repeated) builds familiarity, but focus is not as close due to fatigue and the possibility of distraction. A cycle of the same actions (continuous) reduces attention demand and moves the action towards becoming automatic (autonomous stage of motor learning, see Chapter 3).

TABLE 6.6 Classifying skills

Movement organisation		
Discrete	Serial	Continuous
Definite start and finish	*Number of discrete actions linked*	*No definite start or finish*
Mental or Physical involvement		
Motor	Cognitive	
Less decision making	*More decision making*	
Influence of environment		
Closed	Open	
Predictable environment	*Unpredictable environment*	

Source: From Norris (2013).

Decision-making is also an important consideration. In early rehabilitation (R2), coaching is used extensively to identify unwanted actions and motivate the patient. Cueing is used widely. However, close coaching partially shifts responsibility for the action away from the patient and onto the instructor. Requiring the patient to make decisions shifts responsibility for outcomes back to them in R3 (resilience), and so coaching is gradually reduced in this stage. Decision-making requires analysis of the problem. For example, in a ball catching movement, the patient must analyse to determine where the ball is going to appear (high, low, to the side, etc.) and then explore options (where should I stand to ensure a catch, where should I put my hands). Once decisions are required, one must be chosen (picking the best option), and sometimes this will be right and sometime not. Over time the patient learns which actions are more likely to give a positive result, and the same will be true for daily tasks such as lifting, bending, carrying, for example. Encouraging assessment of potential problems, a task could cause (risk assessment) is an important component of building independence.

CASE NOTE

A 25-year-old female presented with low back pain following a tug-of-war competition. She was a regular gym user but had let the gym training lapse over the last 3 months. On examination she had full range of motion to the spine with some tightness to end of range flexion. She was hesitant to perform flexion as this action had caused discomfort before, and most motion was focused at her thoracic and high lumbar regions. When reassured and encouraged to perform repeated flexion her tight feeling receded and then disappeared. Straight leg raise (SLR) was full and painless and hip mobility was normal. There were no motor or sensory changes detectable. The patient was given progressive range flexion from a standing position as a home exercise initially to a chair back and then chair seat encouraging movement through the whole spine (Pilates roll down action). In addition, she was started on a general spinal re-strengthening programme beginning with a hip hinge action progressing to kettlebell deadlift from a low stool level. After 1 week she was pain free to general spinal movements and had only occasional pain during activities of daily living (ADL) tasks. Her exercises were progressed to deadlifts in her own gym using an Olympic bar, walking, and then running with intermittent floor touch. In addition, she performed band pulls in a tug-of-war stance. Following 3 weeks of rehab she was returned to general tug-of-war team training (twice per week) and continued her progressive training in the gym twice per week. Exercise was progressed to deadlift actions using higher resistance, and she was coached on cleans. She performed sled pulls to build leg and trunk endurance.

References

APA. (2022). American Psychological Association. https://www.apa.org/topics/resilience accessed June 2022.

Babatunde, O.O., Jordan, J.L., Van der Windt, D.A., et al. (2017). Effective treatment options for musculoskeletal pain in primary care: A systematic overview of current evidence. *PLoS One* 12(6), e0178621.

Brabban, A., and Turkington, D. (2002). The search for meaning: Detecting congruence between life events, underlying schema and psychotic symptoms. In Morrison, A.P., Ed., *A Casebook of Cognitive Therapy for Psychosis*. New York: Brunner-Routledge, 74–83.

Bunzli, S., Smith, A., Watkins, R., et al. (2015). Do people who score highly on the Tampa scale of Kinesiophobia really believe? A mixed methods investigation in people with chronic nonspecific low back pain. *Clinical Journal of Pain* 31(7): 621–632.

Cook, J.L., and Docking, S.I. (2015). Rehabilitation will increase the 'capacity' of your …insert musculoskeletal tissue here…" Defining 'tissue capacity': A core concept for clinicians. *British Journal of Sports Medicine* 49: 1484–1485.

Deyo, R.A., Mirza, S.K., Turner, J.A., et al. (2009). Overtreating chronic back pain: Time to back off? *The Journal of the American Board of Family Medicine* 22(1): 62–68.

Dye, S. (2005). The pathophysiology of patellofemoral pain – A tissue homeostasis perspective. *Clinical Orthopaedics and Related Research* 436: 100–110.

Foster, N.E., Hill, J.C., O'Sullivan, P.B., et al. (2015). Stratified models of care for low back pain. WCPT Congress Singapore, May.

Glasgow, P., Phillips, N., and Bleakley, C. (2015). Optimal loading: Key variables and mechanisms. *British Journal of Sports Medicine* 49: 278–279.

Hill, J., et al. (2011). A randomised controlled trial and economic evaluation of stratified primary care management for low back pain compared with current best practice: The STarT Back trial. *Lancet* 378(9802): 1560–1571. https://www.psychologytoday.com/gb/basics/resilience accessed September 2019

Khan, K.M., and Scott, A. (2009). Mechanotherapy: How physical therapists' prescription of exercise promotes tissue repair. *British Journal of Sports Medicine* 43(4): 247–251.

Lagerman, P. (2018). Reasoning exercise dosage for people with persistent pain. In Touch No. 164 Autumn: 30–35.

Lehman, G. (2017). Tissue changes and pain – Explaining their relevance. *Blog*, March 6. http://www.greglehman.ca/blog/2017/3/6/tissue-changes-and-pain-explaining-their-relevance accessed 2022.

NICE. (2016). *National institute for health and care excellence. Nice guidelines: Low back pain and sciatica in over 16s: Assessment and management.* London: National Institute for Health and Care Excellence.

Nijs, J., Meeus, M., Cagnie, B., et al. (2014). A modern neuroscience approach to chronic spinal pain: Combining pain neuroscience education with cognition-targeted motor control training. *Physical Therapy* 94(5): 730–738.

Norris, C.M. (2020). Back rehabilitation – The 3R's approach. *Journal of Bodywork and Movement Therapies* 24(1): 289–299.

Norris, C.M. (2013). *The complete guide to exercise therapy.* Oxford: Bloomsbury.

Norris, C.M. (2017). Injury, tissue capacity and load management. In Touch Spring (edition 158): 10–15.

Norris, C.M. (2019). *Sports and soft tissue injuries.* London: Routledge.

Setchell, J., Costa, N., Ferreira, M., et al. (2017). What constitutes back pain flare? A cross sectional survey of individuals with low back pain. *Scandinavian Journal of Pain* 17: 294–301.

Setchell, J., Costa, N., Ferreira, M., et al. (2019). What decreases low back pain? A qualitative study of patient perspectives. *Scandinavian Journal of Pain* 19(3): 597–603.

Sowden, G., Hill, J.C., Morso, L., et al. (2018). Advancing practice for back pain through stratified care (STarT Back). *Brazilian Journal of Physical Therapy* 22(4): 255–264.

Tan, D., Hodges, P.W., Costa, N., et al. (2019). Impact of flare-ups on the lives of individuals with low back pain: A qualitative investigation. *Musculoskeletal Science & Practice* 43: 52–57.

7

REACTIVE PHASE

In the reactive phase (R1) things are new. A person is suffering a condition which they may be totally unfamiliar with, and the therapist is meeting this person for the first time. We are developing a *therapeutic alliance* and considering the tissues in the acute stage of *healing* (see Chapter 6).

Developing a therapeutic alliance

It is likely that the person will be in pain, fearful, and seeking answers to the many questions they may have. Key to the therapeutic alliance is that the therapist is not seen as an authority figure but more as a facilitator or partner who guides the person to be active in achieving goals which are important to them (patient participation). The focus is very much on the person (person-centred care), but this does not preclude the therapist from using treatment approaches which are proven but may not be popular with the person at the time.

> **Definition:**
>
> The *therapeutic alliance* (working alliance or therapeutic relationship) is the interaction between a therapist and person.

The concept of therapeutic alliance has its roots in the work of Freud in the early 1900s who described unconscious feelings and emotions between the therapist and patient (transference and countertransference). Characteristics of a good therapeutic alliance are empathy and rapport, and two branches have been described, the personal relationship and the collaborative area (Hougaard 1994). The *personal* relationship is a focus of the interaction between the

DOI: 10.4324/9781003366188-7

therapist and person (therapist as friend) while the *collaborative* relationship focusses on tasks and planning how they can be achieved (therapist as coach). Therapeutic alliance ratings between physical therapists and patients have been shown to be associated with improvement in outcomes in the management of LBP (Ferreira et al. 2013).

Everyone has preferences in life, some may like to go to the gym while others prefer to run, for example. One is not better than the other, they are equally effective and a person may prefer one over the other for many personal (psychosocial) factors. The same is true of low back pain. One person may want painkillers while another may prefer not to take tablets but to see if they can cope by resting and using hot showers. *Shared decision making* is a process of respecting and prioritising an individual's choices by considering their views, those of their family and peers, and the whole healthcare team. To make an informed choice, patients need information about treatment options (pros and cons), and a three-step model has been proposed (Elwyn et al. 2012). Step one is a discussion about *choices*. In this stage, the therapist offers support and asks about goals and expectations while describing what treatment approaches are available and noting the person's reaction to these. Step two talks about *options*. Evidence based treatments are listed with the benefits (pros) and potential harms (cons) described. The person's view on each approach is valued, and in step three *decisions* are made about preferences and the order of treatments and a general plan agreed.

CASE NOTE

A 68-year-old female developed low backpain. She searches online and finds that the condition can be treated with drugs, a back brace, a new bed, yoga, or surgery. How does she decide which is best for her? She decides to see a therapist and has a thorough examination which reveals non-specific low back pain potentially brought on by two hours gardening. Her pain is easing, and she is gradually able to do more around her house. She is relieved to know that the condition is common, and she has not badly injured her back. During the discussion she says that one of her major problems is that she thinks she may not be able to take her grandchildren to school and does not want to let her daughter down. She learns that her back pain will ease with time, and she can use exercise to relieve stiffness and strengthen her back and hips even at her age. If she does this, she will be able to garden again, and her back will be less likely to hurt. She does not like exercise classes and does not have any friends who go to the local gym but is told that she can use walking to help her back. This fits in with her wanting to take her grandchildren to school and she agrees on a progressive walking program, gradually building distance up until she can comfortably cover the walk-to-school distance. She agrees to see the therapist again once her backpain has eased and begins an exercise program which she can do at home each day. She has spoken to her daughter and learnt that her daughter has some dumbbells, and they agree to meet twice a week to perform a 20-minute exercise program together.

As we have seen in Chapter 1, the NICE guidelines on the treatment of LBP recommend exercise is a key treatment modality, with manual therapy (MT) only to be considered as part of a treatment programme which includes exercise. Additionally, the focus is on self-management of LBP at all stages of the treatment pathway. In the reactive stage of the 3Rs approach (R1) having established a therapeutic alliance, examined the person to identify or rule out red flags (Chapter 5) and agreed a treatment pathway several treatment options are available.

There is a difference when building a therapeutic alliance between providing information about a condition and using patient education (cognitive reassurance) and showing empathy and building rapport (affective reassurance). Systematic review has shown that cognitive reassurance is more beneficial, giving higher satisfaction and reduced concerns directly after consultation and better symptom improvement at follow-up (Pincus et al. 2013).

> **Definition:**
>
> *Cognitive* (thinking) reassurance provides explanations and education, while *affective* (mood) reassurance creates rapport, and shows empathy.

Do nothing

As strange as it may seem to many therapists, doing nothing is a viable treatment option, as watch and wait is often used in medicine. Within the Startback framework (Chapter 5) we saw that we can identify those individuals at low risk of psychosocial factors who simply require guidance either from personal education or from leaflets or a website. The body will naturally heal itself, and to simply allow that to occur once the person has been assessed and reassured should not be dismissed. This natural process (regression to the mean) enables a person to take charge of their recovery and to progress at their chosen rate.

> **Definition:**
>
> *Regression to the mean* (RTM) is a statistical trend that data which is much higher or much lower than the average will be closer to the average (mean) if it is measured a second time. In therapy terms, it is taken to mean that a body naturally moves towards balance (homeostasis) over time.

However, if healthcare waiting lists are long, the process can be self-selective. Those who naturally will get better often do not present for treatment, and those who have been waiting without guidance may have developed secondary

problems such as deconditioning or fear avoidance beliefs. Not giving intervention (treatment or exercise) is certainly a valid option, but it should be used with
guidance to avoid the potential negative effects mentioned above.

Resting positions, coping mechanisms, and self-management

Lying down

Resting positions are positions which are taken up by a person to minimise their
symptoms, while a coping mechanism is something they can do to lessen the
impact of their condition. Typical resting positions helpful in LBP include lying
rather than sitting. Using a support in the curve of the lumbar spine (lumbar lordosis) can be helpful where lumbar flexion (loss of lordosis) increases symptoms.
Using a rolled towel beneath the back can help when lying supine or using a
towel or cushion under the side when side lying can help. Both will support the
spine in a relatively neutral position (avoiding end range motion) to take some
loading off the soft tissues. These types of supports should only be used for the
time they relieve symptoms and discarded if they no longer modify symptoms,
or the symptoms abate. Using any support for a prolonged period can build reli-
ance on the support and create habitual patterns. Bending the knees when lying
on the back (psoas position) or side can help especially in cases of LBP referred
into the posterior leg as it takes stretch from the sciatic nerve and hamstrings.
Placing the upper leg (bent at the hip and knee) on a cushion will avoid the
weight of the leg pulling the spine into rotation.

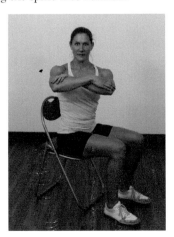

Sitting positions

Sitting can be painful for some people with LBP and varying the sitting position
can be helpful. Lumbar supports, although widely promoted commercially may or
may not help. Where an individual has pain when sitting in flexion due to overload

of tissues (postural syndrome, see below) a firm chair or lumbar support can help. Where extension causes symptoms, sitting in flexion by using a cushion behind the sacrum or sitting on a wedge with the thickest edge forwards can be a better resting position. Generally, varying sitting positions and alternating between sitting and standing positions to avoid accumulated stress is often the most useful approach.

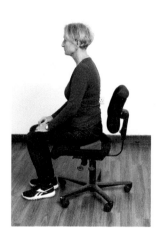 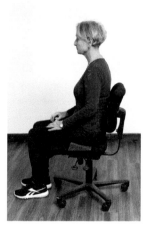 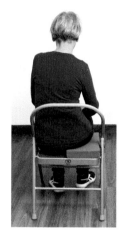

Relaxation

Relaxation training and mindfulness can be helpful in pain conditions in general. However, introducing structured relaxation can be difficult initially when a person is in pain. These techniques can begin simply using mindful breaks. These aim to create a brief gap between pain onset and emotional response to uncouple pain and from suffering (see Table 1.3). The STOP acronym can be helpful (Goldstein 2013) and easy to remember. Stopping (S) and taking (T) a breath initially is useful, and this can be helped by counting down from 10 to 1 and releasing tension with each count. Observing (O) what is happening around you, and within your body is helpful as it can often identify muscle tension in the face and around the shoulders. Finally proceed (P) with something which will support you such as a coping mechanism or distraction.

Later, more structured mindful training such as *progressive muscle relaxation* (tightening and then releasing muscles in sequence), *bodyscan* (mentally travelling through the body noticing tension) and *breath awareness* (noticing in and out breaths and counting them) can be used.

Walking

Walking is a useful method of early exercise but can be used for general fitness throughout the 3Rs approach. As we saw in Chapter 1, walking interventions improve pain, quality of life, disability, and fear avoidance to a similar degree as general exercise in persons with CLBP (Vanti et al. 2019). General advice on walking includes footwear (training shoes rather than hard shoes or heels) and body motion (allowing the arms to swing freely). Walking tall is a good external cue to lengthen through the spine and check for symmetry in cases where muscle guarding has led to a side shift or side flexed position.

Definition:

A *side shift* occurs when the shoulder girdle moves sideways relative to the pelvis creating an S-shaped to the spine. *Side bend* occurs when the shoulder girdle tips to one side towards the pelvis creating a U shape to the spine.

Some people prefer to walk with poles and that is fine. Poles can either be used for support and to help balance (mountain walking pole) or used to help propel you forwards using arm power (Nordic walking pole), as the 3Rs reactive phase (R1) progresses to the recovery phase (R2). Poles need to be correctly adjusted to offer the best function. Where support is the aim (walking stick or mountain walking pole) the stick length is generally measured to the *wrist crease* when the arm is straight by a person's side. Where force (propelling) is the aim, the pole is longer and generally measured to the *elbow crease* with the arm bent to 90°. As with most rehab exercise progression is key and progressive walking programs can vary distance, speed, slope, and terrain.

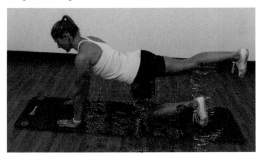

Progressive walking

Starting position:

Begin wearing loose clothing which enable you to move freely. Wear supportive, low, and shock absorbing shoes such as trainers, walking shoes, or simply shoes that you find comfortable.

Method:

Begin walking slowly and when you are comfortable gradually lengthen your pace and speed up until you reach a pace which feels normal for you. Continue this initially for two minutes then build to five minutes and finally ten minutes. Remember to use a circular route rather than walking in one direction and not being able to return due to fatigue.

Points to note:

- It is common to have some pain in your back which will usually ease as you walk. If your pain does not ease but does not increase, you are OK to continue.
- If your pain increases in intensity or begins in your back or buttock and as you walk further gradually spreads down your leg (symptoms peripheralising) stop, rest, and start again the next day.
- As you build up the pace, walk at a speed which is challenging but still allows you to have a comfortable conversation with someone. Do not be so out of breath that you are gasping.

Modifications:

Vary the *distance* (how far you walk) *speed* (how fast you walk), *stride length* (how long each step is) *incline* (walking up or down a slight slope) and *terrain* (smooth surface such as pavement, uneven surface such as a field) for variety.

Postural walking

Starting position:

Begin wearing loose clothing which enable you to move freely. Wear supportive, low, and shock absorbing shoes such as trainers, walking shoes, or simply shoes that you find comfortable.

Method:

Start in standing and keeping your feet on the floor, rock your bodyweight from side-to-side so that you take more weight through one foot and then the other. Stop at a mid-point when you feel you have weight equally through each foot. Lengthen through your spine reaching the crown of your head towards the ceiling as though you were a puppet being pulled upwards on a string. Walk with an even pace (listen to your foot strikes) and swing your arms equally. Aim to stand tall and move freely throughout your walk

Points to note:

- There are no good or bad postures, just one which suits you.
- Aim to reduce your symptoms by moving your spine freely (try not to be stiff).
- You can use any position which reduces your symptoms—experiment and find what works for you.

Modifications:

- Vary your speed and stride length to find what is most comfortable. Once you have done this and found your ideal walking method, stay with it for about one week before you change. Consistency is often a key to recovery.

Keypoint:

Don't underestimate the value of walking as a rehab exercise following low back pain. It can be especially useful in the early phases (Reaction phase R1 and Recovery phase R2).

Exercise therapy in the reactive phase

In the reactive phase (R1) of the 3Rs approach, we are introducing low level exercises which target pain but also act as a starting point to build on. Rehabilitation is a bit like climbing a ladder—you must use the lower steps before the upper ones. We call this progressive exercise therapy (PET).

Sitting twist

Starting position:

Begin sitting on a firm chair (dining chair or stool), with your back clear of the chair back. Sit tall and keep your feet flat on the floor for support. Fold your arms and lift them to chest height to open your chest and lengthen your spine. Reach the crown of your head to the ceiling, rather than looking up or down.

Method:

Turn to your right, pause, and then return to the starting position. Pause again before turning to the left. Keep looking over the centre of your forearms so you turn your head, comfortably but do not strain.

Points to note:

- Lengthening through the spine ensures that the pivot of the twist (your spine) is straight rather than bent as it would be in a flexed sitting position.
- Pause at the end range (full rotation) but do not bounce as this can jar the spine and tissues causing a reaction if the tissues are irritable.
- Asymmetry is normal, with one side being more flexible or stronger than the other.

Modifications:

- The exercise can be progressed by pulling on a resistance band. Hold the band in one hand and attach the free end to a piece of furniture to your right. Perform 5 twists to the left. Stop and re-attach the band to your left and perform 5 twists to your right. Control the movement as you rotate back to the starting position in each case, do not allow the recoil of the stretched band to pull you in an uncontrolled fashion.

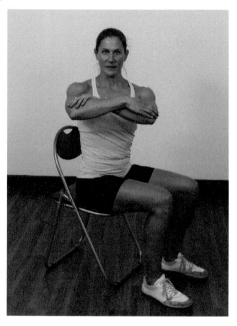

Supported side bend

Starting position:

Begin standing side on to the high table at approximately waist level (kitchen work surface, for example). Place your feet wider than shoulder width apart and have your arms out to your sides.

Method:

Side bend towards the table and place your near arm on the tabletop for support. Take your forearm overhead trying to keep it level with your ear, rather than taking it forwards which can cause your spine to bend (flex). Pause in the fully stretched position for 2–3 seconds and then stand straight again. Perform 5 repetitions to one side, rest and then turn around and perform 5 reps to the other side.

Points to note:

- It is common for one side to be more flexible than the other.
- Mild discomfort/pain to stretch is common, and usually eases with repetition. If pain builds up, stop, rest, and allow things to settle and then try again.

Modifications:

If you do not have a tabletop available, the action can be performed sliding your arm down the side of your leg. Press on your outer thigh to take some weight from your spine. As you progress from the 3Rs reactive phase (R1) into the recovery phase (R2), you will no longer need to take your weight through your arm. When practised without arm support the action works the trunk muscles harder.

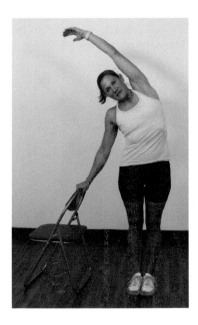

Standing overhead reach

Starting position:

Begin standing with your feet shoulder width apart, arms straight and by your sides.

Method:

Keep your arms straight and reach them forwards and then overhead, pause in the uppermost position and then lower under control.

Points to note:

- Reaching overhead causes your thoracic spine to extend (straighten) as you get to the limit of your shoulder movement. If your shoulders are quite stiff this will occur earlier and if they are flexible, it will occur later.
- At the upper extreme of shoulder range your lumbar (lower) spine will extend and the curve in the spine (lordosis) will increase. Try to feel movement throughout the whole of your spine rather than just the lower spine.
- Looking up at your hands will encourage your upper spine to move more as your neck leads the movement.
- If you feel dizzy looking upwards, keep looking forwards and fix your eyes on a single point in front of you.

Modifications:

- If you feel unsteady in this movement, stand in front of a table, and press your thighs against the edge of the tabletop for support.

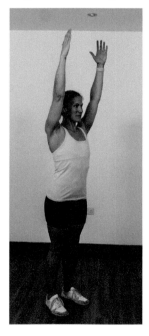

Birddog legs

The Birddog is an exercise performed in the kneeling position where the spine is like a tabletop supported on four corners (two arms, two legs). By removing one or more of the four supports (one leg and/or one contralateral arm) stress is placed on the spine and the muscles surrounding the spine must tighten to maintain alignment. This should happen automatically. Birddog type of exercises have been shown to produce high trunk extensor muscle activity and to reduce relative spinal loading (Callaghan et al. 1998).

Starting position:

Begin kneeling on all fours on a gym mat with your hands beneath your shoulders and knees beneath your hips (box position). Have your knees hip width apart and hands shoulder width apart. Keep your spine relatively straight (neutral) without excessive rounding (flexion) or hollowing (extension).

Method:

Straighten your right leg, leading with your heel and keep your toes in contact with the mat (level 1). Pause in the straight position and then return your leg to the staring position and repeat the movement with your left leg. Perform 5 repetitions with each leg and then rest.

Points to note:

- Leading with the heel rather than pointing your toes should prevent you getting cramp in your calf muscles.
- Try to keep your spine still throughout the movement, try not to arch, hollow, or side bend (laterally flex) your back excessively.

Modifications:

- To progress the exercise, again straighten your right leg, but this time keep your toes off the mat trying to hold your leg horizontal throughout the movement (level 2). Press your heel towards the wall behind you and lock your knee out straight. Pause and then return to the start and perform the same action with your left leg.

Keypoint:

Users who have suffered with low back pain often find the kneeling position comfortable. Their pain may reduce in kneeling but increase in sitting positions.

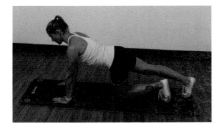 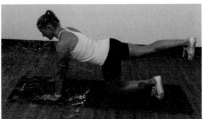

Pharmacological management of low back pain

Many people with low back pain consider pain relief to be a priority, and the use of medication (pharmacology) is widespread. The advantage of using medication in either tablet form or a locally applied cream rubbed into the painful region, is that it is readily available and self-applied. However, the effectiveness of pharmacology and its side effects must be considered.

Many people will have tried over the counter medications as they are instantly accessible. These may have included non-steroidal anti-inflammatory drugs (NSAID) such as *Ibuprofen* or *Diclofenac* which targets pain and fever. However, these can cause stomach upsets, bloating, or nausea. Over time this can progress to stomach ulcers and bleeding, and so long-term usage is normally paralleled with a medication to protect the stomach. An NSAID cream may also be directly applied to the painful area, but care should be taken to avoid broken skin. A systematic review of 35 randomised placebo-controlled trials showed these drugs did reduce pain and disability but this change was clinically unimportant (Machado et al. 2017). In this review six persons would have needed to be treated with NSAIDS rather than placebo for one additional person to gain a clinically important pain reduction, and the risk of gastrointestinal reaction was increased by 2.5 times.

Pain killers such as *Paracetamol* reduce pain at the brain level but are different to NSAIDs as they do not target inflammation. It has fewer side effects and less chance of addiction, but over-dose may lead to liver damage. In a systematic review of its use for spinal pain and osteoarthritis (Machado et al. 2015) high quality evidence showed paracetamol to be ineffective for reducing pain intensity or disability or improving quality of life (QOL) in the short term.

Stronger medications include opioids (found in humans) or opiates (found in plants) which are narcotics—a drug related to opium which dulls the senses. They are effective at targeting acute pain and include drugs such as *Codeine* and *Morphine.*

Where there is back muscle spasm, a benzodiazepine drug such as *Valium* or *Diazepam* may be used which is a sedative or antidepressant (a drug which slows brain activity) and helps relax muscles. Again, this drug has side effects and is normally only prescribed for short-term use. Dependency can occur with long term use and withdrawal symptoms such as anxiety and heart palpitations may occur.

The NICE guidelines for the management of low back pain say that NSAIDS may be used as a pain killer (analgesic) of first choice for back pain and opioids as a second choice providing drug toxicity and person risk factors are considered. NSAIDS should be used at the lowest effective dose and for the shortest period. Weak opioids (with or without paracetamol) may be used for *acute* LBP where NSAIDs are contraindicated or ineffective but should not be used for *chronic* LBP. Anticonvulsants such as *Gabapentin* which are often used to treat neuropathic pain should not be used for managing low back pain according to the guidelines.

Although in research studies the effectiveness of these drugs is questionable, it is understandable that people seek something for short-term pain relief as low back pain can often be debilitating in its acute phase. This is why any treatment which effectively targets pain for a person may be used in the reactive phase (R1) of the 3Rs approach providing it is safe and acceptable to that person. Even if a treatment such as acupuncture (below), manual therapy, massage, or electrotherapies fails to produce clinically significant results in population studies (group research) it may work on a single person for a short time and give them clinically meaningful relief as often described by individual descriptive studies (case histories). Importantly, these treatments must be adjunctive to self-management and exercise and not replace these interventions. It is vital to teach self-management procedures such as the local application of ice or heat, resting positions, relaxation training or self/partner applied massage where these are acceptable to the person as they promote independence and enhance self efficacy.

Use of manual therapy for low back pain

Placing your hands on someone who is in pain or frightened is a natural human response. From childhood, most individuals feel reassured by touch and MT capitalises on this fact. It is important to state, of course, that some individuals recoil from touch. Those who have been victims of abuse or torture, for example, and those who may be very body conscious or body dysmorphic may need special consideration.

MT is essentially communicating with a person through the medium of touch. MT is often categorised as soft tissue or joint based describing where the therapist is focussing. However, an obvious point is that to have an effect on one tissue alone would require that tissue to be removed from the body. Even if a

TABLE 7.1 Manual therapy application framework

Variable	Meaning
Speed	Rate at which the MT force is applied—*e.g. high velocity*
Location within ROM	Is the force applied at the start, middle or end of the motion range currently available to the subject—*e.g. at mid-range*
Force direction	Anatomical and or biomechanical direction of the force—*e.g. lateral glide*
Tissue target	Which joint or part of a joint is moving—*e.g. spinal level*
Relative movement	Which region is moving and which remaining stable—*e.g. tibial glide on femur*
Subject position	Gross body position of subject and limb position—*e.g. supine lying with femur flexed, abducted & externally rotated.*

MT—manual therapy, ROM—range of motion.

Source: After Mintken et al. (2008).

therapist uses a joint based MT technique on a knee joint, for example, they still have to touch the skin and move it together with the tissues which attach to it.

MT techniques categorised as joint based may be applied to both the spinal and peripheral joints. Manipulation (thrust) techniques are generally passive (the person does not move; the therapist applies the force) and applied rapidly (high velocity) to achieve very small movements (low amplitude). Mobilisations are non-thrust techniques which may be applied at various speeds and amplitudes, with or without person movement. The aim in each case is to reduce pain and improve motion, and several variables are involved in the application of joint based MT (Table 7.1).

When originally described, MT techniques where often claimed to apply various forces and potential movements upon the joint, using a standard biomechanical model. However, research disproved and/or modified many of these original claims, and our understanding of the method by which clinical effects are achieved has progressed. Many spinal manipulations, for example, are performed with the joint in close pack position where the joint capsule and collateral ligaments tend to draw the joint surfaces together, so greater movement is unlikely. Cavitation (formation and collapse of bubbles within the synovial fluid) has been demonstrated in both spinal and peripheral joints. However, it occurs both at the level of the manipulation and above or below this point so is non-specific (Ross et al. 2004). Alteration in muscle stiffness through a short-term reduction in tone occurs with a rapidly applied force, but no change has been found between different grades of technique (Dishman and Bullbulian 2001). These findings suggest that the subtleties of grading systems and precision of hand placement once emphasised is less important than at first presented.

The scientific literature in general does not support a biomechanical explanation for MT (McCarthy et al. 2015), leading to the development of a neurophysiological model (Bialosky et al. 2009). The mechanical force imposed through MT can be seen as a noxious stimulus which initiates a cascade of neurophysiological reactions invoking analgesia (pain relief) at local, spinal, brainstem, and higher centre levels. Subjects receiving MT have reduced cytokine levels (blood and serum) and pain biomarkers compared to controls. In addition, temporal summation (a measurement of pain sensitivity) is lessened. A laboratory induced stretch reflex (H-reflex) is decreased following MT suggesting a brief inhibition of the motoneuron pool. Changes in cortical excitability have been observed (Fryer and Pearce 2012), as has alteration in cerebral blood flow (Daligadu et al. 2013). The above effects point to a reduction in pain (pain modulation) and altered muscle tone. In addition, where MT is applied with movement (mobilisation with movement, or MWM techniques), non-associative learning may occur. Here, the response to a stimulus is changed by altering the movement pattern—for example, allowing a greater motion range in the presence of pain. The effect of the MT is to enhance proprioception and increase the subject's body awareness

Definition:

Non-associative learning occurs when a stimulus in separated (uncoupled) from a behaviour.

Although research shows that these effects are statistically significant, the therapist must determine whether they are clinically relevant, and superior to other treatment modalities which could be used.

Classically, MT techniques often claimed that spinal joints were moved individually (for example, L4 motion on L5), or gliding motions were directionally specific (for example, detecting rotation of a spinous process). However, the skin-fascia interface over the spine is essentially frictionless, meaning that any movement of a vertebra which creates a reactive force would not be felt in the overlying skin (Bereznick et al. 2002). Further, many MT techniques while resulting in a change of movement are unlikely to generate sufficient force to enable significant accessory joint movement or tissue changes directly. Neuromuscular factors occurring at the time of MT application are a more likely explanation for any motion change. In addition, motion changes resulting from MT are usually only temporary resulting from a short-term reduction in muscle tone. For this to occur, the MT technique only has to be applied close to the region of pathology for person symptoms to be modified. For example, treating the thoracic spine with MT has been shown to reduce symptoms in the cervical spine (Cleland et al. 2005).

Within the 3Rs framework, an integrated approach of MT is used (Norris 2018a,b,c; Norris 2019). Techniques are largely non-specific (not aimed at a single joint) and performed rhythmically (mobilisation rather than manipulation). In addition, techniques are largely graded in a similar way to the Maitland method (Maitland 1991) but more generalised. Grades (I) and (II) are gentle oscillations aimed at pain reduction while grades (III) and (IV) are more forceful focussed on enhancing mobility (see also Chapter 5).

Example manual therapy techniques used in the reactive phase

PA mobilisation to the lumbar spine

Posteroanterior (PA) mobilisation is aimed at pain reduction and increasing pain free motion range to *extension*.

Starting position:

Most commonly, the person lies prone on a treatment couch with the therapist standing to one side in a walk standing position (one foot in front of the other).

Method:

Contact is made over a spinous process at the desired spinal level. The hand is typically used with the thumb pads (one thumb on top of the other) or the pisiform bone and ulnar surface of hand transmitting force through the fully extended wrist. The other hand supports the first. Force is produced using therapist body sway through the semi- flexed (at the elbow) arms over the selected spinous process (SP). Use only enough force to begin reducing or centralising pain.

Points to note:

- It is normally more comfortable for the therapist if the leg further from the couch is forwards and that closer to the couch is back so that their body is rotated towards the person.
- The semi-flexed elbows absorb some force and soften the technique. Locking the elbows increases force.
- The force is *produced* using a rocking action of the body but *transmitted* through the arms and hands. Force should not be produced by the hands or arms as this increases fatigue on the therapist.

Modifications:

- The PA technique presses the lumbar spine into extension. Where this is too painful, the technique may be regressed by changing the starting position to slight flexion—having the person lie with the abdomen on one or two pillows. Once the mobilisation is painless in this semi-flexed position it can be repeated in full prone lying or progressed to an extended position (see below).

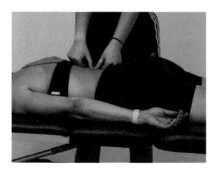 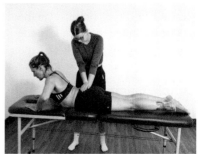

Rotary mobilisation to the lumbar spine

Starting position:

The person is side lying with their symptomatic side uppermost. The couch is adjusted to the therapist's thigh height. The therapist may stand behind the person or in front depending on the precise movement to be carried out. Where a low-grade oscillation is applied, little force is used and the therapist can stand in front of the person guiding the action with their hands. Bend the person's upper leg to 90° hooking the dorsum of their foot into the back of the knee of their lower leg. Draw their shoulders through by gently pulling their lower arm towards the therapist. Aim to keep the spine relatively straight, or in slight extension.

Method:

The therapist places one hand/forearm on the person's lower ribs and the other hand over the person's pelvis or lower spine. The action is to move the arms forwards and backwards against each other using a rocking motion of the therapist's hips.

Points to note:

- Classically, the person lies with their painful side uppermost. However, if pain reduction is better with the painful side down this position should be used.
- Move the person's hip relative to their shoulders to position the lumbar spine into more or less extension.

Modifications:

- When standing behind the person the couch may be lowered, and more force produced by the therapist leaning forwards over their semi-flexed arms. The lower contact point is again over the pelvis, but as force is greater the upper contact point moves to the shoulder. The action is a higher grade (more force) oscillation.
- The technique can be progressed to a high velocity low amplitude (HVLA) manipulation by moving the person to comfortable (mid to end) range rotation to take up tissue slack and locking the therapists' elbows. Perform the thrust using a body drop action where the therapist moves their bodyweight directly downwards by bending their knees suddenly.

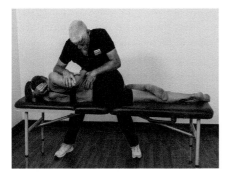 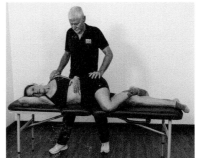

Mobilisation used with movement

MT techniques may also be used during movement in which case a mobilisation with movement (MWM) may be performed. MWM techniques were originally pioneered by Brian Mulligan, a New Zealand based physiotherapist (see Mulligan 2010) and are applied in two main circumstances. Initially, the therapist assesses the person's quality and range of motion into a chosen direction. Where pain occurs, or movement is limited (compared to the non-symptomatic side) and MWM may be used and is continued providing pain lessens or free motion range increases. When originally taught, MWM techniques referred to techniques used in the periphery and when using movements with gliding forces in the spine they were termed SNAGs (sustained natural apophyseal glide), indicating that the MT force was directed in line with the facet (apophyseal) joint line. In this text, the term MWM is used as it more closely describes the gross action which involves a movement by the person being treated (e.g., flexion) and a gliding force imparted by the therapist perpendicular to the person's movement (e.g., spine to abdomen).

MWM to flexion

Starting position:

The person is positioned sitting on the side of a treatment couch with the therapist standing behind. A webbing belt is placed around the therapists' hips and around the person's pelvis or lower abdomen (protected by a folded towel).

Method:

The person flexes their spine to the point of limitation (pain onset or stiffness) and returns to the upright position. The therapist imparts a PA glide in a slightly upward (cephalic) direction. The skin contact is with the ulnar side of the hand. The gliding force is maintained throughout the movement and the person's response monitored.

Points to note:

- The webbing belt is used to avoid pushing the person off the couch as the technique proceeds. It is not used for the glide technique itself.
- Where the technique is performed without person movement it can become a PA mobilisation (see above) performed in sitting.

Modifications:

- The technique can be performed with the person in a slump position, with one leg straight and supported on a chair.

- Rather than flexion, side flexion may be used in which case the gliding force is applied on the convex side of the curve (left side flexion, therapists' hand on the right of the spine). Again, the glide is directed in a PA and cephalic direction.

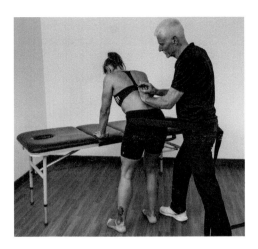

Use of acupuncture and dry needling for low back pain

Acupuncture and DN differ in their technique of application. Acupuncture uses distinct acupuncture points, whose location and needling depth is internationally agreed (WHO 1993). Acupuncture points do not have a distinct anatomical structure, but points may have similarities of structure and response including higher concentrations of microvessels, nerve endings and mast cells, thicker intermuscular or intramuscular connective tissue, lower skin resistance measurements and altered nitric oxide levels (Li et al. 2015). Dry needling (DN) does not use pre-defined points, relying instead on palpation of tissue changes and symptom reproduction. The effect of DN will depend on the target tissue with muscle points often correlated to local trigger points—hypersensitive regions within a muscle or myofascial region. DN may also be used to target tendons or healing tissue within a muscle and point of contact ultrasound (POCUS) may be used to identify target needling points.

Needling into local soft tissue elicits a classic triple response (redness, heat, swelling, and pain) demonstrating the beginning of an inflammatory reaction. The response is due to the release of pro-inflammatory mediators including prostaglandin. Additionally, calcitonin gene related peptide (CGRP) is released as a response to needling giving trophic (healing) effects, and nitric oxide (NO) which relaxes smooth muscle cells to cause local vasodilatation of the capillary bed (Kubo et al. 2010). The physical act of needling also effects the soft tissue mechanically. Stimulating the needle by twisting or thrusting (as is common practice) winds and adheres fascial fibres to the needle shaft to create a whorl

(Langevin 2006) and may change the shape of the fibroblast cells within fascia. This process, in turn, gives rise to remodelling of the cellular cytoskeleton, and extracellular ATP signalling, also called Purinergic signally (Langevin 2013).

Definition:

Purinergic signally is a form of extracellular (outside the cell) communication between cells through the release of chemicals (called purine nucleotides) from the cell membrane. The chemicals are taken up by receptors (purinergic receptors) in adjacent cells.

Pain relief as a result of acupuncture or DN occurs at four levels, local, spinal, brain stem, and higher centre. At a *local* level, the release of opioid chemicals (neuromodulators) has an effect on pain mechanisms. At a *spinal* level, the sensory nerve synapses in the dorsal horn of the spinal cord, and at that point desensitisation occurs, reducing the pain experience. Through interneuron effects at the dorsal horn, the sympathetic nervous system is also stimulated, opening the possibility for effects on internal organs, and changes in skin responses such as sweating. The nociceptive pathway from the dorsal horn ascends in the spinal cord via the spinothalamic tract to the brain stem. In the *brain stem*, pain suppression occurs not just to the injured body part, but to the whole body. This type of 'top down' pain inhibition occurs via several brainstem structures including the Periaqueductal gray matter (PAG) and the rostral ventromedial medulla (RVM). The effect is not especially powerful, but from this region neurons ascend to *higher centres* in the brain to affect the pituitary gland and hypothalamus. Through action on these two centres, and by affecting the limbic system deep within the brain, neurohormonal effects are created which target not the pain sensation per se, but the emotional experience of pain. This later effect is particularly important where long lasting or chronic pain is part of the clinical picture.

Research on the use of acupuncture in low back pain is controversial. Several major scientific trials have shown benefit, including an individual person data meta-analysis (Vickers et al. 2012) which showed acupuncture to be superior to sham acupuncture and no acupuncture (effect sizes 0.20 and 0.46). The German Acupuncture Trail (GERAC) (Haake 2007) showed acupuncture to be superior to standard treatment leading the German healthcare authorities to include acupuncture within their social health insurance system. The NICE clinical guidelines in the UK initially suggested consideration of up to 12 sessions of acupuncture over three months (NICE 2009), however, the updated guidance (NICE 2016) does not recommend the use of acupuncture in the treatment of low back pain. A Cochrane review (Mu et al. 2020) did not find acupuncture more effective than sham but did find it better than no treatment for pain relief and functional improvement immediately after treatment. Acupuncture did not appear to reduce pain clinically significantly but was more effective in improving function immediately after treatment. In this review, the authors commented that the decision to use acupuncture to treat chronic LBP should depend on availability, cost, and person preferences.

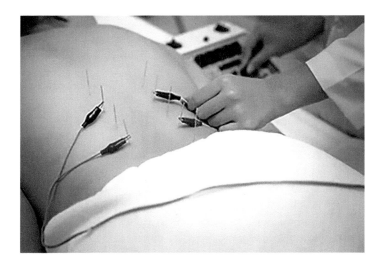

Electroacupuncture treatment of the low back

The use of electrotherapy is not recommended by the NICE (2016) guidelines on the treatment of low back pain. However, self-applied thermal modalities (cold or heat) are easily employed and readily available, and several electrotherapy machines including therapeutic ultrasound and electrical stimulation have been commonly used in the past and are still readily available so will be briefly reviewed.

Therapeutic ultrasound (TUS) is a type of mechanical energy which does not travel through air but will travel through water or tissues containing water. A TUS machine produces ultrasonic waves from a transducer head which changes electrical energy into mechanical energy using the piezo-electric effect.

> **Definition:**
>
> A *Piezoelectric effect* is the ability of a material to generate an electric charge in response to applied mechanical stress and vice versa.

TUS produces three main non-thermal effects in tissues. First, *cavitation* produces bubbles which either vibrate (stable cavitation) or collapse (unstable cavitation). Second unidirectional movement of fluid (*acoustic streaming*) occurs in tissue within the ultrasound field. Finally *standing waves* are produced at tissue interfaces, where the oncoming wave combines with the wave reflected from the neighbouring tissue and the new combined wave is more powerful than the two originals.

TUS mainly has tissue effects during the inflammatory phase of tissue healing (Watson and Nussbaum 2021) with effects are cellular level. The modality acts as an inflammatory optimiser moving healing on through the healing cascade. Although these changes have been documented in animal and laboratory studies (Young and Dyson 1990, Ng 2011), the clinical effect of TUS on low back pain is generally poor. A Cochrane review (Ebadi et al. 2020) concluded that "there is little to suggest that ultrasound is an effective treatment for people with non-specific low back pain".

TENS (transcutaneous electrical nerve stimulation) and NMES (neuromuscular electrical stimulation) and both forms of electrical stimulation given through the skin which activate nerves. Both have the advantage that they are portable battery powered units which are readily available and easily applied by a person themselves after training. TENS is used predominantly for pain relief (analgesia) stimulating *sensory* nerves and activating the pain gate mechanism and endogenous opioid chemical release. NMES stimulates muscle contraction by depolarising *motor* nerves. Depending on the electrical frequency either a twitch (separate) or tetanic (continuous) muscle contraction is stimulated. NMES may be used to strengthen and re-educate muscle and to enhance circulation by instigating a muscle pump action when voluntary contraction is weak. Neither TENS nor NMES is recommended by the NICE back pain guidelines.

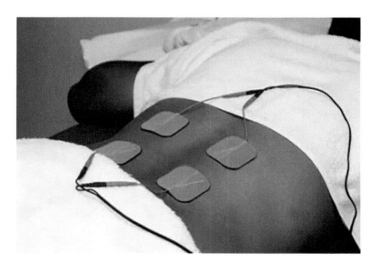

Use of TENS for low back pain

Thermal therapies again have the advantage of ready availability and self-application. Common types include cold (packs, sprays, gels, cold immersion, crushed ice) and wet or dry heat (packs, lamps, whirlpool). Although both cold and heat have biological effects in the laboratory, these techniques often do not penetrate deeply enough to affect tissue directly in real world situations. Heat from an infrared lamp will penetrate to a maximum depth of approximately 3 mm with some heat transfer from superficial to deeper tissues (Watson and Nussbaum 2021). Rapid heating from a whirlpool bath may not be maintained for long enough to pass through the insulating subcutaneous fat layer. Topical application of cold can have an analgesic effect and whole-body cryotherapy (WBC) may have an effect on inflammation and healing. In terms of low back pain management, thermal therapies may give some short-term pain reduction and make a resting position more comfortable. The application of a standard hot water bottle or microwavable moist heat pack is often reported by persons to reduce their pain and suffering and gives them some control over their symptoms.

Pain neuroscience education (PNE) in the management of low back pain

Education is essential in the management of LBP because people typically have negative beliefs and expectations about the condition and its treatment. In a survey study of over 400 participants, 4 main negative beliefs have been identified. People believed that having back pain meant they would always have weakness in their back, that the conditions would get progressively worse, that resting was a good form of management, and that X-rays or scans were necessary to ensure the best medical care (Hall et al. 2021).

As we have seen in Chapter 1, psychological interventions used by themselves have shown equal results to active exercise interventions (Hoffman et al. 2007). When used in combination with exercise or MT however, the effect can be enhanced. PNE is a clinical technique which teaches a person to rethink how they view pain. It aims to reconceptualise pain relating it to an alteration of central nervous system processing ('software' metaphor) rather than a direct result of tissue damage ('hardware' metaphor). In this way, PNE aims to reduce the threat value of pain and separate it from suffering.

These effects may be achieved by increasing pain thresholds (the point at which pain is experienced), decreasing fear of movement, and modulating brain activity in regions associated with the pain experience. Both PNE and exercise show *strong* evidence of benefit on pain and function in musculoskeletal conditions generally, compared to only *moderate* benefit (modest effect sizes) for NSAIDs and opioid drugs, for example (Babatunde et al. 2017).

Keypoint:

Pain neuroscience education (PNE) helps people to rethink how they view pain.

Essential messages

Whilst PNE can be very detailed and back school approaches can cover many weeks, only essential messages are used in the 3Rs approach to facilitate learning. Three messages are used as these have been shown to be valued by people themselves (Leake et al. 2021). *First*, that pain does not necessarily mean the body is damaged (hurt and harm message), *second*, that thoughts, emotions, and experience can affect pain, and *third* that the overprotective pain system can be retrained. Practically, this can take several steps (Smith et al. 2019). As with any consultation (subjective examination, see Chapter 5) we must first find out what the person knows. Why do they think they have pain and what is their understanding of pain? From this discussion, any unhelpful beliefs may be identified and challenged by words or actions. For example, if they believe flexion will cause pain or hurt them, can we use pain free limited flexion to confront this? Progressive exercise and graded exposure can help with this process and enhance self efficacy. Reassurance can make the person feel safer and have a positive effect on the pain experience. Providing guidance on pain and activity levels forms part of the coaching process during rehabilitation.

> **CASE NOTE**
>
> A 42-year-old female primary school teacher presented with a history of enforced rest following an acute onset low back pain which resulted in a microdiscectomy 5 years ago. Following the surgery, after a period of initial recovery pain levels were not reducing so the procedure was repeated 1 year later with the aim of removing scar tissue. See had received no structured rehabilitation believing that movement of her spine was pulling on the injured area causing pain and had stopped working. Listening to her story, she mentioned that she really missed exercise, so we discussed beginning a walking programme. I emphasised that this was likely to give her some reaction, but it was unlikely that the reaction would be from her previously injured tissues, as a portion of disc and scarring had been removed, more likely that the reaction would be from prolonged deconditioning. When she felt a reaction, we agreed that she would continue walking for another 2 minutes. The person was very conscious of bending and sat straight up in her chair throughout our discussion. I asked her to stand and experiment with bending (rolling) her spine down to touch a chair back and after two sets when she did not get pain, she tried the chair seat. Again, I emphasised that any discomfort was likely due to tight tissues stretching rather than the return of her original injury. Through a programme of graded exposure and graded exercise she eventually returned to normal activities.

Use of metaphor and analogy

We have seen in Chapter 3 how metaphor and analogies can be used when cueing an exercise. Now, we will look at some examples of using metaphors in

TABLE 7.2 Useful metaphors in pain neuroscience education

Metaphor	Topic
Overactive alarm system	Pain as a warming of threat
Bee sting & sparking electricity	Peripheral and central sensitisation
Computer keyboard, cable, & CPU	Input, transport, processing faults
Stress and feeling down	Biopsychosocial factors,
Nosy neighbours	Symptoms spreading to other areas.
Past experiences	Fear avoidance, kinesiophobia, catastrophising
Calming a barking dog	Relaxation, mindfulness, addressing fear
Feeling the burn	Hurt and harm—sore but safe
The body's pharmacy	Endogenous pain control,
Bends in the road	Flare up and setbacks

PNE (Table 7.2) which are useful to facilitate person understanding of sometimes complex neuroscience principles (Zimney et al. 2019). Using the alarm system metaphor is helpful to distinguish between nociception and pain, and to introduce the possibility that the system may be overactive and so creating pain (alarm going off) when a minor fault occurs—

> The smoke alarm in your house can save your life if there is a fire downstairs when you are in bed, but it sometimes also goes off when you are in the kitchen and you burn the toast.

Using a desktop computer set up of keyboard, cable, and CPU (central processing unit) can be helpful to illustrate targets for therapy

> If you see fuzzy letters on your computer screen it could be that you spilt coffee on your keyboard (input – skin), the dog under your desk just bit through the cable (transport – nerve), or your computer program has a virus (processor – brain)

Connecting pain and suffering with psychosocial factors is important to separate the link between pain and purely mechanical factors. The use of the barking dog metaphor is helpful with this, as is the alternative of screaming young children.

> If you come across a barking dog you don't shout at it and threaten it because it might bite you. Instead to try to calm it down and talk quietly. It's the same when your back flares up. Don't rub it or try to work the pain off, talk a breath and try to relax. Perhaps count from 10 down to 1 slowly, releasing tension with each count.

Gradually it becomes more obvious that the body can treat itself and each person has the capability to heal. When this realisation surfaces, it is useful to talk about the body's pharmacy, and this can be linked to exercise or MT being a catalyst for the body to release pain relieving chemicals.

It is important in the reactive phase (R1) of the 3Rs approach that PNE is not introduced too soon. The person must be listened to (person story) and their thoughts and feelings about pain are *validated*. Many people who have been in pain for a long time (chronic pain) or have seen several practitioners often feel that they are not understood or that the practitioner believes they are making their symptoms up. Many times, they can doubt themselves and think there is something wrong with them as there may be no outward signs of their condition.

Definition:

Validation occurs when a practitioner communicates that a person's thoughts and feelings are understandable and *genuine*.

From the perspective of PNE, it is important that validation does not mean that a therapist agrees with the speaker's perspective (they simply accept it) and the therapist must make sure that they don't encourage maladaptive beliefs (Edmond and Keefe 2015). For example, if a person states that

> My scan shows wear and tear and I realise it won't be possible for me to get back to activity

Simply to say that you understand how frustrating that must be and will see how you can help validates the persons' feelings without necessarily strengthening their argument.

Manual therapy as pain neuroscience education

One of the criticisms often waged against MT is that it disempowers the person, encouraging them to be dependent on their therapist and so less reliant on themselves—effectively eroding self efficacy. However, the technique itself is unlikely to instigate this but the way in which it is presented may do so (Langridge 2017). Giving the message that a person's pain results from a stiff joint which is 'blocking a movement' is likely to result in the person coming back to see a therapist time and time again. Seeing pain and lack of movement as a temporary barrier to recovery and using MT to instigate rehabilitation, enables the person to manage their own treatment outcome. Using MT as part of a progressive rehabilitation programme can lead to increased self efficacy enabling the person to move further along the recovery timescale when previously their recovery had plateaued.

In the person's mind, there is often a link between pain and the severity of an injury or the degree of tissue damage (hurt and harm). The more something hurts, the worse it is. However, PNE aims to break this link and the use of touch in MT can help this through the process of graded exposure (see below). Using a MT technique which pushes slightly into pain reinforces that pain is not always harmful as the person is in a secure environment of the treatment session (sore but safe). Additionally, MT techniques such as joint mobilisation use repeated oscillations which engage descending inhibition as a form of analgesia (the body pharmacy). The use of MT in this way can form an experiential type of PNE (Louw et al. 2017). Essential to this process is communication between the therapist and person and reinforcing that it is the person's body which is responding as it is unlikely that the therapist can exert sufficient force to directly affect human tissue.

Graded activity and graded exposure

Exercise therapy may also be given in a form which creates a bridge between psychological and physical interventions to enhance PNE. Cognition targeted exercise focusses on stopping an exercise at a specific time (time-contingent) rather than as the result of discomfort or pain (symptom-contingent). Typically following pain or injury a person will stop an action when it begins to hurt, and this can reinforce that pain is important and should limit their activities. Continuing to move safely through pain can break this link and is a form of graded exposure.

Graded exposure introduces activities which a person fears (e.g., flexion or lifting) in a hierarchical fashion (least feared progressing to most feared) to gradually increase confidence and capability. Usually, pain acts as an alarm system to notify a person about threat. For example, taking a tissue to its full limit, pain should occur just before tissue failure begins. However, in cases of central sensitisation pain may occur too soon, for example, when load is initially put on a tissue. Using graded exposure, the system is gradually re-set so that pain occurs at the correct point.

Definition:

Central sensitisation is the increased reaction in the central nervous system (CNS) to a normal nociceptive stimulus.

Graded activity is more physical in its aims, as it progresses components of an exercise (e.g., strength, range of motion, aerobic fitness) applying overload with the aim of achieving tissue adaptation. Graded exposure has been shown to be more effective than graded activity in decreasing catastrophising (viewing a situation as considerably worse than it is) in the short term (Lopez-de-Uralde-Villanueva et al. 2016).

Symptom modification

Movement may be used to modify symptoms identified as aggravating or easing factors during the subjective examination (Chapter 5). This approach underlies the McKenzie method of mechanical diagnosis and therapy (MDT) originally developed by New Zealand physiotherapist Robin McKenzie (see McKenzie 1981). Some of the fundamental features of this method are adapted in the 3Rs approach as they focus on empowering the person by encouraging self-management. The McKenzie approach uses subgrouping based on classification by symptom behaviour. There are four categories, derangement, dysfunction, postural syndrome, and non-mechanical syndrome (Table 7.3). Essentially *derangement* syndrome focusses on finding a direction of movement (dynamic) or position (static) which *centralises* or abolishes symptoms, a feature termed *directional preference*. Directional preference (DP) differs from a resting or accommodating position (see above). An accommodating position is often a position we take up instinctively which gives temporary relief (it feels good), while a DP gives a more permanent change (helps to make the condition better). Whilst not present in all cases, centralisation has been found to be more common in acute cases (prevalence 74%) than chronic (prevalence 42%) while that of DP was 70% (May and Aina 2012).

> **Definition:**
>
> *Centralisation* is defined as progressive and stable reduction of the most distal presenting pain towards the spine midline in response to standardised spinal loading strategies (Chorti 2009).

Dysfunction aims to identify adaptive shortening of tissue which when placed on stretch causes symptoms. The aim is to enhance mobility (range and quality of

TABLE 7.3 McKenzie mechanical syndromes

Syndrome	Characteristics
Derangement	Directional preference—a repeated movement or posture eases or centralises symptoms
Dysfunction	Pain results from deformation of impaired tissue such as adaptive shortening, scarring
Postural	Pain from mechanical deformation of normal soft tissue held at end range for prolonged periods
Non-mechanical	Other pathologies

movement) by using repeated end range motion into pain which should reduce in intensity, emphasising a 'hurt not harm' approach. *Postural syndrome* results from end range loading of pain sensitive structures and requires person education and postural modification to allow tissue irritability to settle. Non-mechanical syndromes consist of pathologies which do not change consistently with repeated movements and may require further investigation (McKenzie and May 2003).

Prone passive spinal extension

Starting position:

Begin lying on your front (prone). If you are unable to do this because of pain or stiffness, place one or two pillow under your abdomen to bend (flex) your spine slightly. As your symptoms settle or centralise (move from your leg or buttocks towards your low back), remove one pillow and try again. Let your symptoms settle and then remove the final pillow so that you are lying flat. This may take 5–10 minutes to achieve if your back is very irritable and to begin with (day one after pain onset) this is enough. As symptoms ease and you can lie flat without the need for pillows, you are ready to begin the exercise (day two or three after pain onset).

Method:

Begin the movement by trying to extend your spine passively (without using your back muscles). This may be achieved in two ways. The first (static) is to raise your chest above the level of your hips. On a treatment couch this is achieved but angling the couch end, but at home this can be done by making a wedge shape from several firm cushions (try the cushion from your armchair or sofa). Maintain this extended position for 2–5 minutes allowing your symptoms to centralise.

The second passive extension method (dynamic) is to use the power of your arms but to keep your back relatively relaxed. Place your arms to the side of your shoulders, hands flat. Press with your arms and lift your chest up so you look to a point about 0.5 m in front of you. Lower from this position and then repeat, gradually trying to get a little higher with each push. Try to keep your back as relaxed as you can and keep your pelvis on the floor. Perform 5–10 reps and then rest. Repeat for three sets.

Points to note:

- The power for this action must come from your arms. The aim is to keep your back muscles as relaxed as you can.
- Try not to hold your breath as you focus closely on the action. Breathe normally through the action.

- Spinal extension from a prone position is a common movement in several exercise types. In yoga it is called the Sphinx pose, and in Pilates the Swan, where less lumbar extension is used, and the focus is more on the thoracic and cervical spines.
- Sometimes it is more comfortable to offset your chest and pelvis slightly (chest slightly to the right and pelvis to the left or vice versa), so that your hips are off-centre. If this works for you, it is fine to begin with. As you improve, you will be able to keep your spine in a straight line.

Modifications:

- If you are unable to take weight on your wrists, press from your flat forearms instead, fingers pointing forwards.
- To help keep your pelvis down you can use a belt or folded towel, or a partner's hands to keep you down and to act as a pivot to move around. (i) In a clinic, a therapist can fasten a webbing belt around your low back just above your pelvis. (ii) At home, lie on the floor and place a wide strap or towel folded lengthways across your spine. Have your partner hold the towel down by placing one foot on each end of the towel. (iii) In the clinic or gym, a therapist or trainer can perform an extension mobilisation (PA glide) by pressing their hands down onto the lumbar spine as the person has pushed up into extension. The effect is to encourage further movement into extension (local vertebral rotation and shear).

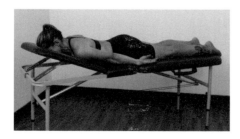
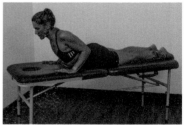

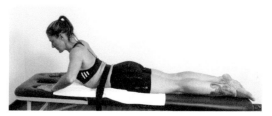
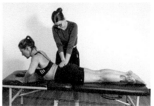

Standing active spinal extension

Starting position:

Method:

Begin standing with your feet apart. Place your hands flat on the top of your buttocks. Lean backwards to look at the ceiling, taking some of your upper body-weight through your hands onto your buttocks. Pause briefly and then move back to the straight standing position. Repeat the action five times and then rest.

Points to note:

- As people may not be able to lie down through the day (especially if they are working) standing spinal extension may be used. This is an active movement (the spinal muscles are involved) and the spine is vertical and so subjected to more loading than when lying.
- If you feel dizzy, do not look up but keep looking straight ahead, and rather than focussing on bending your back, press your hips forwards—your spine will bend naturally.

Modifications:

Some people find they form a deep crease (hinge) in their lower spine, and this can be painful. Try leading the movement by lifting your breastbone (sternum) upwards towards the ceiling and maintain the feeling of length through your spine as you bend. This method of a standing backward bend is popular in yoga where it is known as a standing backbend pose *(Anuvittasana)*.

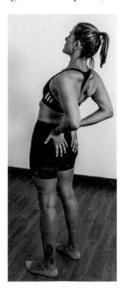

Sitting spine extension

Starting position:

Begin sitting on a firm chair, at the front of the seat. Part your knees, and have a towel rolled lengthways handy.

Method:

Feel yourself taking your weight through your two sitting bones in your buttocks. Rock your pelvis backwards (posterior tilt) to take your weight onto your tailbone, and then rock your pelvis forwards (anterior tilt) to take your weight onto your pubis (front pelvic bone). Keep your spine lengthened but rock your pelvis back and forwards to flex and extend your lower back (lumbar region).

Points to note:

*   If you find it difficult to hollow your back (anterior pelvic tilt), place the towel folded lengthways into your lower back just above your belt. Grip both ends and pull it forwards and upwards (aiming for shoulder level) to gently pull you spine into a hollow position.

Modifications:

*   If you find the pelvic tilt position difficult, use a sitting wedge. With the thick end placed to the chair back it will encourage anterior pelvic tilt (back hollowing). With the thick end at the front of the seat it will encourage posterior pelvic tilt (back rounding).
*   To focus on thoracic spine extension, place the towel just under your armpits. As you pull it forwards and upwards focus on lifting your breastbone (sternal lift action) and pulling your shoulder blades downwards (scapular depression).

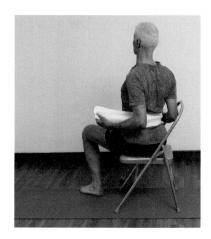

Lying spinal flexion using overpressure

Starting position:

Begin lying on a mat on the floor. Draw your legs up, bringing your knees to your chest. Grip around your knees (or under them if you have knee pain).

Method:

Draw your knees in towards your chest and upwards towards your shoulder so that your tailbone (sacrum) lifts off the mat. Hold this position for 1–2 seconds and then lower your tail back onto the mat but keep holding your knees in preparation for the rest of your reps.

Points to note:

- If your hips are quite stiff, your lower back will bend (flex) earlier in the exercise. If they are very flexible, your knees will touch your chest and you will need to pull more towards your shoulders.

Modifications:

- If you find this action difficult, lie on a wedge or rolled towel to lift your tailbone from the mat (posterior pelvic tilt). Now, the action will be much smaller as the back is already rounded as you begin.

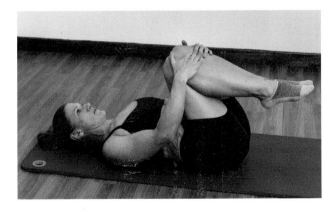

Support standing spinal flexion

Starting position:

Begin by placing a chair with its back against a wall. Stand with one leg on a chair seat. If you have pain referred into your leg, place the painful leg on the chair.

Method:

Bend your spine as though trying to put your forehead onto your knee.

Points to note:

- Repeat the action to allow your spine to stretch out. You should notice pain reducing or symptoms centralising.

Modifications:

- Perform the action standing without chair support. Keep your feet shoulder width apart and roll your spine as though trying to put your nose close to your belly button (umbilicus) and finally look between your knees. In Pilates, this is called a roll down exercise.

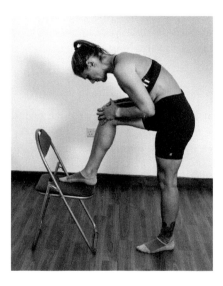

Side support pelvic shift

Starting position:

Begin standing side on to a wall with your right arm bent to 90°, forearm on the wall at shoulder height.

Method:

Keeping your right arm still (do not shrug your shoulder) press your right hip in towards the wall. Repeat the action several times, gradually easing into the movement until you can perform the action to the same degree on both sides.

Points to note:

- If one side of your spine is tight, it can pull you into a side shift position where your shoulders are not directly over your pelvis.
- If you are side shifted to the left (left shoulders further over than your pelvis), place your left arm on the wall and press the side of your pelvis to the wall to correct the shift.

Modifications:

- This is used as a self-practice exercise. However, it can also be performed by a therapist holding your pelvis and pressing your shoulders with their body as a MT technique.

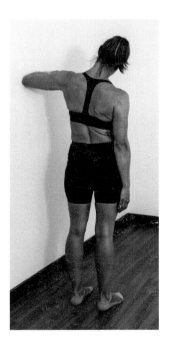

References

Babatunde, O.O., Jordan, J.L., Van der Windt, D.A., et al. (2017). Effective treatment options for musculoskeletal pain in primary care: A systematic overview of current evidence. *PLoS One* 12(6), e0178621.

Bereznick, D.E., Ross, J.K., and McGill, S.M. (2002). The frictional properties at the thoracic skin-fascia interface: Implications in spine manipulation. *Clinical Biomechanics* 17(4): 297–303.

Bialosky, J.E., Bishop, M.D., Price, D.D., et al. (2009). The mechanisms of manual therapy in the treatment of musculoskeletal pain: A comprehensive model. *Manual Therapy* 14: 531–538.

Callaghan, J.P., Gunning, J.L., and McGill, S.M. (1998). The relationship between lumbar spine load and muscle activity during extensor exercises. *Physical Therapy* 78(1): 8–18.

Chorti, A. (2009). Towards a uniform definition for the centralisation phenomenon. PhD thesis. Coventry: University of Warwick.

Cleland, J.A., Childs, J.D., McRae, M., et al. (2005). Immediate effects of thoracic manipulation in persons with neck pain: A randomized clinical trial. *Manual Therapy* 10: 127–135.

Daligadu, J., Haavik, H., Yielder, P.C., et al. (2013). Alteration in cortical and cerebellar motor processing in subclinical neck pain persons following spinal manipulation. *Journal of Manipulative and Physiological Therapeutics* 36(8): 527–537.

Dishman, J.D., and Bulbulian, R. (2001). Comparison of effects of spinal manipulation and massage on motoneuron excitability. *Electromyography and Clinical Neurophysiology* 41(2): 97–106.

Ebadi, S, Henschke, N., Forogh, B., et al. (2020). Therapeutic ultrasound for chronic low back pain. *Cochrane Database of Systematic Reviews*. Issue 7. Art. No.: CD009169.

Edmond, S.N., and Keefe, F.J. (2015). Validating pain communication: Current state of the science. *Pain* 156(2): 215–219.

Elwyn, G., Frosch, D., Thomson, R., et al. (2012). Shared decision making: A model for clinical practice. *Journal of General Internal Medicine* 27(10): 1361–1367.

Ferreira, P.H., Ferreira, M., Maher, C., et al. (2013). The therapeutic alliance between clinicians and persons predicts outcome in chronic low back pain. *Physical Therapy* 93(4): 470–478.

Fryer, G., and Pearce, A.J. (2012). The effect of lumbosacral manipulation of corticospinal and spinal reflex excitability on asymptomatic participants. *Journal of Manipulative Physiology Therapy* 35(2): 86–93.

Goldstein, E. (2013). Stressing out? S.T.O.P. https://www.mindful.org/stressing-out-stop/ accessed 2022.

Haake, M. (2007). German acupuncture trails (GERAC) for chronic low back pain. *Archives of Internal Medicine* 167: 1892.

Hall, A., Coombs, D., Richmond, H., et al. (2021). What do the general public believe about the causes, prognosis and best management strategies for low back pain? A cross-sectional study. *BMC Public Health* 21(1): 682.

Hoffman, B.M., Papas, R.K., Chatkoff, D.K., et al. (2007). Meta-analysis of psychological interventions for chronic low back pain. *Health Psychology: Official Journal of the Division of Health Psychology, American Psychological Association* 26(1): 1–9.

Hougaard, E. (1994). The therapeutic alliance–A conceptual analysis. *Scandinavian Journal of Psychology* 35(1): 67–85.

Kubo, K., Yajima, H., Takayama, M., et al. (2010). Effects of acupuncture and heating on blood volume and oxygen saturation of human Achilles tendon in vivo. *European Journal of Applied Physiology* 109(3): 545–550.

Langevin, H. (2006). Connective tissue: A bodywide signalling network? *Medical Hypothesis* 66: 1074–1077.

Langevin, H.M. (2013). Effects of acupuncture needling on connective tissue. In Dommerholt, J. and Fernandez, C. Eds., *Trigger point dry needling*. Edinburgh: Churchill Livingstone.

Langridge, N. (2017). Manual therapy – Feeling for cracks in the theories and practices. *Podcast*. http://chewshealth.co.uk/tpmpsession38/

Leake, H.B., Moseley, G.L., Stanton, T.R., et al. (2021). What do persons value learning about pain? A mixed-methods survey on the relevance of target concepts after pain science education. *Pain* 162(10): 2558–2568.

Li, F., He, T., Xu, Q., et al. (2015). What is the Acupoint? A preliminary review of Acupoints. *Pain Medicine (Malden, Mass.)* 16(10): 1905–1915.

López-de-Uralde-Villanueva, I., Muñoz-García, D., Gil-Martínez, A., et al. (2016). A systematic review and meta-analysis on the effectiveness of graded activity and graded exposure for chronic nonspecific low back pain. *Pain Medications* 17: 172–188.

Louw, A., Nijs, J., and Puentedura, E. J. (2017). A clinical perspective on a pain neuroscience education approach to manual therapy. *Journal of Manual & Manipulative Therapy* 25(3): 160–168.

Machado, G.C., Maher, C.G., Ferreira, P.H., et al. (2015). Efficacy and safety of paracetamol for spinal pain and osteoarthritis: Systematic review and meta-analysis of randomised placebo-controlled trials. *BMJ (Clinical Research ed.)* 350: h1225.

Machado, G.C., Maher, C.G., Ferreira, P.H., et al. (2017). Non-steroidal anti-inflammatory drugs for spinal pain: A systematic review and meta-analysis. *Annals of the Rheumatic Diseases* 76: 1269–1278.

Maitland, G.D. (1991). *Peripheral manipulation* (3rd ed). Oxford: Butterworth Heinemann.

May, S., and Aina, A. (2012). Centralization and directional preference: A systematic review. *Manual Therapy* 17(6): 497–506.

McCarthy, C., Bialosky, J., and Rivett, D. (2015). Spinal manipulation. In Jull, G., Moorse, A., Falla, D., et al., Eds., *Grieve's Modern Musculoskeletal Physiotherapy* (4th ed). London: Elsevier.

McKenzie, R. (1981). *The lumbar spine: Mechanical diagnosis and therapy*. Wellington, New Zealand: Spinal Publications.

McKenzie, R., and May, S. (2003). *The lumbar spine. Mechanical diagnosis and therapy. Volume one*. Waikanae, New Zealand: Spinal Publications.

Mintken, P. E., Derosa, C., Little, T., Smith, B., & American Academy of Orthopaedic Manual Physical Therapists (2008). A model for standardizing manipulation terminology in physical therapy practice. *The Journal of Manual & Manipulative Therapy* 16(1): 50–56.

Mu, J., Furlan, A.D., Lam, W.Y., et al. (2020). Acupuncture for chronic non-specific low back pain. *Cochrane Database of Systematic Reviews* Issue 12. Art. No.: CD013814.

Mulligan, B.R. (2010). *Manual therapy: Nags, Snags, MWM* (6th ed). New Zealand: Orthopedic Physical Therapy and Rehabilitation.

Ng, G.Y. (2011). Comparing therapeutic ultrasound with microamperage stimulation therapy for improving the strength of Achilles tendon repair. *Connective Tissue Research* 52(3): 178–182.

NICE Guideline on Low Back Pain. (2009). http://guidance.nice.org.uk/CG88.

NICE Guideline [NG59] (2016). Low Back Pain and Sciatica in Over 16s: Assessment and Management, Published: 30 November 2016. Last updated: 11 December 2020.

Norris, C.M. (2018a). Clinically effective manual therapy for the hip. *Co-Kinetic Journal* 78: 33–36.

Norris, C.M. (2018b). *Sports and soft tissue injuries* (5th ed). Oxford: Routledge.

Norris, C.M. (2018c). *Sports and soft tissue injuries: A guide for students and therapists* (5th ed). London: Routledge.

Norris, C.M. (2019). Clinically effective manual therapy for the knee. *Co-Kinetic Journal* 79: 33–36.

Pincus, T., Holt, N., Vogel, S., et al. (2013). Cognitive and affective reassurance and person outcomes in primary care: a systematic review. *Pain* 154(11): 2407–2416.

Ross, J.K., Bereznick, D.E., and McGill, S.M. (2004). Determining cavitation location during lumbar and thoracic spinal manipulation: Is spinal manipulation accurate and specific? *Spine* 29(13): 1452–1457.

Smith, B.E., Hendrick, P., Bateman, M., et al. (2019). Musculoskeletal pain and exercise-challenging existing paradigms and introducing new. *British Journal of Sports Medicine* 53(14): 907–912.

Vanti, C., Andreatta, S., Borghi, S., et al. (2019). The effectiveness of walking versus exercise on pain and function in chronic low back pain: A systematic review and meta-analysis of randomized trials. *Disability and Rehabilitation* 41: 622–632.

Vickers, A.J., Cronin, A.M., Maschino, A. C., et al. (2012). Acupuncture for chronic pain: Individual person data meta-analysis. *Archives of Internal Medicine* 172(19): 1444–1453.

Watson, T., and Nussbaum, E.L. (eds) (2021). *Electrophysical agents* (13th ed). Oxford: Elsevier.

WHO. (1993). *Regional office for the western Pacific. Standardized nomenclature for acupuncture.* Manila: World Health Organization.

Young, S.R., & Dyson, M. (1990). Effect of therapeutic ultrasound on the healing of full-thickness excised skin lesions. *Ultrasonics* 28(3): 175–180.

Zimney, K.J., Louw, A., Cox, T., et al. (2019). Pain neuroscience education: Which pain neuroscience education metaphor worked best? *South African Journal of Physiotherapy* 75(1): 1–7.

8

RECOVERY PHASE

We have seen in Chapter 2 some of the principles of exercise therapy, and in Chapter 3 some of the features of teaching. Now, we will see how these can be put into practice. The person being managed has passed through the reactive phase (R1) and so their pain has reduced, and irritability settled. They can perform common daily activities and are able to walk 10 minutes without pain and to perform the sit-to-stand action for 3–5 reps (see Chapter 6). Now it is the time to gradually increase fitness relative to the back and compensate for deconditioning which will have occurred during their painful period (R1) where rest has been enforced through need.

It is important to remember that although exercises are listed and described below, the selection of exercises and the order in which they are performed and progressed must be person/user specific. Some users will favour certain exercises because they appeal to them or may find others less convenient due to lifestyle factors or facilities. Remember that no exercise type is universally superior to another when it comes to the management of low back pain (LBP).

Core stability—is it still relevant?

Core stability was the leading fashion in the fitness industry in the 1990s, originally stemming from physiotherapy research out of Australia (Hides 1994, Jull and Richardson 1994). It was popularised in the UK (Norris 1995) and entered the public domain on the back of fashionable exercise classes such as aerobics and Pilates within the burgeoning fitness industry. The original concept was that the trunk muscles, especially those more deeply placed such as the Transversus abdominis and internal oblique were able to support the spine and offset loads placed on spinal tissues (see Chapter 4) while at the same time local spinal

DOI: 10.4324/9781003366188-8

TABLE 8.1 Abdominal hollowing starting positions

Starting position	Advantage	Disadvantage
Kneeling (4 point)	Abdominal wall placed on stretch to facilitate AH action Unfamiliar pattern to athletes so avoids 'sit-up' motor programme Comfortable for LBP patient and during pregnancy	Stress on wrists and knees Difficult for obese subject
Prone lying	Easier to avoid spine movement Good cueing to pull abdominal wall away from table AH can be measured using pressure biofeedback	Inappropriate for obese or pregnant subject due to abdominal compression
Supine lying	Good for self palpation Surface EMG (sEMG) and pressure biofeedback used easily Link to PF contraction easier as patients often learn PF work in this position	Position may lead to sit-up muscle strategies in athletes (rectus dominance)
Standing (wall support)	Cueing to pull abdominal wall away from waistband of trousers useful for home exercise Appropriate for obese and pregnant patients Functional for daily activities	Weight bearing may not be suitable for disc patients Those with extreme postural abnormalities may find position uncomfortable
	AH = abdominal hollowing LBP = low back pain PF = pelvic floor	

From Norris, C.M. (2008) *Back Stability*. Human Kinetics, Champaign Illinois. With permission.

muscles such as the Multifidus could stiffen the spine and offer a resistance to bending. Although this was proven in laboratory settings (efficacy) in clinical settings (effectiveness) the concept was less clear-cut. People often found the (sometimes complex) stability exercises difficult to perform and several studies showed outcomes from stability training programmes to be no better than those from other exercise forms (Smith et al. 2014, Gomes-Neto et al. 2017). As a result, core stability is often demonised on social media in favour of simple weight training programmes. However, as we looked at symptom modification in the reactive phase of the 3Rs approach (Chapter 7) there will be individuals (or possibly sub-sets of people) whose symptoms may be reduced using a stability approach. In addition, this type of approach with its close focus on body position (alignment) can be helpful as a starting point for some during the initiation of progressive exercise therapy (PET) to increase body awareness. Finally, as core stability is still popular in commercial gyms, practicing something which is familiar can provide a security to a fearful person. These actions are by no means essential, but if people like them or favour them, then as with any exercise form, they can be useful.

> **Definition:**
>
> *Efficacy* is the degree to which something works under ideal (laboratory) conditions. *Effectiveness* is how well something works in a real-world (general population) setting.

Traditional core stability exercises

It is essential when teaching these exercises that they are used as a starting point with expressions such as "the first rung on the rehabilitation ladder", for example. Once mastered these types of exercises can be dropped, and the person moves on (progresses) to more challenging actions. Importantly, we must be careful not to instil a sense of fear or guilt around lack of core stability.

Each of the example starting positions covered below may be extended into exercise sequences and progressed or regressed depending on person needs. As we have seen in Chapter 2, progression is key to ensuring tissue adaptation with any aspect of fitness and this is the case also for rehab.

> **Keypoint:**
>
> Training trunk stability is not essential, but it can be a useful starting point.

Abdominal hollowing and bracing

Abdominal hollowing (pulling the abdominal wall inwards towards the spine) was traditionally said to be a key action for core stability training. The view was that the action (visceral compression) increased intra-abdominal pressure (IAP— see Chapter 4) and so was an important component to stabilisation. Although IAP is undoubtedly important, its voluntary control is unlikely to be crucial to rehabilitation in all individuals. It may help those who have poor abdominal floor control or visceroptosis, however.

> **Definition:**
>
> *Visceroptosis* is the downwards displacement of abdominal organs brought on through loss of abdominal muscle tone. It can be associated with abdominal distension, indigestion, and heartburn.

The action of abdominal hollowing (AH) is to draw the abdominal wall inwards. The action is a muscle isolation, so the rib cage should stay relatively inactive, and the spine does not move significantly. Additionally, the movement should be performed without the person holding their breath or taking a deep breath to avoid breathlessness or hyperventilation. Several starting positions may be used, and four have been selected as examples (Table 8.1).

Abdominal hollowing in kneeling

Starting position:

Begin kneeling on all fours on a gym mat with your hands beneath your shoulders and knees beneath your hips (box position). Have your knees–hip width apart and hands–shoulder width apart. Keep your spine relatively straight (neutral) without excessive rounding (flexion) or hollowing (extension).

Method:

Focus your attention on your tummy button (umbilicus) and pull your abdomen inwards towards your spine. Think of drawing your abdominal wall in as though you had been hit in the stomach. Hold the inwards position for 1–2 seconds and then release. Perform 5 reps and then rest.

Points to note:

- Try to keep your spine still throughout the movement, try not to arch, or hollow your back.
- Breathe normally throughout the exercise, do not hold your breath or breathe too deeply.
- The action can be more difficult to perform after abdominal surgery

Modifications and coaching:

- Fastening a belt around the abdomen is a useful cue. It gives you something to pull away from (external cue) rather than focussing on pulling your own muscles inwards (internal cue).
- Where this action alleviates symptoms, it can be used in the reactive phase (R1) of the 3Rs approach. It is used here in the recovery phase (R2) as it is an action which requires close focus and does not usually relate directly to pain or irritability.
- Where a person finds it difficult to avoid bending (flexing) the spine, using a pole or half foam roller (D roll) balanced along the spine can help. Back movement becomes more obvious as the pole will also move (external cue), and the focus can be on pulling the abdominal wall in towards the pole.

Sequencing

The kneeling core training position can be progressed using limb movement. In four-point kneeling the trunk is supported on four corners (two arms, two legs), so removing one support is challenging as it knocks us off balance. Moving one arm by bending it and trying to avoid the shoulder on the unsupported side dipping down challenges the core (a Pilates exercise called cat paws). Taking this further by moving the arm forwards or to the side alters and increases the overload. Performing a similar action with the knee, lifting it slightly above the ground (referred to as hovering the knee) begins to knock us off balance and this increases with leg movement. Eventually, combining opposite arm and leg actions take us to the birddog exercise (Chapter 7) which may be progressed using hand and ankle weights.

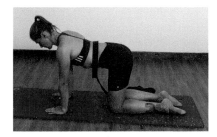 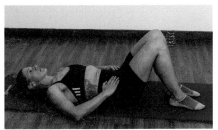

Pelvic floor contraction and abdominal hollowing in sitting

Starting position:

Begin sitting on a firm chair (dining chair or stool), with your back clear of the chair back. Place your feet shoulder width apart and flat on the floor. Sit in a mid-position, neither back on your tail nor forwards on your public bone, but central on your sitting bones.

Method:

Focus your attention on the area between your legs (pelvic floor) and pull it upwards away from the chair (female) or try to lift your penis (male). Try to hold the upward position of for a count of 2 and then lower. Repeat 3 times and then rest. Perform a second set of pulls trying to hold each for a count of 5. Rest and then repeat the action trying also to pull your lower abdominal region (the part below your tummy button) inwards towards your spine. Hold both contractions for a count of 5.

Points to note:

- These two actions are normally linked. If you cough or sneeze you should not wet yourself (urinate) unless you have poor pelvic floor control after childbirth, surgery, or injury.

- It can be easier to learn the two actions separately (part task training) and then when each is learnt to combine them.
- Practise the two contractions simultaneously as soon as you can.

Modifications and coaching:

- If you find sitting upright uncomfortable, either sit back in a firm lounge chair. Alternatively turn a dining chair around, place a cushion over the back, and sit forwards resting your folded arms on the cushion.
- In cases of low back and pelvic pain following childbirth or prostate surgery, this exercise can be used in the reactive phase (R1) of the 3Rs approach.
- Visualise an elevator (lift) lying in your low abdomen. Contract the pelvic floor by feeling a lifting action (elevator moving upwards). Grade the contraction by lifting to the 1st, 2nd, 3rd floors, for example.

Sequencing

As with the kneeling position (above) sitting core work can be progressed with arm and leg movements and then loading. Additionally, an unstable base may be used to sit on (sit-fit cushion or Swiss gym ball) which increases balance challenge. Sitting can then move to sit-to-stand (STS) actions controlling both sitting up (concentric) and sitting down (eccentric) which are especially useful to those with lower limb actions and older people who may lose confidence with STS actions following injury.

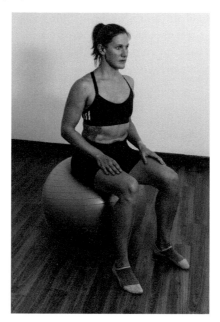

Abdominal hollowing in wall support standing

Starting position:

Begin standing with your back against a wall, feet forwards by 20–30 cm to allow your bodyweight to fall back against the wall. Either place a belt around your waist, or draw the waistband of your trousers out by 3–5 cm,

Method:

Focus your attention on your tummy button (umbilicus) and pull your abdomen inwards towards your spine. Think of drawing your abdominal wall in as though you had been punched in the stomach. Hold the inwards position for 1–2 seconds and then release. Perform 5 reps and then rest.

Points to note:

- Initially, there may be little movement occurring, but eventually you should feel a small gap forming between your waistband and your abdominal wall.
- The action is one of muscle contraction and is not directly related to obesity or abdominal girth. People with a 'big belly' can often still draw it inwards and those who are lean can sometimes not. It's all about muscle control.

Modifications and coaching:

- Once this action is learnt in standing, it can be used in walking (see postural walking, Chapter 7). When walking, draw the abdomen in for five steps and then relax and breathe normally for five steps.
- Repeat the action for 2–3 minutes to build muscle endurance.
- Cueing 'suck your stomach in' can help providing the person does not hold their breath but continues to breath normally.
- If a person finds it difficult not to hold their breath, have them count out load (1–10) while holding the abdomen away from their waistband.

Sequencing

Standing actions may progress again to limb loading, with a focus on gait. Control of pelvic level can be an important feature following lower limb injury. Side tilt of the pelvis (positive Trendelenburg sign) is often seen following hip or knee pathology and the standing action can be sequenced to improve this. Progressing to single leg standing actions with leg movement (flexion /extension/abduction) and then stepping (low/high step) and walking actions can all be useful.

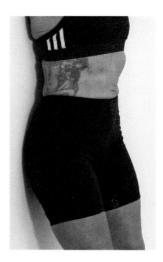

Abdominal hollowing in crook lying

Starting position:

Begin lying on your back on a gym mat with your knees bent and feet flat (hook lying or crook lying). Have your feet and knees shoulder width apart and place your hands on your lower abdomen (below your tummy button), fingertips pointing toward your groin.

Method:

Draw your abdominal wall inwards towards your spine and feel it gently tighten beneath your fingertips. Keep your rib cage relatively still (do not allow your lower ribs to push down as though performing a sit up) and breath normally.

Points to note:

- This was one of the classic positions to teach AH as it could be used with a self-monitored EMG attached to the lower abdomen at the retro aponeurotic triangle. Additionally, the depth of the lumber curve (lordosis) was often monitored using a pressure biofeedback cuff.

Modifications and coaching:

- Several cues are useful to separate the hollowing action from lumbar flexion. "Imagine water is lying on your tummy, now allow it to be drawn downwards and into your tummy button".
- Using the visualisation 'draw the ribs down' can help prevent rib flare where a person gains a flatter abdominal contour simply by expanding the rib cage.

Definition:

(i)   *Electromyography* (EMG) is a machine which measures the electrical response of a muscle. It is traditionally used with surface electrodes (stuck on the skin) or needle electrodes (puncturing through the skin and into the muscle).

(ii) The *retro aponeurotic triangle* is the most superficial portion of the transversus abdominis. At this point, the external oblique is said to be largely aponeurotic and so not electrically active. It is often used as the location of an adhesive EMG electrode used to monitor contraction of the transversus abdominis and internal oblique.

Sequencing

Limb movements of the leg (bent knee fallout, heel slide, straight leg lift) or arm (single arm raise, double arm raise or arm scissors) are traditionally used in exercise types such as Pilates. In addition, the crook lying position can progress to trunk curl actions (flexing the spine) or V sit exercises (balancing on the buttocks with the arms and trunk off the mat).

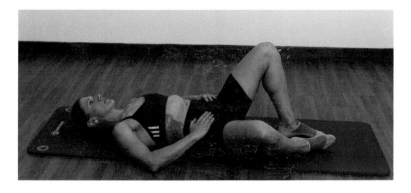

CASE NOTE

A 45-year-old person sought treatment for persistent abdominal pain following inguinal hernia surgery. The person had received an open surgical technique using mesh repair under local anaesthetic. He had a 6 cms healed scar over the region of the hernia and described pain to this local region which he stated was like that from the hernia prior to surgery. He had been re-examined by his surgeon who confirmed that there had been no complications and the surgical technique had been successful. The person was instructed to perform an abdominal hollowing technique to engage the lower abdominal muscles in the region of this scar. The muscle contraction was monitored using surface EMG comparing the affected and unaffected sides. EMG feedback confirmed that he was able to perform abdominal hollowing on his non-affected side and tighten and relax the abdominal muscles at will. On the affected side he was able to tighten his abdominal wall but was not able to relax the muscles at will. It took 30–60 seconds of close focus before he was able to relax his muscles using EMG feedback (audible tone). Practicing daily initially using EMG feedback and then simply self practice the person was able to use the abdominal hollowing action to contract and relax his lower abdominal muscles voluntarily and his abdominal pain lessened and then disappeared. It is hypothesised that a low-level persistent muscle contraction was occurring which gave local ischaemic muscle pain. Teaching the person to switch the muscles off targeted the pain producing action.

Select some S factors

We have seen in Chapter 2 that there are a variety of aspects to the term fitness, with the S factors an easy way of viewing these. As we move from the reactive phase (R1) to the recovery phase (R2) our aim is to enable the person to return to their chosen activities pain free, confident, and without limitation. Enhancing physical fitness is one of many ways to achieve this, although as we saw in Chapter 1 improvement in symptoms of LBP is often unrelated to physical fitness changes directly. We have also seen that the act of performing an exercise may be more important than the physical adaptations it achieves. In general, if we can find exercises which reduce symptoms and/or make the person more confident to perform activities of daily living (ADL) or a chosen sport or pastime these can be used. They will influence general health and perhaps in parallel with this their spinal health as well.

In terms of performance in either sport or recreation, physical fitness attributes may be enhanced to improve execution of a task.

In this section, we will select some of the many hundreds of exercises which can be used to load the back directly or indirectly. Often in both therapy and the exercise professions, a mistake which can be made is to choose too many exercises or to change them too often. This can be confusing for people and erodes consistency which is a key component to training.

Keypoint:

Consistency is often the key to successful training. Don't change things too much or too often.

Strength

Hip hinge

Starting position:

Begin standing with your feet shoulder width apart. Your feet can be turned out slightly and your knees unlocked (soft knees).

Method:

Bending from your hips (keep your spine straight) angle your whole body forwards to 45° and then stand up straight again.

Points to note:

- The aim of this action is to learn to lower your shoulder towards the floor without bending your spine but moving instead from your hips.
- The pivot for this action is through the hips rather than the lower spine.
- This action can be used as a precursor to deadlift actions (see below).

Modifications and coaching:

- If you find it difficult not to bend your spine, place a pole (or foam roller) along the length of your spine holding it behind your head with one hand and behind your tailbone with the other. If your spine begins to bend, you will feel it against the pole.
- Placing your hands behind your back at the level of your tailbone (back of your hand, one on top of the other on the tail) can be a good method of cueing. When you begin, your fingers will point downwards to the floor, as you angle forwards to 45° your fingers should point to the wall behind you. If they are still pointing to the floor, you have not anteriorly tilted your pelvis.
- Visualising a waiter bowing can help avoid spinal flexion

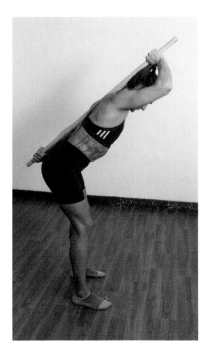
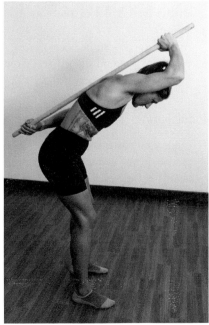

Lifting from the floor

Lifting from the floor is a common requirement. Ever since we evolved from quadrupeds to bipeds, we have needed to reach downwards for our food. We have seen in Chapter 4 that we can do this by bending the knees (squat lift), bending the spine (stoop lift) or a combination of the two which feels natural to us as individuals (free lift).

Starting position:

Begin by placing a tall (mid shin or knee height) object such as a rucksack or bag on the floor and stand with your feet either side of the bag, roughly shoulder width apart. If you don't have a suitable bag, place a box/stool or several cushions on the floor and put the object on top.

Method:

Bend forwards, bending from both your knees and your spine to lift the object. Stand up straight, pausing in the standing position before you bend down again to place the object on the floor or stool. Try to get more bend from your knees than from your spine.

Points to note:

*   The aim of putting the object on stool or using a taller object is so that you don't have to bend down as far. As you get used to the action you can bend all the way down to the floor using both knees (squat) and back (stoop) actions.
*   As you start to lift heavier objects, try to use your legs more, but still allow your back to bend slightly so that it is springy and not rigid as this reflects a more natural or functional action.

Modifications:

*   Once you master this action it can also be used with either a single dumbbell placed on end between the feet and lifting with both hands, or a dumbbell placed outside each foot and lifted in each hand.
*   When lifting two dumbbells, the exercise can change from strength (best in R2) to power (more suitable for R3) by using a jumping action.
*   If a person finds it difficult to bend from the hips, regress the exercise to a hip hinge (above) and perform that to begin. Move on from the hip hinge to hinging with the arms forwards, hands sliding on the thighs (called a *Monkey squat* Pilates exercise). Once the action is learned, the arms move off the thighs and the object can be grasped.

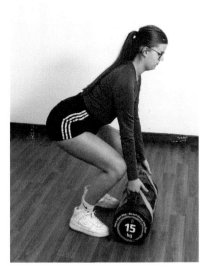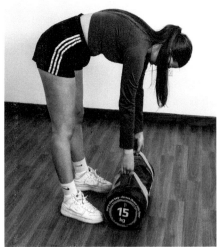

Classic deadlift

Starting position:

Classically this action is performed using an Olympic barbell, but it can also be performed with adaptation using two dumbbells or a single kettlebell and this may be more suitable in the early recovery (R2) phase for those unfamiliar with barbells.

Begin standing close behind a barbell resting on the floor. The bar will normally be loaded with Olympic plates which are typically 45 cms in diameter. Begin with it slightly forwards from your shins. Classically coaches say the bar should start over the front lace holes of your shoes, so it will rest against your mid shins as you bend down to grip it

If you are using smaller diameter weight plates (discs), you can rest them on blocks to bring them up to the same shin height. Your feet should be hip width apart and turned out slightly. The precise foot position should be made for comfort, and sometimes you will find one foot naturally turns out more than the other and that is fine. Grip the bar with your hand outside your legs knuckles on top (over-grasp). Again, the precise width is dependent on your body proportions and comfort.

Definition:

An *over-grasp* (overhand) grip is performed with your knuckles facing upwards, an *under-grasp* (underhand) grip with your knuckles facing downwards.

Method:

If you are lifting a heavy weight (more likely in the resilience phase R3 of the 3Rs approach), classically you would inhale deeply and hold your breath (Valsalva manoeuvre) but with lighter weights you can breathe in as you take hold of the bar and then out as you lift.

As you lift the bar, keep your arms straight and keep the bar in towards yourself as though trying to rub it against your shins. Try to lift the bar and your hips at the same time, do not lift your hips first.

Points to note:

- Your body angle should be roughly 45° to the floor as you grip the bar and will reduce on 0° (vertical) as you lift. If your body angle increases as you lift the bar from the floor, your hips have lifted before the bar.

Modifications and coaching:

- As the weight you lift increases, grip strength can limit this action so three methods may help. The first is to use an alternate grip, with one hand over grasp (knuckles up) and the other under grasp (knuckles down). The second is to use a hook grip where you grip the bar with the thumb first and then wrap your fingers on top of your thumb and around the bar. Finally, you can use lifting straps which hook around your wrist and wrap around the bar so that the bar is fatter and softer to grip.
- Placing your feet wider (usually about 1.5–2.0 times shoulder width) enables you to grip the bar inside your legs. This is them called a *Sumo deadlift* and changes the muscle action slightly.
- With a straight bar it is in front of you, but an alternative is to use a hex bar (trap bar) which is a frame you stand within. Now, the weight is aligned closer to your posture line and so there is less chance that you will be pulled into a flexed spine position.
- Where a subject leans over the bar or holds the bar too far forwards, the cue "pull up and in" can help.
- Where a subject bends their arms, have them lock their arms at the start and use the cue "push into the floor" creating an external focus.

Stiff legged deadlift

The stiff legged deadlift (also called a Romanian deadlift or RDL when modified) is a modification of the standard deadlift where the legs are held relatively immobile.

Starting position:

Begin standing close behind a barbell resting on the floor as above. Your feet should be shoulder width apart and normally not turned out so far as with a classic deadlift, but the precise foot position should be made for comfort. Grip the bar with your hands outside your legs knuckles on top (overgrasp). Your knees may be either locked out completely or bent slightly to unlock them.

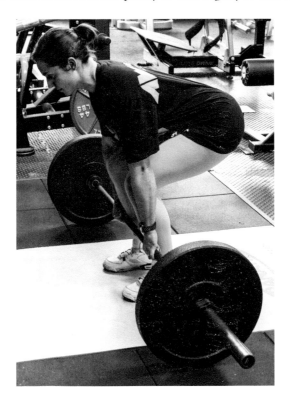

Method:

Keeping your knee stiff (don't increase their bend) hinge from your hips to lift the bar and then lower it back to touch the floor before lifting again.

Points to note:

- The action of hinging (see hip hinge exercise above) should occur at the hips and not the spine. Try to keep your spine rigid throughout the exercise.
- You require a high degree of flexibility in your hamstrings to enable you to lift from the floor with your knees locked. Build up to this by using a weight on blocks to begin with and gradually lower the blocks as your flexibility increases.
- In the classic RDL, the action begins from the standing position, and you hinge at the hips and lower the bar to below knee level, flexing the knees slightly. Before the bar touches the floor, stand back up again to avoid releasing the tension from the posterior chain muscles.

Modifications and coaching:

- If you are very flexible, you can do this action standing with a light weight on a box (wooden plyometric or 'plyo' box) with the weight discs touching the floor.
- Where a subject takes the weight too far forwards and begins to lift their heels, the cue 'wiggle your toes' or 'lift your toes' can help to throw the bodyweight back over the heels.

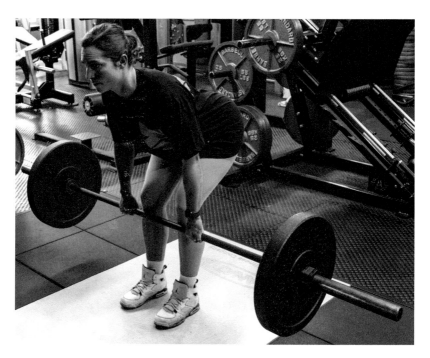

Roll down

Flexion, is often a co-factor in the instigation of LBP, be it flexing to lift, sitting in flexion, or combining flexion with side bending (lateral flexion). Little surprise then that many back-care programmes in the past have focussed on reducing the amount of flexion. We now know however that the spine has adapted to flexion and can be as resilient to this action as to any other (see Chapter 4). People are often fearful of flexion, partly because it may be painful in the early stages of recovery but also because popular health messages often demonise the action. Using flexion actions progressively throughout the 3Rs approach allows recovery and then builds resilience (mental and physical) to this action. The roll down is a useful exercise to introduce flexion in a controlled manner from a standing position and is often practised as a Pilates movement (partial or full roll down, see below).

Starting position:

Begin standing with your feet shoulder width apart and turned out slightly, arms by your sides. Allow your knees to unlock (soften) but keep them still (legs stiff) throughout the action.

Method:

Begin bending your spine from top down. Flex your neck as though trying to put your chin into the hollow at the top of your breastbone (jugular notch), continue the bend by aiming the tip of your nose towards your belly button (umbilicus). As you bend further aim to look between your legs so that the crown (top) of your head is pulled towards the floor. Hang in this low position for 1–2 seconds and then roll back beginning with the low back, middle back, upper back and finally the head. Pause is the standing position for 5 seconds to allow any light headedness to settle before repeating.

Points to note:

- To emphasise the trunk flexion (spine bending) action and distinguish it from the hip hinge (spine straight) stand close to a wall so that the bend prevents you from brushing your head against the wall (constrains based coaching—see Chapter 3).
- Imagine a sheet of glass in front of you. You must bend your trunk to avoid your head touching or going through the glass.
- As your bodyweight is taken forwards, your pelvis and hips will naturally move backwards to balance you. As your spine bends past the horizontal and into the lower position, your hips should come forwards again so that your hips are above your ankles in the final resting position with your head down.
- At the beginning of the exercise your weight should be taken equally between your toes and heals. As your weight shifts back, you will feel your weight move towards your heels. In the final position with your head down make sure you can again feel weight equally between your toes and heels.
- If you are uncomfortable having your head downwards or have a condition (such as glaucoma or hypertension) which makes this unsuitable, avoid using this exercise regularly.

Modifications:

- If you feel unsteady with this movement, stand in front of a firm chair (dining chair) or gym bench and place your hands on the bench as you bend down.
- As you gain confidence, slide your hands down the front of your thighs and then progress to the full movement with your hands hanging free.

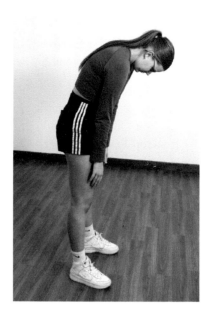

Jefferson curl

The Jefferson curl is really just a weighted roll down (above) which works both the spinal musculature and overloads the hamstrings in the final position. It is also a useful eccentric action to stretch the hamstrings, described as a *loaded stretch*.

Starting position:

Begin standing with your feet shoulder width apart and turned out slightly. Grip an unloaded barbell in both hands, with your arms by your sides. Allow your knees to unlock (soften) but keep them still (legs stiff) throughout the action.

Method:

Begin a roll down action with your spine (see above) bending your spine from top down. Flex your neck, upper spine, mid spine, and finally lower spine and hips aiming to look between your legs so that the crown (top) of your head is pulled towards the floor in the lowest position. Hang in this low position for 1–2 seconds and then roll back beginning with the low back, middle back, upper back and finally the head. Pause in the standing position for 5 seconds to allow any light headedness to settle before repeating.

Points to note:

- Using an Olympic barbell with 45cms weight on will stop you in the low position as the weights touch the floor. If you want to go further, begin the action standing on a firm box.

Modifications:

- This movement may also be performed using a single dumbbell or weight disc held in front of you.
- Hold the low position (full range) to focus the exercise as a *loaded stretch*. This type of stretching induces tensile strain on the muscle and can elicit muscle hypertrophy and architecture change (Nunes et al. 2020).

Definition:

A *loaded stretch* is essentially an eccentric contraction followed by an isometric contraction (holding) at full end range to form a type of static stretch.

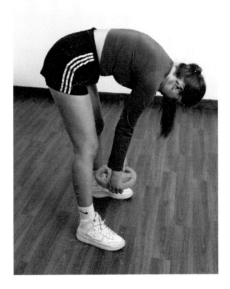

Stretching (flexibility)

Both the roll down and Jefferson curl are eccentric actions and so work for stretch and strength combined. However, sometimes you may want to work just for stretch with less load. This may be to alleviate pain or stiffness, or because your sport involves this type of held (static) stretching with bodyweight only. Here, we will look at some classic static stretches to affect the lumbo–pelvic region.

Kneeling arch and hollow

Starting position:

Begin kneeling on all fours, with your hands below your shoulders, and your knees below your hips (box position).

Method:

Focus your attention on your pelvis and tilt your pelvis backwards drawing your tummy button inwards and rounding your back. Pause, and then tilt your pelvis forwards, hollowing your back. Try to avoid moving your hips forwards and backwards, restrict the movement to your pelvis alone. As you progress, increase the range of motion to take in your whole spine. As your back hollows point your tail to the ceiling and look upwards. As your back rounds your point your tail downwards to the floor and look down towards your knees.

Points to note:

• This is a *voluntary* action which is easy if your spine is quite flexible. However, if your spine is very stiff you may need a partner to assist you with this movement in which case it changes is from a voluntary to a *passive assisted* movement.

• It is common to note stiffer regions within the spine. For example, some people find they are very mobile in their upper spine but quite inflexible in their lower spine. If this is the case, try to focus on the stiffer region to increase its flexibility over time.

Modifications:

• If you find this movement difficult to control work with a training partner.

• Have your partner loop a belt around your waist and stand above you. As you round your spine your partner pulls on the belt to increase the amount of spinal flexion and as you hollow your spine, they relax the belt to allow the increase in spinal extension.

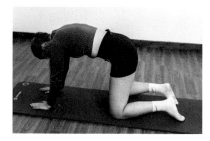 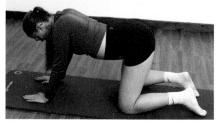

Standing pelvic tilt

Starting position:

Begin standing with your feet hip width apart and place your right hand flat on your lower tummy and your left hand flat on your lower back, to monitor movement.

Method:

Tilt your pelvis forwards dropping your tummy and pelvis down so that you increase the hollow in your low back. Pause and then tilt your pelvis up decreasing the hollow in your back so that you flatten the region.

Points to note:

- Initially you may feel little movement occurring but with each repetition try to increase the range of motion.
- Try to avoid thrusting your whole pelvis forwards instead limit the movement to pelvic tilt alone.

Modifications:

- If you find it difficult to limit the movement to the pelvis, perform the action with your back towards a wall. Place both hands in the small of your back and as you tilt your pelvis backwards you should feel your low back squeeze onto your hands. As you tilt your pelvis forwards you should increase the hollow between your back and the wall.
- Visualising your pelvis as a saucer or basin can be a useful internal cue. Tip the saucer forwards (anterior tilt) to allow the water to flow out of the saucer, pull back (posterior tilt) to stop the water.

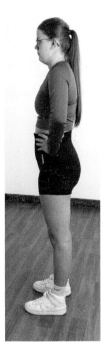

Lying active knee extension

Starting position:

Begin lying on your back on an exercise mat on the floor.

Method:

Draw your bent leg up towards hip level and grasp your hands behind your knee. Keep your thigh still by bracing your arms and try to straighten your leg leading with your heel. When you get to the maximum movement hold that position (breathing normally) for three to five seconds.

Points to note:

- If you point your toes with this exercise, you may get cramp in your calf muscles. For this reason, it is important to lead the movement with your heel (foot dorsiflexed).
- This action stretches the posterior thigh tissues including the hamstrings and sciatic nerve. Where the nerve movement is restricted or it is recovering from irritation or impingement, you can sometime get tingling in the leg. Providing these eases with repetition, it is fine.

Modifications:

- If you are unable to reach your hands around your thigh, loop a belt around instead and grip the ends of the belt in each hand.
- Alternatively, perform the exercise lying in a door frame. The straight leg on the floor passing through the door space, the lifted leg is placed on the door frame, and you slide your heel upwards taking leg weight on the frame. Shuffle your whole body forwards or backwards to allow for different movement ranges.

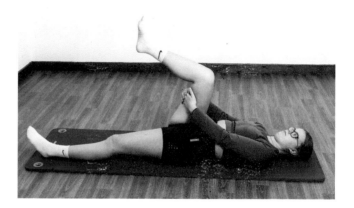

Slump stretch

Starting position:

Begin sitting on the edge of a treatment couch or gym bench with your feet off the ground.

Method:

Bend your trunk forwards as though putting your nose towards your tummy button and link your hands behind the small of your back. Straighten your right leg drawing your toes towards you. Hold this position for two seconds and then relax.

Points to note:

- Flexing the trunk winds up the spine and placing the hands behind the small of the back places stretch on the upper limb nerves. As you straighten your leg and dorsiflex your foot, you give the neural system a final wind up in the leg.
- You can split this movement up into three components. Perform the action just with the trunk and arms but without the leg. Perform the action just with the leg and trunk but without the arms. And finally, keep the trunk straight while you perform the action with your arm and leg simultaneously.
- This movement can be performed to stretch nerve (*extender* neural mobilisation) or to slide it (*slider* neural mobilisation).

> **Definition:**
>
> A *neural mobilisation* (neurodynamics) is a movement aimed at mobilising a nerve largely independent of other tissues.

Modifications:

- Place your foot on the floor on a shiny piece of paper (or skateboard!). Slide your heel forwards as you straighten your leg so that the leg weight is taken through the floor.
- Work with a partner to monitor and help control your movement.

Lying straight leg raise

Starting position:

Begin lying on the floor on a gym mat with both legs straight, arms by your side.

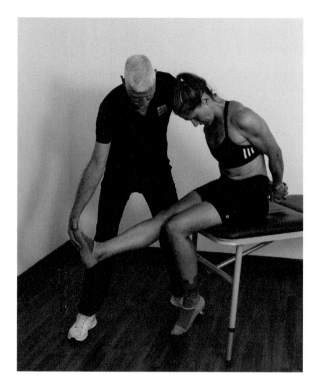

Method:

Keep your right leg straight and raise it (hip flexion) pointing your heel towards the ceiling. Hold this position for two seconds and then lower.

Points to note:

- This is an active movement of the hip flexors which through a reflex action will encourage the hamstrings (hip extensors) to relax further.

Modifications:

- The exercise can also be performed as a passive movement by looping a long belt (yoga belt) around the foot. Grip the belt in each hand and use your arm strength to lift the leg rather than your leg muscles.
- This action may also be performed with a partner as a passive stretch where the subject relaxes their leg and their partner lift the leg and performs the action.
- The passive action (above) may be changed to a *neural mobilisation* to reduce focus on the hamstrings muscles and increase focus on the sciatic nerve. Perform the straight leg action with ankle dorsiflexion and hip adduction.

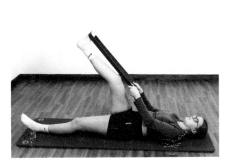 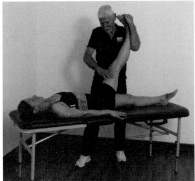

Mind-body exercise types

The popular exercise forms yoga and Pilates are often termed mind-body exercises. This is because they are claimed to involve more inner focus. Rather than exercising in a gym and listening to music or watching a video on a TV screen, for example, in a mind-body exercise the aim is to focus on the quality of each movement. For this reason, the movements are often slow and deliberate and there is a focus on breathing throughout the action. There are several similarities between yoga and Pilates and we will initially look at the exercise types themselves and follow this with some examples.

Originally based on Hindu teaching, yoga nowadays often represents an activity which combines both physical exercise and a mindful approach to movement. Participants are typically encouraged to pay attention to the sensations in their body during exercise with special attention to the breath, these two aspects often being central to mindfulness approaches used in stress management, for example.

> **Definition:**
>
> *Mindfulness* is a psychological term inherited from the Buddhist tradition. It is paying attention to the present moment in a non-judgemental way.

A typical yoga class often begins with a centring activity designed to act as a brake between the ADL and the focus required in the yoga class. The body of the class uses exercises or postures typically practised on a non-slip (sticky) mat and often uses basic props such as foam blocks, wooden bricks, and webbing belts. Exercises are practised in a number of starting positions including lying, floor sitting, chair sitting, kneeling, and both free and wall support standing. A yoga class will involve several postures progressing in intensity and finishing with a relaxation and/or meditation session. The postures are often held for a number of seconds and clients encouraged to relax and breathe normally. Postures are normally practised symmetrically with emphasis on good alignment as well as range of motion. In addition, counter poses are often used to prevent stress accumulation within the tissues. For example, postures emphasising spinal flexion are often countered by those emphasising extension. Body alignment when performing yoga is usually compared to an idealised version typically presented by a yoga book, organisation, or senior practitioner. Sometimes the reasoning behind the idealised postures lacks clear scientific evidence, so be prepared to vary a posture to suit your body.

Pilates is a method of exercise instruction whose popularity closely parallels the use of core stability in the rehabilitation of LBP. Originally developed by Joseph Pilates in the 1920s, the *classical* technique was mainly confined to the rehabilitation of dancers. These initial movements were modified and developed into a more widely available *contemporary* fitness form in the 1980s. Many of the exercises used will be familiar to any therapist using core stability work. Pilates exercises often use a number of key elements although normal breathing (avoiding breath holding), light tension within the core, and a focus on body alignment are most commonly emphasised. Many of these are similar to those used in yoga and there is much overlap between the two exercise forms (Table 8.2).

As we have seen throughout this text, LBP is a biopsychosocial condition with several interrelated co-factors. Mind-body exercises can be helpful, first because being popular they are often widely available, but second, by involving a component of mindfulness they are often useful forms of stress reduction which do not require separate practice. The action of mindful movement being sufficient and acting as a type of experiential learning.

Definition:

Experiential learning is the process of learning through experience and involves the user reflecting on what they are doing. It is the opposite of learning through direct instruction (Didactic learning).

TABLE 8.2 Key elements of Pilates and yoga practice

Pilates	*Yoga*
• Alignment	• Alignment
• Breathing	• Extension
• Centring	• Direction
• Concentration	• Stability
• Coordination	• Precision
• Precision	• Mindfulness
• Flow	

Source: Data from IYUK (2013), Modern Pilates (2017).

Triangle yoga pose

Starting position:

Begin standing on a yoga mat with your feet approximately one leg length apart toes facing forwards. Stretch your arms out sideways (shoulder abduction) keeping your elbows straight and palms facing the floor.

Method:

Turn your right leg outwards from your hip, so that your toes face the short edge of the mat. Reach your right hand out and downwards placing it onto your right shin, while at the same time reaching your left hand upwards towards the ceiling. Repeat the action on the left side of the body.

Points to note:

* Avoid allowing the left side of your pelvis to roll forwards. Keep the pelvis level so that the hip joints are stacked (right and left joints aligned in a vertical position).
* Open your chest (rib cage) and extend your thoracic spine.
* Reach with your left arm upwards and press with your right hand onto your shin to come out of the pose—do not just release the pose and collapse!

Modifications:

* Perform a limited range action taking the right hand down to a chair, placing your hand in the centre of the chair and keeping your arms straight.
* To increase range, further use a wooden yoga block placed with its long edge aligned vertically. The block should be aligned with your centre shin.

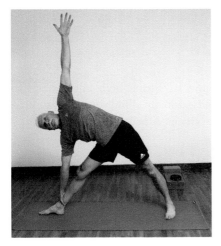
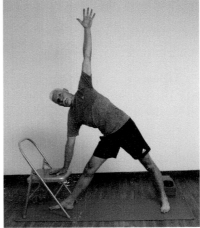

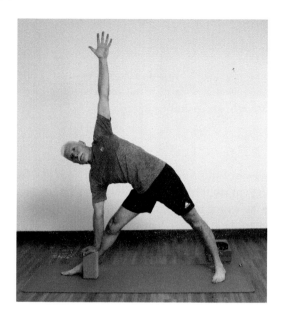

Downward dog yoga pose

Starting position:

Begin lying on your front on a yoga mat. Position your hands at the sides of your chest palms flat, as though preparing to do a press-up. Tuck your toes under tightening your quadriceps muscles to straighten and brace your legs.

Method:

Simultaneously press with your hands and feet driving your hips upwards. Keep pushing until your arms are straight and level with your ears, and your hips are as high as possible.

Points to note:

- Tighten your quadriceps and calf muscles lifting high onto your toes. Maintain this high pelvic position and gradually allow your heels to lower downwards placing a stretch on your calf and Achilles.

Modifications:

- Perform the action with your hands against a wall. Turn your arms outward (external rotation) so your thumb and index finger rest against the skirting board. Press hard against the wall to straighten your arms.

- Perform the action with a partner and have them loop a yoga belt around your waist (at hip level within the hip crease). Get them to stand behind you and assist by pulling upwards with the belt to emphasise a high hip position to straighten your spine and extend your arms.
- Pace your feet on blocks angled to 45° against a wall to reduce calf stretch and encourage pressing through your arms.

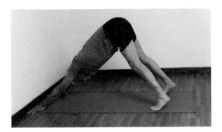 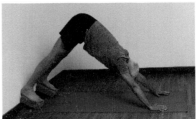

Cobra yoga pose

Starting position:

Begin lying on your front on a yoga mat with your feet together. Place your hands at the side of your chest with your palms downwards, as though beginning a press-up action.

Method:

Begin the exercise by drawing your shoulder blades back and down (retraction and depression). Extend your upper (thoracic) spine to lift your breastbone (sternum) from the mat. Press with your arms to continue the movement extending your spine throughout its full length. Hold the upper position for three breaths and then lower under control.

Points to note:

- The aim of this action is to move equally through the full length of the spine. Visualising lengthening the tailbone can help with this.
- Ensure that the lower back and buttocks (gluteals) remain relaxed to reduce muscle tension in this area.

Modifications:

- To help with the pushing action, work with a partner. Have your partner stand over you and place their hands beneath your armpits to assist you as you lift your chest and shoulders.

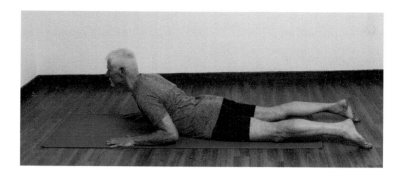

Bridge yoga pose

Starting position:

Begin lying on your back with your knees bent and feet flat, arms by your sides, palms facing downwards.

Method:

Press down with your hands and feet and lift your hips so that you form a straight-line from your shoulders through our hips, thighs, and knees. Hold the position for three breaths and then slowly lower under control.

Points to note:

*   Try to press equally with each foot so the pelvis is even at the highest point of the lift and not dipping to one side.

Modifications:

*   To reduce the work on the arms, lift into the bridge position and place several foam blocks or a single wooden block (standing on end) beneath your pelvis or tailbone (sacrum).

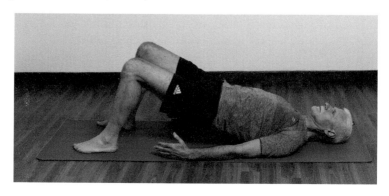

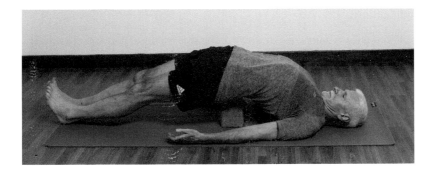

Standing body sway

The body sway (often simply called the Sway in Pilates) is a useful exercise to begin Pilates practice and is typically used at the start of a beginner's class. It teaches the subtleties of balance and encourages an internal focus to enhance body awareness.

Starting position:

Begin standing with your feet hip width apart and knees just short of full extension (knee soft). Hands by your sides.

Method:

First, sway your bodyweight forwards towards your toes, and then backwards towards your heels (*toe-heel sway*). Stop in the mid position when you have weight equally distributed between toes and heals. Next, sway your bodyweight from side to side taking more into your right leg and then more into your left (*side sway*). Again, stop in the mid position when you have equal weight distributed between both feet.

Points to note:

- It is common in the swayback posture to favour your dominant leg and take 80% of your bodyweight through this leg leaving only 20% through the normal dominant side.
- The aim of this exercise is to increase awareness of weight distribution so that there is some overflow into day-to-day activities to improve postural awareness and postural control.
- A useful visualisation is for the person to imaging they are standing on a rocking boat with the feet glued to the floor.

Modifications:

*   If you feel very unstable or dizzy doing this exercise, perform the movement against a wall with your arms out in front of you, hands flat on the wall (wall support standing).

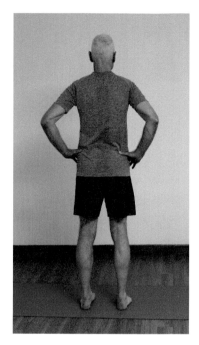 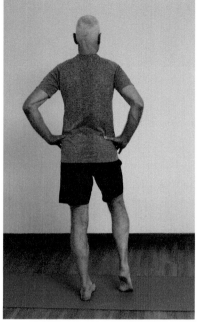

Partial roll down

Starting position:

Begin in a standing posture with your feet hip width apart hands by your sides.

Method:

Bend forwards moving from your spine, vertebra by vertebra initiating the movement from your neck and thoracic spine. Pause in your hands reach mid-thigh level and then roll your spine back up again moving vertebra by vertebra (*partial roll down*).

Points to note:

*   Try to get an even movement throughout your whole spine.
*   The upper thoracic spine is often very flexible, so try to reduce the contribution of this region and increase flexion in the lumbar spine.

- A useful visualisation is to imaging bending (flexion) the body over a beachball.

Modifications:

- Perform the partial roll down (above) and continue the movement reaching your arms down towards the floor allowing your pelvis to tilt as you do so. Aim to move throughout your whole spine vertebra by vertebra keeping your body close to your legs. Pause at full range without straining, and then reverse the movement rolling back up leading with the posteriorly pelvic tilt followed by spinal extension (*full roll down*).
- If you have very tight hamstrings, it is fine to unlock (soften) your knees to allow greater pelvic tilt.

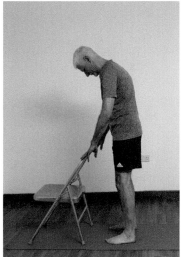 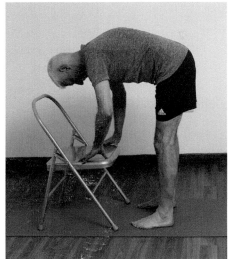

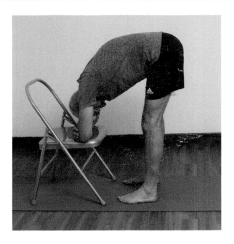

Dart

Starting position:

Begin lying on your front on a gym mat with a folded towel placed beneath your forehead. Hold your arms by your sides, palms facing inwards.

Method:

First, perform a *scapular squeeze* action by drawing your shoulder blades down (depression) and together (retraction). Lift your arms off the ground but keep your head on the floor. Hold the arm raise position for two seconds and then lower.

Points to note:

- This first action is called Dart preparation (prep)
- There is a tendency to hold your breath with this action. Try to avoid this and breathe normally throughout.

Modifications:

- Perform the scapular squeeze and arm lift as above and lift your trunk into minimal extension so your head and upper breastbone (sternum) clear the floor, but your lower sternum stays on the floor. This is the full Dart exercise

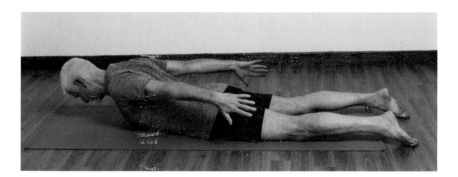

Threading the needle

Starting position:

Begin kneeling in the box position with your hands beneath your shoulders and knees beneath your hips.

Method:

Take your weight off your right hand (cat paw action), and then keeping your arm straight, move it outwards and upwards (abduction and extension) keeping your hand in line with your shoulder. Watch your hand as it goes upwards to provide rotation through the whole length of the spine. Pause in the upper position and then lower your hand back to the floor and across your chest between your left arm and left knee. Watch your hand throughout the movement to rotate your spine evenly. Rest and repeat the action with the left arm.

Points to note:

- The focus of this exercise is the spinal rotation. By watching the hand, the users' attention is taken away from the spine towards the moving arm. Ensure that spinal alignment is maintained, as there is a tendency to hyper extend the spine as the arm moves backwards and hyperflex it as it moves beneath the body.

Modifications:

- It is sometime easier to split this exercise into two separate actions, performing the arm in the air action, resting, and then performing the arm across the chest action.

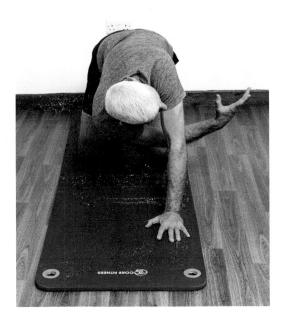

Shell stretch

Starting position:

Begin kneeling on all fours with your knees hip distance apart, hands slightly in front of your shoulder line.

Method:

Sit back towards your ankles, keeping your hands in position. As you rest your buttocks onto your ankles relax your head and place your forehead onto the mat. Move your arms to the sides of your body, palms upwards. Relax in this position focussing on lateral breathing.

Points to note:

- Where your ankles are very stiff, place a rolled towel beneath so that you do not need to flatten then completely (passive plantarflexion) as you sit back.
- Where your knees are stiff, place one or more cushions on your calves to raise your hips up when you sit back.

Modifications:

- Modify the position by widening your knees to 1.5 hip width and placing your toes closer together. Sit back onto your heels so that the sides of your rib cage rests on your knees, but your breastbone (sternum) passes between your knees. Reach your arms forwards placing your hands 1.5–2.0 times shoulder width apart, palms downwards.

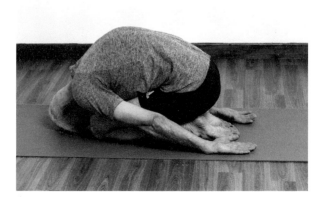

Balls and bands

Gym balls (Swiss gym ball) and bands are useful pieces of exercise equipment as they are relatively simple and widely available. They can be used for both resistance and to create instability by challenging the bodies balance. Many exercises (and indeed classes) can be offered using this type of equipment, but we will look at a few basic examples.

Sitting knee lift on gym ball

Starting position:

Begin sitting on a gym ball with your knees and hips at 90 degrees. Keep your feet shoulder width apart and flat on the floor. Sit tall, lengthening through the spine.

Method:

Initially, begin with your arms out into a T-shape to the side. Lift your right leg, maintain the balance, and then lower it back to the floor. Lift your left leg and repeat the movement aiming to keep sitting tall and to avoid rocking to the side as you lift your leg.

Points to note:

- If you find you wobble excessively perform the exercise next to a wall with one hand placed on the wall for support.
- The ball can be prevented from rolling and made more stable by placing in onto a support ring.

Modifications:

- Lift your legs repeatedly as though walking or running and pump your arms at the same time.

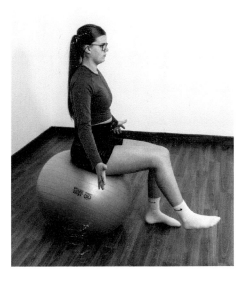

Gym ball bridge

Starting position:

Lie on the floor on a gym mat with a gym ball at your feet. Place both calf muscles on the gym ball with your knees 10 cm apart. Place your arms to your sides at a 45-degree angle to your body.

Method:

Press down with your calf muscles on to the gym ball to lift your hips. Maintain your stability by pressing your straight arms into the floor. Try to avoid your hips dipping, instead keep your hips level.

Points to note:

- This exercise gives intense work to the gluteal muscles and spinal extensors.
- As a useful teaching aid, work with a partner and pass a ball beneath your hips/buttocks in the high lift position. Progress endurance by passing the ball several times.

Modifications:

- Folding your arms will make your body less stable and so increases the challenge.
- When you are in the raised position, try rapidly pressing harder with one calf and then the other in a flutter action.

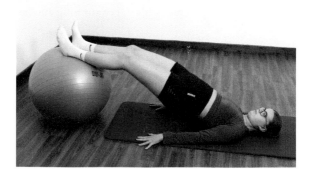

Gym ball wall squat

Starting position:

Begin with a gym ball placed on the wall behind you. Place your back on the gym ball with your feet flat on the floor. Keep your knees and feet shoulder width apart and turn your fee outwards slightly for comfort.

Method:

Perform a squat action (hack squat) rolling down the ball until your legs are at 90 degrees knee flexion and then push back up again.

Points to note:

- Keep your bodyweight pushing back into the wall throughout the action.
- You will need to shuffle up and down until you find the ideal position of the gym ball on your back.

Modifications:

- Perform a single leg gym-ball hack squat but placing one foot closer to your midline and straightening the other leg.
- Move your feet further forwards (away from the wall) or further back (towards the wall) to vary the work intensity in your leg muscles.

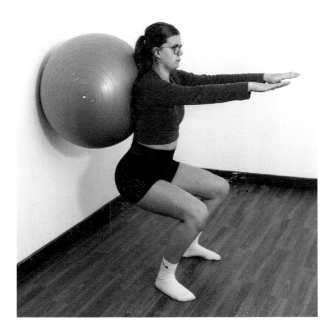

Pallof press

Starting position:

Begin standing side on to an exercise frame with a resistance band knotted around a frame upright. Hold the band in both hands and step away from the frame to pretension the band. Keep your feet shoulder width apart and knees slightly bent.

Method:

Maintain tension on the band and push your arms forwards and backwards in a pumping action. Aim to keep your trunk upright and do not allow the band to pull you in towards the frame.

Points to note:

- Standing further away from the frame will stretch the band further and increase resistance
- As the band pulls you towards the frame, it is important to perform the exercise facing in both directions.

Modifications:

- The Pallof press can also be performed in a kneeling position (high or 2-point kneeling).

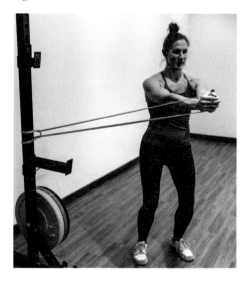

Band resisted trunk rotation

Starting position:

Begin standing in front of a gym rack with a band looped around the frame up right. Hold the band in both arms and keep the arms stiff throughout the movement.

Method:

Keep the knees slightly bent (soft) and turn the hips and shoulders as one unit to the right, hold the position and then turn to the left.

Points to note:

- Ensure that the arms move with the trunk as a single unit rather than simply performing a cross body shoulder action.
- This action can also be performed from a sitting action with the feet firmly on the floor to give the body purchase, or in kneeling.

Modifications:

- Perform the action using an adjustable pulley set at chest height.

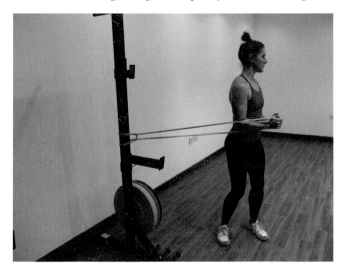

Yes, but is it functional?

Functional training mimics everyday activities and includes actions such as pushing, pulling, bending, lifting, and carrying. In reality, any movement may be functional depending on the daily requirements of an individual. However, functional movements are typically whole body and rarely use weight training machines. They may be introduced at any stage of a programme, but in the 3Rs approach they tend to begin in the recovery (R2) phase and their use is continued into the resilience phase (R3). Actions such as the deadlift may be termed functional, but here, the same action is used with a bag lift.

Functional lift

We saw when looking at lifting techniques we could perform a *squat* lift where the back was straight, or a *stoop* left where the back was flexed. A more functional or realistic version is a freestyle left which combines movements at the leg and spine. In a *freestyle* left the person decides on the optimal body position for their own comfort.

Starting position:

Begin the lift with a weight (bag or kettlebell) positioned on the floor between your feet or on a lift on one side of you.

Method:

Bend over and lift the weight from the floor to chest height. Walk four or five paces and then place the bag back down on the ground again.

Points to note:

- Initially this action is performed slowly, but as confidence builds the speed of the movement can increase as can the number of repetitions to build endurance

Modifications:

- Practise lifting with the bag at one side of the feet or positioned at different heights such as a step bench or low stool.
- Practise lifting down from/to a high point such as a shelf or cupboard top at head height.

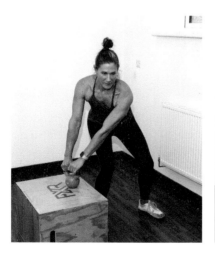 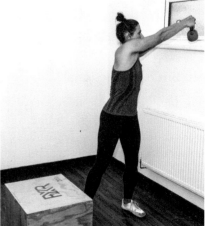

Bear hug carry

Starting position:

The bear hug carry exercise is essentially a bag lift where the bag is carried in a position held against the chest. Begin with the bag on the floor.

Method:

Lift the weight bag to waist and then chest height gripping the bag closely onto the rib cage. Walk forwards by 10 paces turn and walk back placing the bag back onto the floor once again.

Points to note:

- The lift action is performed a split second separately to the carry initially. Eventually, both actions may be carried out simultaneously.

Modifications:

- Perform the same action but weave in and out between cones or climb up and down a short staircase.

Wall push

Pushing and pulling actions should see the force for the movement created by the legs, transferred through the spine and torso and delivered by the arms and hands. However, if the spine lacks stability and moves as you push or pull, some of the force created by the legs is lost and the action becomes less effective. The analogy here is a car tyre sliding on ice. If you put your foot on the car accelerator and the tyres grip against the road surface, you will move forward efficiently. However, if the car tyre grips on an icy road surface, however hard you push your foot on the accelerator much of the forward motion will be lost as skidding. The key here is that in this movement you need both stability and force production and the same is true for pushing and pulling.

> ### Keypoint:
>
> When pushing or pulling, trunk stability provides a firm base for the limbs to act upon.

Starting position:

Begin standing in front of a wall with your right foot back. Place your hands flat on the wall, fingers pointing upwards and lock your arms out straight.

Method:

Use your legs to drive your body forwards into the wall, ensure that your hips are kept low and that the power for the movement comes from your legs alone.

Points to note:

- Your back should stay relatively straight and stiff throughout the movement do not allow your spine to extend as you produce the power from your legs.
- Change legs placing the left foot back and repeat the action.

Modifications:

- Place a cushion or Swiss gym ball on the wall and press into that rather than the hard wall.

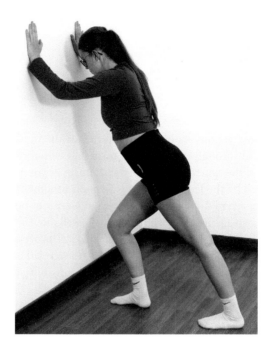

Resisted walk on the spot

Starting position:

Stand in front of a gym rack with a resistance band fastened around a rack support. Hold the gym band in both hands against your body or place it around your waist.

Method:

Place your right foot forwards and sit back slightly to pretension the band. Walk on the spot lifting your right and then left legs maintaining your body position. Perform 5 repetitions and then reverse the movement placing your left foot forwards.

Points to note:

- The aim of this action is to mimic a pulling movement driving with your legs and maintaining a stable core as you push with your legs. Try not to flex and extend your spine.

Modifications:

- Once you can perform this action with good technique using the resistance band, you are ready to progress to a sled all prowler machine (Chapter 2).

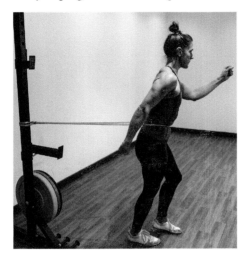

References

Gomes-Neto, M., Lopes, J. M., Conceição, C.S., et al. (2017). Stabilization exercise compared to general exercises or manual therapy for the management of low back pain: A systematic review and meta-analysis. *Physical Therapy in Sport* 23: 136–142.

Hides, J.A., Stokes, M.J., Saide, M., et al. (1994). Evidence of lumbar multifidus muscle wasting ipsilateral to symptoms in people with acute/subacute low back pain. *Spine* 19(2): 165–172.

IYUK (2013). *Teacher training manual. Iyengar yoga UK*. East Sussex: Southview Close.

Jull, G.A., and Richardson, C.A. (1994). Rehabilitation of active stabilization of the lumbar spine. In Twomey, L.T. and Taylor, L.T., Eds., *Physical therapy of the low back* (2nd ed). Edinburgh, UK: Churchill Livingstone, 34–41.

Modern Pilates. (2017). *Diploma in teaching Pilates (YMCA award). Professional fitness and education*. New York: Leeds.

Norris, C.M. (1995). Spinal stabilisation 2. Limiting factors to end-range motion in the lumbar spine. *Physiotherapy* 81: 4–12.

Nunes, J.P., Schoenfeld, B.J., Nakamura, M., et al. (2020). Does stretch training induce muscle hypertrophy in humans? A review of the literature. *Clinical Physiology and Functional Imaging* 40(3): 148–156.

Smith, B.E., Littlewood, C., and May, S. (2014). An update of stabilisation exercises for low back pain: A systematic review with meta-analysis. *BMC Musculoskeletal Disorders* 15: 416.

9

RESILIENCE PHASE

The resilience phase (R3) of the 3Rs approach is the stage where we build toughness, both physical and mental (see Chapter 6). It is a progression on the reactive and recovery phases, but resilience is built from the very first meeting with a person as part of the therapeutic alliance, as confidence and self-efficacy is enhanced. In this chapter, we are looking at resilience as part of an ongoing rehabilitation process where we have progressed from treatment (targeting a pathology) to wellness (targeting the whole person). The approach underlies the biopsychosocial (BPS) model of healthcare.

By now, the subject has returned to normal daily function, and it is time to increase movement variability, boost confidence, and push for independence. In the resilience phase the subject is self-paced and self-correcting exercise. They may be coached, but the coach will be motivating and teaching advanced exercise techniques where required.

We will introduce more of the 'S' factors having built sufficient training effect in the three basic components, strength, stretch (flexibility), and stamina (endurance). The subject has regained their former motion range of the spine and hips, can perform exercise for an extended time (typically greater than 15 minutes) and rebuilt strength to pre-injury levels. Now, we can introduce speed and skill-based actions and use drills such as change of direction (COD) having introduced lifting, pushing, and pulling in the recovery phase (R2).

Exercises in the resilience phase (R3) build on the functional aspects of the recovery phase (R2) and activity choice will reflect person demands in terms of lifestyle and/or sport. In addition, building confidence develops from graded exposure to fear producing actions revealed in previous phases.

DOI: 10.4324/9781003366188-9

Deadlift variations

We saw the deadlift in the recovery phase (R2) in Chapter 8. Now, in the resilience phase (R3) we continue training using the deadlift to enhance posterior chain performance and introduce further deadlift variations.

Definition:

The *posterior chain* consists of soft tissues on the back (dorsum) of the body creating active and passive force. It consists of muscles (calves, hamstrings, gluteals, erector spinae, latissimus dorsi, trapezius, cervical extensors), ligaments (supra & infraspinous and posterior longitudinal ligaments) and fascia (thoroco-lumbar fascia [TLF] and its connections).

Deadlift variations are shown in Table 9.1. As we saw in Chapter 8, when performing a deadlift, the upper body (chest and arms) and lower body (legs) should move at the same speed. A common mistake is to move the hips first and "leave the bar behind" meaning that the trunk angles further towards the horizontal. Alternatively, if the upper body moves first forming a hinge action, power from the legs is reduced. As heavier weights are lifting now in the resilience phase (R3) the back stays straighter and braced throughout the action. Lifts from the floor where the back bends (Roll-down and Jefferson curl) are performed with bodyweight or lighter weights and target strength and flexibility. Now, we are aiming to build strength, so the weight lifted is heavier.

As the chest lifts, the breastbone (sternum) should lead the movement. A common mistake is to look up and lead with the head. The action should be to tuck the chin in (skull rock action) and keep the head still. Further, as the chest lifts, the back should remain fairly wide rather than drawing the shoulder blades together.

TABLE 9.1 Deadlift variations

Name	Overview
Conventional	Feet hip width apart, hands just outside feet
Sumo	Wide stance with hands inside the legs
Hex/Trap bar	Specialist frame keeping barbell closer to posture line
Rack pull	Lift from higher point—bar off ground
Deficit	Stand on blocks to lift from lower point—feet off ground
Romanian (RDL)	Legs straight initially, knees bend as bar passes below knee. Barbell stays off the floor
Stiff leg (SLDL)	Legs stay stiff (knee unlocked) and barbell touches the floor
Snatch grip	Wider hand grip on bar

Starting position:

For the *conventional* deadlift, place your midfoot beneath the bar so that your shin is about 2 cm behind the bar (this will allow the bar to stay close, but not strike the shin during the lift and roll the bar forwards). The grip is overgrasp (pronated) or alternate undergrasp (supinated) on the one hand and overgrasp on the other.

Method:

With a heavy weight it is common to inhale deeply and hold the breath (Valsalva manoeuvre). Although widely taught and used in competitive powerlifting, there are considerations for less fit individuals or those who have pathologies such as hypertension (high blood pressure), glaucoma (high pressure within the eye), or respiratory conditions so this action can be varied. Take up slack in your body by initially pulling against the barbell without trying to lift it.

To begin the lift, drive the heels into the ground and sit back into the lift (weight over heels rather than onto toes). The first part of the lift aims to start the static barbell moving (break its inertia) and this should be a squeeze rather than a jerk. Aim to keep the barbell moving in a vertical path, and once it moves past your knees drive your hips forwards and into the bar while raising the chest. Lower the bar under control to touch the weight plates on the floor in preparation for your next repetition (rep). Do not bounce the bar on the floor to make the next rep easier!

Points to note:

- Your shoulders will move back naturally and there is no need to shrug (elevate) or drive your shoulders back (retract).
- If you have held your breath, exhale at the end of the rep and inhale again. Do not hold your breath for several reps.

Modifications and coaching:

- For the *Sumo deadlift*, take a wide stance (width dependent on comfort) and turn your feet out. Your arms are straight so there is a vertical line from shoulders through your elbow to your wrist and hand, and your arms are between your legs.
- For the *Hex bar deadlift*, you stand within a specially shaped bar rather than behind it, and your hands grip handles facing forwards which are usually higher up providing a reduced motion range to the lift. As a result of the improved mechanics of the lift, generally heavier weights can be lifted compared to the conventional deadlift.
- For the *Romanian deadlift (RDL)* begin at the top of the lift (standing) and allow the barbell to slide down the thighs until it is below your knees and

then flex (unlock) the knees slightly. The barbell is lifted again before it touches the floor, so the motion range is less than the SLDL (below) but the time under tension (TUT) greater.

- With the *Stiff legged deadlift (SLDL)* the knee is locked straight or unlocked but held immobile and the action is a hinge of the hips with no knee movement. In contrast to the RDL the barbell touches the floor, allowing muscle recovery before the next rep.
- For the *Rack pull deadlift* the barbell is placed off the ground on the pins of a rack to reduce the range of motion. For the *deficit deadlift,* the lifter stands on a platform (typically weight discs) to raise them up from the floor and increase the range of motion.

Definition:

Time under tension (TUT) is the amount of time a muscle is loaded (under tension) during a movement. Longer TUT works the muscle harder.

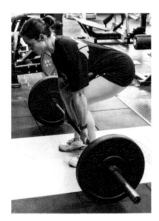
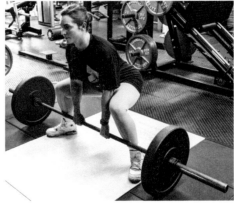
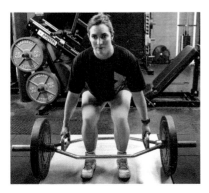
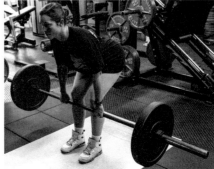

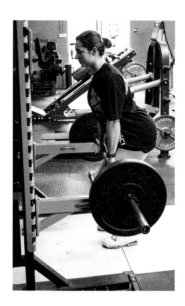

Squat variations

The squat action simply involves bending both knees simultaneously from a standing position and may be performed in several variations (Table 9.2). The *bodyweight squat* (also called a free squat or air squat) is a squat without resistance. It is often used as part of an aerobic circuit or warm up prior to performing a resisted action. As with any squat the range of motion (ROM) may be varied. A conventional depth is where the thigh is parallel to the floor and the kneecap (patella) level with the hip crease (inguinal crease), while a full squat involves the user going lower until they make soft tissue contact between the thigh and calf (colloquially termed 'arse to grass'). Practically, it is often better to be guided by comfort as a person will often find their optimal alignment themselves.

Foot position is again guided by comfort, but normally taught with the feet shoulder width apart and feet turned out. Be aware that due to hip dysplasia it is

TABLE 9.2 Squat variations

Name	Overview
Bodyweight	Squat action without additional loading
Back	Barbell across shoulders and behind neck
Front	Barbell across front of shoulder and in front of throat
Hack	Barbell behind legs with arms straight
Goblet	Dumbbell held at chest height and positioned vertically
Box	Squat to touch buttocks onto box
Overhead	Barbell held overhead. Wide (snatch) grip with arms locked.

common for one hip to turn further than the other, and equal ROM should not be forced. As the knee is bent the aim is to guide the knee over the foot to avoid a pronounced valgus (knock knee) knee alignment which can place medial stress on the joint. This can cause irritability in novice users, but where it has been used consistently adaptation will have occurred, so it is not usually a problem.

Once the bodyweight squat has been used, the progression can be to a *goblet squat* where a dumbbell or kettlebell is held on the chest in both hands. The forearms as aligned close to vertical, and the elbows dropped inwards so they will not strike the inside of the knee as the squat is performed.

The back squat

The *back squat* is probably one of the most used techniques in a gym and is traditionally performed with an Olympic barbell held across the back of the shoulders. It is one of the three lifts used in competitive powerlifting (squat, deadlift, and bench press) so is often considered a fundamental exercise.

Starting position:

Stand with your feet shoulder width apart the turned out to approximately 20°. Place the bar across your shoulders. If you find the bar digs into your skin, use a pad (folded towel or foam pad).

Method:

Grip the bar 1–2 hand widths wider than your shoulders and pull the bar down onto your shoulders to brace. Take a deep breath and hold it (Valsalva manoeuvre). Bend your knees aiming to keep the bar over the middle of your foot (mid-foot). Descend until your thighs are parallel with the ground (kneecaps level with hip crease), and then ascend by driving your shoulders into the barbell and pressing your feet into the floor.

Points to note:

- In the lower position, do not stop but instead create a small bounce using the stretch of the muscles (stretch reflex) to initiate the ascent.
- Pull the barbell firmly onto your shoulders as though trying to bend the bar.

Modifications and coaching:

- Hold the bar either level with the lower neck (high bar position) resting on the Trapezius muscles or help over the upper thoracic spine (low bar position) resting over the rear Deltoids.

- When taking the bar from a rack, the initial movement is to lift the bar upwards and off the rack J hooks. Pause and then step back using two definite steps and pause again to set your balance before performing the squat.
- Taking too many steps back or initiating the squat when you are recovering from the step back risks overbalancing.
- Perform a *box squat* by having a wooden plyometrics box or gym bench behind you. Touch your thighs (hamstrings) onto the box (but do not sit back onto your gluts) in the lower position and then stand back up again.
- Where you find the bar position uncomfortable even with padding due to shoulder flexibility or spine conditions, use a squat safety bar (SSB) which is an angled bar with forward facing handles to grip.

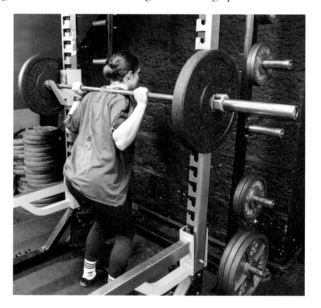

The front squat

The front squat is an alternative to the back squat and for some people, a more technical movement. It has its roots in Olympic lifting where it is receiving position (front rack) following execution of the clean action (pulling the bar from the floor to the shoulders) prior to the jerk (pressing the bar from the shoulders to an overhead position).

Starting position:

Begin with the bar on the front of your shoulders. Your hands are positioned just outside shoulder level, palms under, and elbows raised (called the front rack position). The bar rests on your open fingers and anterior deltoid muscles.

Method:

Lift the bar off the rack by dipping your knees and then pressing upwards. Take a deep breath and hold and then initiate the squat by bending your hips and pressing your hips backwards. Guide your knees over your feet and as with the back squat above, use a small bounce at the bottom of the movement to initiate the ascent.

Points to note:

- The advantage of the front squat over the back squat is that the front squat allows you to remain more upright (spine vertical, chest raised) and there is less tendency to hinge at the hips.
- Drive your feet into the floor and lead with your upper chest (sternal lift action) and you move upwards.

Modifications and coaching:

- The front rack position requires a fairly high degree of shoulder flexibility to obtain. Where this is uncomfortable substitute a cross-arm position for the front rack hold.
- As an alternative, keep your arms outstretched forwards and balance the bar on your shoulders (*Zombie squat*). As you squat, your arms should stay horizontal (chest held high) to avoid the bar slipping forwards out of the shoulder crease.

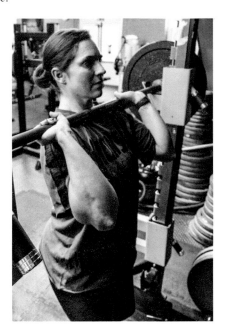

Overhead squat

Starting position:

The *overhead squat* is essentially the standard back squat but with a bar held over-head in a snatch position. It demands quite a high degree of shoulder flexibility and because of this, is often performed with a pole or PVC pipe to establish the technique before a bar is used.

Begin hold a pole or bar in a snatch width grip. This is a wide grip usually measured so the bar rests at your hip crease (just above your pubis) with your arms are straight and held downwards.

Method:

Begin with your feet shoulder width apart and feet turned out (Back squat position—see above). Press your hands into the bar to lock out the elbows and keep pressing towards the ceiling as you bend your hips and knees to your maximum position. Aim to keep your torso upright (vertical) throughout the movement.

Points to note:

- If your grip is too wide, it can place stress on your wrist due to the altered wrist joint angle. Experiment with the optimum grip for your comfort.
- Begin by squatting to a point where your hip remains above your knee. Progress to a lower squat as you improve. Eventually, the full Snatch position is with the thighs and calves in contact.

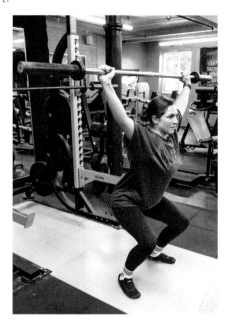

Modifications and coaching:

- Using the cue "stretch the bar" can be helpful to keep the elbow locked.
- Using the external cue "push through the ceiling" helps to maintain body length and upright trunk angle.

Lunge actions

A lunge is performed with one leg forwards (unilateral action) compared to a squat where the legs are alongside each other (bilateral action). The exercise is performed by taking a single step into a stride position. A *forward lunge* steps forwards, while a *lateral lunge* steps sideways. A *split squat* is a similar action, but rather than stepping forwards using load, the action is to lower the loaded body downwards. If the rear foot is placed on a gym bench or step, this is a *rearfoot elevated split squat* or Bulgarian split squat.

Starting position:

Begin standing with your feet shoulder width apart. Either have your hands by your sides or behind your head (bodyweight lunge). Alternatively hold a dumbbell in each hand or a single dumbbell or kettlebell at your chest (loaded lunge).

Method:

Step forwards with your right foot and lower your left knee to the ground. Stand back up and step your right foot back to the starting position. Step forwards with your left and lower your leg knee to the ground, stand back up and return to the start.

Points to note:

- Keep your feet apart as you step. Imagine standing on the short edge of a rectangle, and as you step, move along the long edge, do not cross the mid-line.

Modifications and coaching:

- Rather than stepping back and then stepping forwards again, step forwards as you stand. This is a *walking lunge*, and the length of your pace can be varied to alter flexibility requirements and for comfort.
- Using a lightweight bar across your shoulders (back squat position) is an alternative way of adding resistance. Keeping the bar horizontal is an additional method of feedback.
- Staying in one place and performing several reps moving down each time (not changing legs) changes the lunge into a *split squat*. Perform the same number of reps with each leg.

- For variation, either the front foot or back foot may be elevated by placing it onto a step bench or gym bench. Elevating the rear foot (*Bulgarian split squat*) focusses on the gluteal muscles, while elevating the front foot enables the front shin to remain more vertical.
- A *step-up* is performed by placing one foot flat onto a bench and stepping up with the other. Step down with the first leg and repeat.

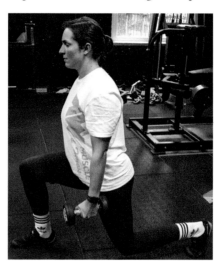

Bridge actions

Starting position:

The bridge action is performed from a lying position with the knees bent (crook or hook lying). In Chapter 8 (recovery phase), we used the shoulder bridge in several phases and eventually moved to the single leg bridge.

Method:

Lie on the floor with your knees bent and feet flat on the floor. Have your knees hip width apart. For the standard bridge lift your hips and keep your arms on the floor for support. Progress the exercise by raising your arms and reaching towards the ceiling. Finally, straighten one leg and keep the other bent but place your foot more central. Now, the action is to push with one leg only to perform a *single leg bridge*.

Points to note:

- Progress the exercise by holding a weight disc on your tummy.
- Make the exercise harder by placing your foot on an unstable surface such as a balance board or Bosu.

Modifications and coaching:

- Perform the action with your shoulders on a bench and a barbell placed across your hips, to perform a *hip thrust* (glute bridge) exercise. Use a pad or folded towel beneath the bar for comfort.
- A similar bridging action may be performed in prone on a specialist machine called a glute-hamstring-deck (GHD) or spinal extension unit (see below).

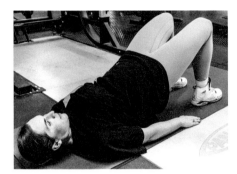
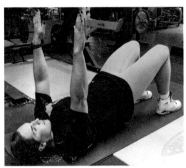

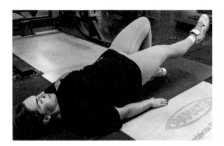
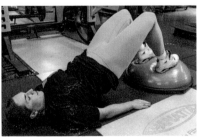

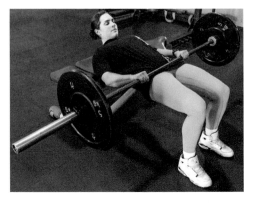
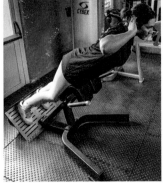

Chopping actions

Chopping actions combine trunk rotation with a pulling action. They can be performed with a pulley machine or resistance band. The woodchop action pulls from above head height (*standard wood chop*) or from the ground (*reverse woodchop*). Torso twist actions (see below) are similar to chopping but the arms do not move relative to the body.

Starting position:

Begin facing left side on to a high pulley machine with your feet shoulder width apart and knees slightly bent (soft). Turn your trunk towards the machine and grip the D handle with both hands, taking any slack out of the cable by adjusting your body position and moving your feet slightly.

Method:

Keeping your elbows stiff (slightly flexed but immobile), turn your torso to the right (away from the machine) while at the same time pulling the handle down and across your body towards the floor to your right side. Pause briefly and then reverse the action to lower the weight again. Perform the same number of reps facing in each direction.

Points to note:

- The action combines torso rotation with shoulder movement and movement at the hips. The knees and ankles flex slightly to accommodate the movement.
- When using a pulley machine, rapid movement builds momentum in the weight stack, so it is important to lower the weight under control and not allow it to drop.
- When using resistance bands, the resistance is greater as the band is stretched. For this reason, it is important to control the movement and torso angle as you turn back and release the chopping action. Failure to do so can cause your body to be pulled towards the machine (lateral flexion).

Modifications and coaching:

- For the *reverse woodchop*, grip the D-handle of a low pulley machine and pull upwards to a point at the ceiling away from the machine.
- The woodchop can also be performed using a dumbbell or heavy club. This changes the emphasis as trunk rotation is no longer resisted by the pulley or band. Instead, the momentum of the heavy object must be controlled as it is a ballistic action.

Definition:

A *ballistic action* is a rapid explosive movement which features acceleration and deceleration phases. Between these two phases, the object moves through its own momentum requiring less muscle force.

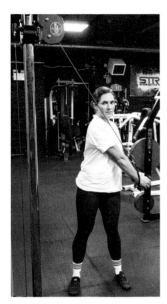 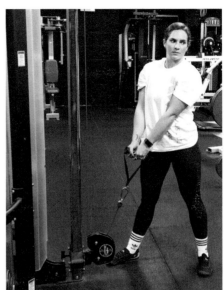

Pulling up actions

Pulling actions either lift the bodyweight from a hanging position or reverse the action by pulling a weight from above you downwards to your body. The *pull-up* (forearms pronated, knuckles facing user) and *chin-up* (forearms supinated, knuckles facing away from user) are the most common bodyweight actions. The *lat pull down* (lateral or latissimus pull) also called a wide grip pulldown and its modifications are the most common machine pulldown exercise. This type of action works the latissimus dorsi (which attaches into the thoroco-lumbar fascia or TLF) and posterior shoulder muscles and so is a good upper core action.

Starting position:

Where the exercise is performed using a lat pull machine, adjust the seat height for comfort and the thigh grips to fit your leg bulk and knee angle. Grip the bar using a comfortably wide grip, forearms pronated, and fingers closed. Either sit down on the seat of a lat pull machine or kneel in front of the high pulley where not using a specialist machine.

Method:

Keeping the torso relatively still (do not rock) pull the bar downwards to your upper chest. Pause in this position and then lower the weight under control. Repeat the action to perform your reps.

Points to note:

- When you pull to the upper chest, there will be a slight backward trunk angle throughout the movement.
- As an alternative, you can lean forwards and pull the bar behind your head. This requires greater motion range (lateral rotation) at the shoulder. Ensure that long hair is tied back so it cannot catch around the bar, and do not strike your neck with the bar.
- Alternative grip width may be used to vary the training effect. A chin-up (pronated) or pull-up (supinated) grip is slightly wider than shoulder width. A narrow grip (approximately 20 cms) may also be used with a straight bar or a specialist row bar.

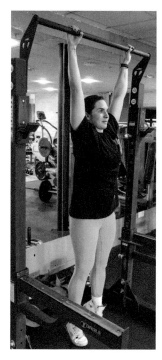 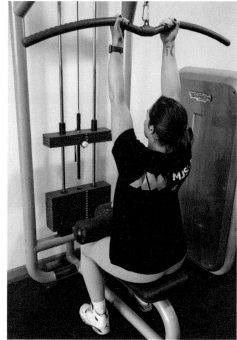

Modifications and coaching:

- Using a *wide grip* keeps the elbows away from the side of the torso, while a *narrow grip* brings the elbows in to brush the side of the ribs.

- Where gripping the bar with a narrow grip is uncomfortable, an alternative is to loop a hand towel around the cable and centre of the wide bar in a U-shape. You can then grip the towel which varies the hand position and prevents the hands from slipping.
- When performing a *chin-up* or *pull-up* step on a stool to reach the bar and grip it at the required width. Where you cannot lift your bodyweight, use a *resistance band* looped around the bar and stretch it down to place around your knee or loop around your foot. As you descend, the band is stretched, and its recoil assists your ascent (banded pull-up).

Rowing actions

Rowing actions pull a bar or pulley from in front of you towards your chest. The *barbell bent over row* using a hinge position, while the *one-arm dumbbell row* is performed with the trunk supported on a bench. *Seated rows* performed on a low pulley machine or using a resistance band.

Starting position:

For the bent-over row stand with your feet shoulder width apart. Grip the bar with a pronated grip, hands slightly wider than shoulder width apart. Hinge from your hips (hip hinge action Chapter 8) angling your body to approximately 45°. The torso angle is usually mid-way between vertical (standing) and horizontal (torso flat) but should be varied for comfort as body height and arm length variations dictate the optimum torso angle.

Method:

Maintaining your torso angle (do not sway excessively) pull the bar towards yourself, touch it to your lower chest or upper abdomen. Allow the bar to lower to the straight arm position and repeat your reps.

Points to note:

- When using lighter weight, you can pull the bar higher up your body to touch your lower chest or breastbone (sternum).

Modifications and coaching:

- When performing the *seated row*, sit with your knees bent and torso upright. If using a specialist machine place your feet on the footplates, but if performing the action using a low pulley or resistance band attached at floor height, place your feet flat on the floor. Pull towards your chest, drawing your elbow outwards to contact your breastbone.

- For the *single arm dumbbell row* grip a dumbbell in one arm and lean over a bench supporting your upper body weight with your other arm. Your knees can be slightly bent, or you can place one knee on the bench to allow your torso to be straight. Pull the dumbbell towards yourself brushing the side of your ribs with your elbow.

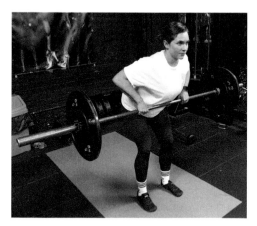 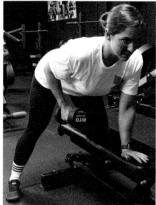

Overhead pressing

Overhead pressing actions involve pushing a weight or resistance band into an overhead position. The classic *military press* is a push from the top of the chest with the knees locked out straight. Bending (dipping) the knees gives momentum to the bar to assist the action and is called a *push press*. If the bar is held behind the neck, the shoulder motion range (lateral rotation) is greater, and this is the *press behind neck*.

Starting position:

Begin with the barbell on the upper chest, hands gripping to the outside of the shoulders. Use a loose (false) grip so the barbell rests on the base of your palm and your fingers are curled but not gripping. Drop your elbows so your forearms are closer to a vertical pushing position.

Method:

Press the barbell directly upwards, pulling your chin inwards slightly to enable it to pass your chin. Do not allow the barbell to move forwards to avoid your chin as it creates a less effective push. Lock your elbows and hold the bar overhead, before lowering under control back to the starting position.

Points to note:

- The width of the hands is best judged by comfort. If they are relatively narrow (close to the ear) the push direction is directly upwards (vertical). A wider grip (closer to the weight discs) takes the action to a snatch position (called a *snatch press*). This is harder as the push is more oblique but does represent the position in which a snatch is performed, so it is perhaps more functional for this action.

Modifications and coaching:

- Placing the bar behind the neck in a back squat position demands greater lateral rotation range at the shoulder. However, it gives a more direct press without having to avoid the chin and is classically used for the *snatch press* and snatch dip positions.
- The overhead press may also be performed using dumbbells (*dumbbell press*). The action is similar, but the hand position can begin with the dumbbell facing end on to the wall in front of you. Consequently, the hand is positioned knuckles to the side rather than for the barbell overhead press where the knuckles face back and down. As the dumbbell is pressed overhead, you can allow the arm to rotate naturally so the knuckles face backwards. Some users find the dumbbell alternative more comfortable, and if this is the case experiment with the starting hand position to optimise the action for the user.

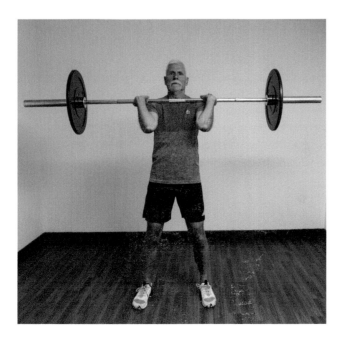

Quadruped training

There is much evidence for the physical benefits of exercise (Momma et al. 2022, Reid et al. 2022), but less emphasis on the psychological benefits. Cognitive wellbeing has been shown to improve with dance exercise (Kim et al. 2011) and a link established between quadrupedal (QDP) exercise used in the rehabilitation of people with movement disorders in children (Dietz 2011). What is less known is the effect of QDP on adults, but it has been argued that crawling actions which involve coordination across the midline may stimulate the brain to organise itself and has been shown in initial studies to have a beneficial impact on cognitive flexibility (Matthews et al. 2016).

In addition, QDP exercises move the limbs with the trunk in a horizontal alignment thus working trunk stability and potentially lessening compressive loading on the spine due to gravity. This type of action also introduces novel challenges and variety to a training programme.

Several kneeling QDP exercises have already been introduced in Chapter 8, we can now progress this type of exercise from kneeling (staying in one place) to crawling (moving across the floor).

Lizard

Starting position:

Begin on all fours (hands and knees) and lift off your knees so you are balanced on your hands and balls of your feet.

Method:

Initially (level one), reach your right-hand forwards and place it on the ground. Then, reach your left leg forwards and place it on the ground. Progress across the floor forwards moving first the hand and then the foot. When you have performed five reps, reverse the action leading with the foot and following with the hand. As a progression (level two) move one hand and opposite side foot at the same time. Again, move forwards and then backwards.

Points to note:

- As you move the knee, it should stay in line with the hand, keeping to the box position which you started in. However, if you have very long legs, it may be more comfortable to move the leg to the side slightly and drop the knee closer to the floor (flexion, abduction, and external rotation at the hip).

Modifications and coaching:

- If you find the position painful on your wrist to begin, make sure you practise on a soft mat.

- Alternatively take your weight through your forearms instead of your wrists.

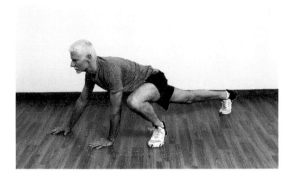

Crabwalk

Starting position:

Begin sitting on the floor with your knees bent and feet flat. Place your arms behind you with your fingers facing to the side.

Method:

Crabwalk forwards placing one foot forwards and then the hand on the opposite side of the body. Once you master the action move the hand and foot at the same time. Perform the same action crab walking backwards.

Points to note:

- The exercise becomes harder if you lift your abdomen high aiming to form a tabletop shape rather than dipping in the middle.

Modifications and coaching:

- Practise the *side crabwalk*, moving the arm and foot sideways across the floor for lateral movement emphasis.

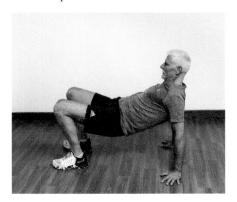

Olympic weightlifting drills

The two classic Olympic lifts are the *Snatch* and *Clean and Jerk*. Although these actions are specialist competitive techniques requiring close coaching, parts of each technique are useful in general training and rehabilitation. Some of these portions (weightlifting derivatives) are discussed below.

Weightlifting actions can offer advantages when working for power training compared to more traditional training with weight resistance, jumps, or kettlebells, for example. The triple extension action is similar to that seen in competitive sprinting and jumping actions (Suchomel et al. 2020) and this may not be present in other forms of training. *Triple extension* is extension at the knee (straightening), hip (leg moving backwards relative to trunk) and ankle (plantarflexion—foot moving downwards).

> **Definition:**
>
> *Power* is the rate of performing work and combines force (how hard) and velocity (how fast). *Speed* is how fast a limb moves. *Strength* is the ability to exert a force against a resistance.

In addition to lower limb action, weightlifting derivatives involve both rapid pulling (joint traction force) and catching actions (joint compression force) which both represent upper limb load absorption.

Snatch balance

We have seen (above) how the overhead squat is performed. The Snatch balance uses a similar position, but involves a greater movement variety.

Starting position:

Begin standing with a barbell across your shoulders (back squat position). Position your hands wide apart using a snatch grip position.

Method:

Press the bar overhead by *straightening* your arms, and at the same time lower/drop into a squat position by *bending* your legs.

Points to note:

- As your knees and hips bend at the same time as your arms straighten, the bar should remain in roughly the same position vertically.

Modifications and coaching:

- Perform a drop snatch by beginning in the same pressing starting position with your feet hip width apart (pulling stance). Lift your feet off the ground and move them outwards slightly (pressing stance) at the same time punching the bar overhead.

Clean

The clean is the first part of the competitive clean and jerk lift. The aim is to lift the bar from the ground using triple extension (see above) through the legs. The bar is received onto the shoulders (front rack position) and the user dips down into a squat position to cushion the weight. In training the clean derivative involves a pull from the floor, triple extension and a small dip as the bar is received in the front rack position when a light weight is used. This is sometimes referred to as a *muscle clean* action.

Starting position:

Begin with your feet hip width apart and the bar lying over your mid-foot. Grip the bar (overgrasp) with your hands shoulder width apart. Bend your knees and hips to sink down and keep your back straight. Tighten (pre-tension) your body to take the slack out of your muscles and breathe in and hold your breath (Valsalva manoeuvre).

Method:

Push your feet into the floor to raise the barbell relatively slowly but deliberately until it passes the knee (first pull). Once past your knees speed the movement up and explosively extend your knees and hips, lifting onto your toes (triple extension), shrugging your shoulders, and raising your elbows (second pull). Allow the bar to lift upwards through its own momentum and at the top of its lift dip under the bar, turn the bar over by reversing your hands to receive the bar in the front rack position (see above) with your elbows flexed and pointing forwards, palms upwards (catch). Lower the bar under control and repeat your reps.

Points to note:

- At the end of the first pull as the bar passes your kneecaps there is often a small dip (double knee bend) which occurs naturally. This is called the *scoop* and provides a counter movement to the rapid second pull.

Modifications and coaching:

- Perform a *power clean* by receiving the bar in the front rack position and moving down into a squat to absorb the bar weight and recover. Keep the trunk upright as you lift out of the squat position to standing.

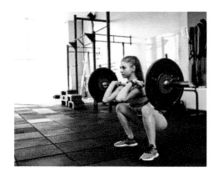 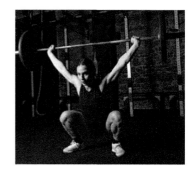

Hinge actions

We looked at the hip hinge action in Chapter 8 and saw that it can be combined with leg movement or performed with stiff legs. Hinging with leg movement has been covered (above) when looking at deadlift actions. Here, we will look at hinge actions which keep the spine straight, legs stiff, and aim to isolate movement to the hips alone. The most common action is the *good morning exercise* and its derivatives.

Starting position:

Begin standing with your feet shoulder width apart. Place a light barbell across your shoulders in the back squat position and grip the bar at a comfortable width to steady it.

Method:

Hinge forwards from your hips, keeping your back flat (straight) and your knees soft. Lower into a comfortable position, usually about 45° to the horizontal and then return to the start.

Points to note:

* As the action occurs at the hip rather than the spine, the pivot point (axis) is through the hip, not the lower spine.
* To help open the chest, perform the first set of exercises with your hands behind your neck or behind the small of your back.

Modifications and coaching:

* Use a "proud chest" cue to open the chest. However, if the user simply takes a deep breath change this to "point your chest at the mirror in front".

- The action may also be performed with a resistance band. Loop the band around your upper back and shoulders and then beneath your feet to stand on the band. As you straighten back up push into the band to retract your shoulders and extend your spine.
- Perform a *kettlebell good morning* holding a kettlebell in front of you at arm's length. This action is similar to a SLDL using a kettlebell, but there is a greater emphasis on the spine staying straight and maintaining the lumbar lordosis (neutral position) as best as possible.
- The good morning movement is also a useful rehab exercise following hamstring injury as it emphasises the upper portion of the hamstrings (knees are slightly bent) and is a closed chain exercise.

Definition:

A *closed chain* is present when the end of the limb (hand or foot) is fixed on a surface (floor or wall). An *open chain* is present when the end of the limb is free to move (hand in space as with throwing or foot off the floor in the swing phase of gait).

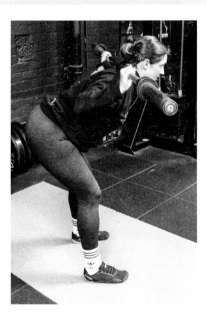

Activities of daily living

Although many people enjoy participating in structured exercise, some absolutely hate it, and as therapists and exercise professionals, we must be able to give people the benefits of training without the need for specific exercise or gym attendance. To do this, we must be able to adapt activities of daily living (ADL)

TABLE 9.3 Activities of Daily Living (ADL) used as exercises

ADL	Exercise
High reach	Reach to top shelf of kitchen cupboard using small heavy object
Chair	Sit to stand using bodyweight or a bag held on chest
Stairs	Climb up then down 5 stairs repeatedly
Walking	Walk 3/5/10 mins in a circuit
Lifts	Lift two heavy bags (one in each hand) from the floor repeatedly
Balance	Stand on one leg (arms out, facing a wall) for 10/20/40 seconds
Bending	Bend down to touch low object then reach up to touch high object
Activity	Dance to a track on the radio until it finishes

and use them at an intensity sufficient to give a training effect and progress from the recovery phase (R2) to the resilience phase (R3) of the 3Rs approach.

ADLs are skills required to manage personal needs and daily life. Primary ADLs are related to basic needs in the home and include such things as gait, feeding, toileting, personal hygiene, and dressing. Secondary ADLs may be task or occupation dependent and can include things such as lifting and carrying, sitting, and driving, stair climbing, gripping, and reaching.

Any of these actions can be used as an exercise and repeated (reps) and overload varied (progressed or regressed). For example, a simple shoulder exercise might be reaching up to the middle shelf of a kitchen cabinet for 10 reps, resting, and then reaching up to the top shelf for 10 reps. Repeated daily, this can enhance ROM and repeated using an item for resistance (e.g., a can of food or bag of sugar) strength may be built up. Sit to stand actions using a high level (kitchen bar stool or arm of a sofa) and then a lower level (dining chair) can provide overload which is progressed by holding a heavy bag in the arms. Table 9.3 shows several ADL ideas for exercise usage at home.

Trunk performance tests

While any torso exercise can be used as a measure of performance by simply recording performance scoring (resistance, holding time, sets & reps) several tests have been validated and normal values issued for a studied population. Clinically, tests of this type are of less value but may still be used to monitor symptom onset or progression through rehabilitation. The tests can be used as part of test batteries (see Chapter 5) and as before/after assessment through a training block or sports season.

Sorensen test

The Sorensen trunk extensor endurance test (Biering-Sorensen 1984), measures hip and back extensor muscle endurance in an unsupported upper body position. The subject lies on a gym bench or treatment couch with their legs supported and the edge of the bench level with their pelvis (iliac crest). The legs and buttocks are held by webbing straps and the time measured until failure (dropping upper body below the horizontal) or to a maximum of 240 seconds. Time values of less than 176 seconds has been shown to be predictive of low back pain (LBP) occurrence within the next year (Demoulin et al. 2006). The test position may be mimicked in training by the subject lying over a gym bench with their feet held by a training partner or using a GHD or Roman chair (see above). In each case, holding time is built up (muscle endurance).

McGill side bridge

The side bridge (side plank) endurance test has the subject lying on their side with their feet apart and upper placed leg forwards. They support their upper body on their forearm (elbow flexed to 90°) with the upper arm placed against the side of their chest. The pelvis is raised from the floor until the spine is straight (no side bend) and the position held until alignment is lost (thigh touches the floor or the subject drops the pelvis for a second time). Side to side differences are noted and mean values of 84.5 seconds have been quoted (McGill et al. 1999). Side bridge actions are commonly used in Pilates and bodyweight training in gyms and endurance times may be built up.

Sit-up test

The sit up exercise may be used repetitively or as a static hold. As a repetitive test it is performed with the ankles fixed. The sit-up action is performed until the hand (thenar pad) touches the patella (superior pole) and repeated at a rate of 2–3 seconds per repetition. The maximum number achieved is counted (with a maximum cut off of 50) with typical mean values of 20–30 being seen, reducing with age (Alaranta et al. 1994). Values greater than 30 (male) or 25 (female) are viewed as excellent in youth sport (Davis et al. 2004). When performed as a static test the subject flexes knees and hips to 90° and is supported on a wedge at a fixed ankle of 50 degrees. The wedge is withdrawn, and the position held for a maximum value. Mean values of healthy individuals have been quoted at 134 seconds (McGill et al. 1999).

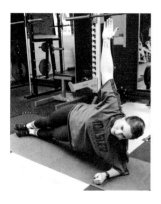 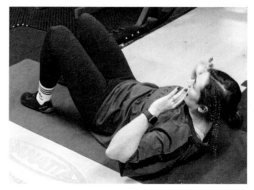

Advanced core training exercises

We have seen in Chapter 8 what core training involves, and both the positive and negative effects of this type of training. In the resilience phase (R3) it is likely that some individuals will be exercising in advanced classes, gyms, or playing competitive sports. In this section, we will look at examples of advanced core exercises which target the trunk muscles and load the spine.

Dead bug variations

The Deadbug exercise begins with the subject lying on their back on a mat. Arms and legs are then moved to give limb loading while the spine stays still (stable). Use of leverage and limb movement combinations gives exercise progression.

Starting position:

Begin lying on your back on a gym mat with your knees bent and feet flat. Reach your arms towards the ceiling so they are vertical. Consider engaging your core muscles by gently drawing them inwards and breathing normally.

Method:

Initially, lift and lower your right leg keeping it bent. Once you have performed five reps, rest and then perform the same leg lift movement but at the same time reach your left arm overhead. Alternate the movement lifting one heel from the mat which reaching the opposite side arm overhead.

Points to note:

- Breathe normally throughout the movement, do not hold your breath.
- The initial setting of the core muscles is only important when you are learning the exercise or if your abdominal muscles bulge. With practice the muscles will work automatically to prevent excessive spinal movement (lumbar hollowing) or abdominal wall bulging.

Modifications and coaching:

- Progress the exercise by starting with your hip and knee flexed to 90°. Straighten your leg initially to touch your heel to the floor as you reach your opposite arm overhead.
- Progress further by keeping your leg off the ground throughout the movement. Do not touch your heel to the mat but hover your straight leg 2 cms above the ground in the lower position.

- The final progression (very demanding) is to bend and straighten both legs together (right angle to fully straight) as you reach both arms overhead simultaneously.

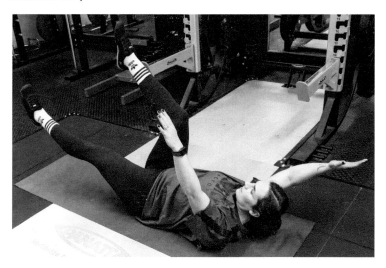

Leg raise variations

Leg raise actions are a common type of trunk muscle exercise and may be performed from several starting positions. Functionally, they are often seen in gymnastic-based sports and gym training programmes. When performed from supine (lying on your back), they typically begin from a bent knee (crook or hook lying) position (see Chapter 8) and progress to straight legs with single or double leg actions or advance to the deadbug exercise above. Performing the exercise from a hanging position has several differences compared to supine. The spine is placed under traction when hanging and single and double leg actions may be performed with or without extra loading by simply holding a weight (dumbbell) between the feet. The disadvantage of a hanging position is that grip my limit the exercise and so using straps to support the forearms or a tower (power tower) unit where the forearms rest on pads are alternatives.

Starting position:

Begin hanging from a high bar, using a hook grip. Use a bench/stool so your feet rest when your legs are vertical.

Method:

Initially, raise one knee at a time, placing the foot back down on the rest between reps. Progress to raising both knees and then single and double straight legs.

Points to note:

- Having your feet rest on a stool (or the floor depending on your height) allows you to relax slightly between reps. Keeping your feet lifting is a progression, but also works the grip hard.
- If you have longer legs, leverage is greater so you may find the exercise harder to perform than your training partner if they are shorter.

Modifications and coaching:

- When lifting both legs, the speed and ROM may be varied to change overload. Lifting with a greater range (just off the floor/45°/90°/to shoulder height) increases the exercise intensity as does slowing the exercise.
- Combine a leg and arm action by pulling on the bar (pull-up action) slightly to begin your leg raise.

Definition:

A *hook grip* involves wrapping the thumb around the bar first and then curling the fingers over the thumb and around the barbell. Pressure from the fingers presses the thumb tighter around the bar and can increase grip effectiveness by 20%.

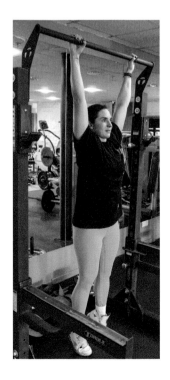

Sit-up variations

Sit-up exercises involve moving from a supine to sitting position and are a functional action used daily when getting out of bed, and often used in some variation when getting up from the floor. They may be performed with the back straight (isolated hip flexion) or by flexing through the spine (trunk curl). By convention, a sit-up involves the lumbar spine leaving the floor while a trunk curl keeps the lumbar spine on the floor.

> **Keypoint:**
>
> In a *sit-up* the lumbar spine lifts off the floor, in a *trunk curl* the lumbar spine remains on the floor. The two actions are often combined with hip flexion and spine flexion occurring together.

Starting position:

Begin lying on your back on the floor (supine lying) on a mat and bend your knees so your feet are flat (crook lying). Have your hands by your sides.

Method:

For the trunk curl, bend the spine and slide your arms along the floor towards your feet. Aim to look between your legs at the far wall.

Points to note:

- The action is a smooth curling (spinal flexion) trying to move each part of the spine. Often the upper thoracic spine is very flexible to flexion while the lumbar spine is quite inflexible.
- Sliding the hands along the floor rather than lifting the arms focusses on the trunk curl action

Modifications and coaching:

- For the sit-up as you get to the end of the curl action, raise the (now flexed) trunk off the mat. As you sit back down aim for the lumber spine to touch the mat first, followed by the thoracic spine and finally the head.
- Perform a straight leg sit-up by lying with the legs straight. Curl the trunk (neck, thoracic spine, and finally lumbar spine) until you can lift your trunk off the mat.
- If you are taller, you have greater leverage of your trunk and legs and so may find this exercise more difficult. If you have heavier legs, it is often easier for you.

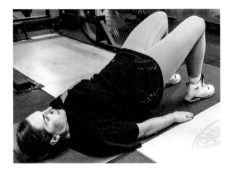 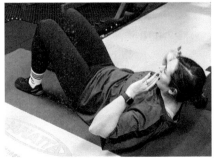

Gym ball exercises

Using a gym ball (Swiss ball) can provide low-cost variation to exercise and may be used both in the gym and at home. Ideally, a gym ball should be sized so that your knees and hips are at 90° when you sit on it. It is too large if your thighs (femur) are angled downwards and too small if they are angled up.

Tuck and Pike

Starting position:

Begin in a press up position with your shins on the gym ball.

Method:

For the *tuck*, draw your legs in towards your body (hip and knee flexion) and then re-straighten them. As the ball rolls towards you your legs will also roll over it so if you begin with the ball on your thighs, it will often end up on your calves. For the *pike* the action is similar, but you keep your legs straight and as you roll the ball towards your body, lift your hips high to create a 'V' shape with your body.

Points to note:

* As you lift, some users find it helpful to tighten their core muscles (performing an abdominal hollowing action) prior to initiating the rolling movement.

Modifications and coaching:

* The press-up position places stress on the wrist and some users find it more comfortable to have their fingers facing outwards to the sides (lateral rotation at the shoulder) rather than forwards.

Superman

Starting position:

Begin lying on your front with the gym ball beneath your abdomen, arms out to the side at shoulder height and hands on the floor (loose press-up position).

Method:

Keeping your feet on the floor (slightly apart for balance and comfort). Lift your arms up keeping your elbows flexed to 90° (surrender position) and at the same time draw your shoulder blades down and inwards. Extend your thoracic spine aiming to lift your breastbone (sternal lift action).

Points to note:

*   Aim to lift your hands to the level of your ears. Keep your head looking downwards to maintain your neck in a neutral position (neither maximally flexed nor extended).

Modifications and coaching:

*   Progress the exercise by straightening your arms once they are lifted to ear level.
*   Reverse the action to perform *Superman legs* by keeping your hands on the floor and lifting your legs up straight. You may need to adjust the ball position for balance depending on your body proportions.

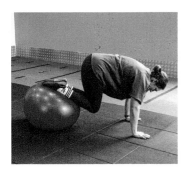 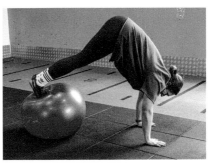

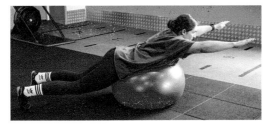

Jumping actions

Jumping actions involve stability of the trunk and lower limb combined with balance on landing. Initiation of the jump is acceleration (force production), and landing is deceleration (force acceptance), and both are vital for unhindered performance of daily manual tasks and competitive sport. In addition, the rapidity of movement requires a focus on the task (external focus) rather than the body (internal focus) and can improve confidence and self-efficacy. Jumps may progress along the floor (horizontal or lateral jumps) or aim for height (vertical jumps) and often combine the two (hurdle jumps, hops, bounds).

Horizontal jump

Starting position:

Begin standing with your feet hip width apart. Pay attention to your footwear! Make sure your shoes are laced firmly and the laces are not overhanging to avoid your shoe slipping around your foot or you tripping over a dangling lace.

Method:

Begin standing still. Take your arms back and then swing them forwards and jump at the same time. Land on your whole foot (heels and toes) with your knees unlocked (slightly soft). Allow your knees and ankles to bend as you land, to absorb shock. Once you have recovered your balance turn, readjust your stance, and jump back.

Points to note:

- Initially, this action is about timing and confidence. The jump does not have to be long or high. As confidence improves, both can increase.

Modifications and coaching:

- This is a *broad jump* (jumping and landing on both feet at the same time). It may be progressed to a *bound* where you jump off one foot and land on the other, and then to a *hop* where you jump off one leg and land on the same leg.
- A lateral jump involves jumping to the side, again on both feet or one.
- Perform a countermovement jump by dipping the knee rapidly (1/4 squat position) and then jumping back up again immediately to engage the stretch shortening cycle (SSC).
- Perform *hurdle jumps* by setting up a line of low (± 20cms) plastic hurdles and jump over them in a continuous action using either both feet or one leg.

Definition:

The *stretch shortening cycle* (SSC) is an active stretch (eccentric muscle contraction) followed immediately by an active contraction (concentric action). The SSC capitalises on muscle reflexes and elastic recoil of non-contractile parts of the muscle.

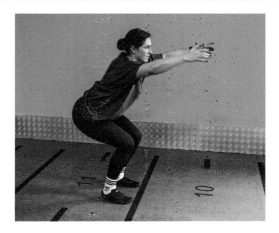

Vertical jump

Starting position:

Begin standing with your feet shoulder width apart and your arms by your sides.

Method:

Swing your arms backwards and dip your knees before jumping up as high as you can. Land and regain your balance before repeating.

Points to note:

- Aim to land equally on both feet (right and left weight distribution equal).
- Land through your whole foot rather than staying on your toes. Try to flex at your ankle, knee, and hip (triple flexion) to absorb the load of landing.
- Time the ankle, knee, and hip flexion to heel contact.

Modifications and coaching:

- Perform the action standing side on to a wall and mark your jump height by placing a mark on the wall (chalk mark) with the fingertips of your outstretched arm. Tap the walk to mark again at the top of your jump. This is the basis for the *vertical jump test*.

- Perform a *countermovement jump* by dipping down into a squat position and then springing up immediately into a vertical jump position.
- Perform a *box jump* by jumping from the ground to a low bench or box (plyometric box) or a *depth jump* by standing on a bench and jumping off to land on the ground and absorb your bodyweight.

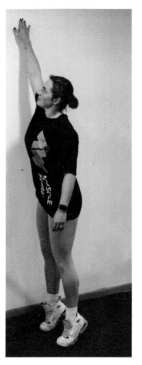

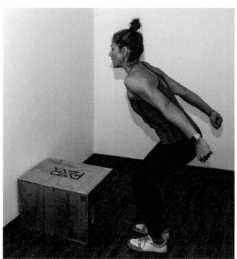

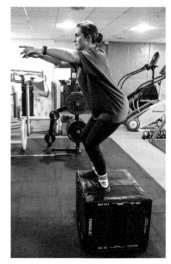

Loaded carrying

Carrying an object is a functional activity for most people. Whether it is a shopping bag in a supermarket, a suitcase on holiday or a large object when gardening carrying loads the spine and most other body regions.

Straight arm carry

Carrying a heavy object with a straight arm holding a handle is one of the most common carrying acts. The *farmer's carry* is performed when holding a heavy object in both hands, and the *suitcase carry* when holding an object in one hand.

Starting position:

Begin standing side on to the object to be lift. Grip the handle making sure you wrap all of the fingers around the handle to ensure a secure hold—you may need to consider padding (rolled cloth or folded piece of foam rubber) if the handle digs into your skin.

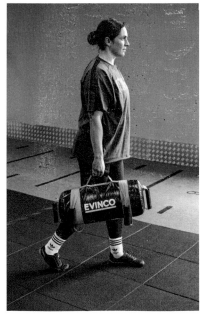

Method:

Bend your knees to provide power to lift and once you have your balance walk forwards using even, measured steps to avoid shuffling or tripping. Practise walking forwards and turning as well as lifting from the ground and placing the object down again.

Points to note:

- For heavy training weights, Farmer's walk handles are available either to hook around a barbell or as a self-contained unit.
- Asymmetry is common, so you may find one arm/leg stronger than the other.

Modifications and coaching:

- When using sub-maximal or lighter weights vary the task by setting up cones and walking in and out or around them.
- Set up hurdles to step over and use steps to practise climbing and descending.

Shoulder carry

Starting position:

Begin standing with your feet shoulder width apart and the object to be carried (power bag) on the floor in front of you.

Method:

Lift the bag from the floor, either directly to your shoulder (light object) or first to your waist, then chest, and then shoulder (heavy object). Hold the object firmly on your shoulder with arm and hand wrapped around it. Walk forwards using measured steps, turn and then walk back to your starting position.

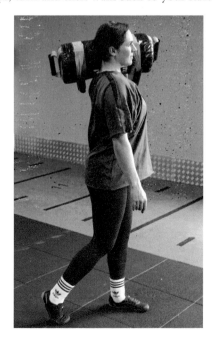

Points to note:

- The shoulder carry on one shoulder is sometimes called the *log carry* and on both shoulders a *fireman's carry*, the latter sometimes being a requirement for military entry.

Modifications and coaching:

- With lighter loads this action can be practised over hurdles, up and down steps, or using ladders to reflect actions used in manual occupations.
- Holding the object and carrying it on the chest (rather than the shoulder) is sometimes referred to as a *bear hug carry* or baby carry (see Chapter 8).

Overhead carry

Starting position:

Begin standing with your feet shoulder width apart. Grip a weight disc (bumper plate) or weight bag in both hands.

Method:

Lift the weight overhead, either directly if light, or to your chest, then shoulder and finally press it overhead (shoulder press action). Lock your elbows and when balanced walk forwards. Stop, turn, and then walk back.

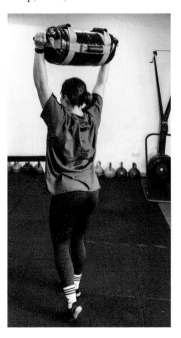

Points to note:

- As the weight is held overhead any slight movement will unbalance you, so a light weight is all that is usually needed.
- Make sure you grip the weight firmly and if you feel it slipping, stop immediately and lower the weight. Do not risk the weight falling and striking you on the head.

Modifications and coaching:

- As with other loaded carries this can be practised walking around objects, up and down steps, or over hurdles to vary the requirement.

Plyometrics

Plyometric exercise uses the stretch shortening cycle or SSC (see above) commonly seen in jumping as a form of power training. There are three phases, *eccentric* (lengthening), *concentric* (shortening), and *amortisation* (transition between eccentric and concentric). The eccentric phase acts as a pre-stretch. The amortisation or transition phase should be kept as short as possible (the user should not take a long pause) to prevent dissipation of the energy stored within the eccentric phase. The concentric phase is a rapid contraction in the opposite direction to the eccentric phase. Plyometric training results in changes in both the contractile and non-contractile elements of muscles. The rapid stretch invokes the stretch reflex on the muscle but also stretches the elastic framework of the muscle which recoils.

> **Definition:**
>
> The *stretch reflex* (myotatic reflex) is the contraction of a muscle in response to rapid stretching. It involves sensors within the muscle (muscle spindles) which send signals to the spinal cord, but not all the way to the brain hence the reaction is faster.

Most actions can be made into plyometric exercises. However, typically hops, jumps, and bounds are used for the lower limb and throwing and striking actions for the upper limb. Specific trunk exercises are rarely truly plyometric; however, the trunk is generally involved in all limb plyometric actions to provide a firm base for force production.

We have covered vertical and horizontal jumps above, with mention of single leg and double leg actions. Here, we will take this further to use three examples of plyometric exercises.

Depth jump

Starting position:

Begin standing with your feet shoulder-width apart on a bench or plyometric box, arms by your sides.

Method:

Step off the box and land on both feet simultaneously. Absorb the jump by flexing at your ankles, knees, and hips keeping your arms to your sides. From the squat position, immediately jump upwards reaching your arms up for balance. Land, remount the box and repeat.

Points to note:

* Do not pause in the squat position (amortisation phase) but jump up straight away, to minimise ground contact time (GCT).
* Do not jump off the box, moving upwards first. Instead step outwards and off the box.

Modifications and coaching:

* Upon landing instead of jumping upwards (vertical) jump forwards (horizontal) performing a *depth jump to standing long jump*.

Definition:

Ground contact time (GCT) is the amount of time in milliseconds (ms) that the foot is in contact with the ground. Elite level sprinters generally have shorter GCTs.

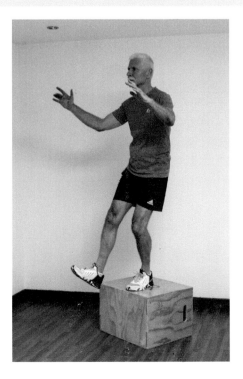

Two handed overhead throw

Starting position:

Stand with your feet shoulder width apart gripping a ball (light medicine ball) in both hands. Face a wall, 45° rebounder, or training partner.

Method:

Keeping your arms fairly straight (stiff). Reach your arms overhead and backwards (cocking position) and then immediately bring them forwards and down to throw the ball either at a wall or to your training partner.

Points to note:

* Bending the arms transfers emphasis of the training effect from the shoulders to the elbow.

Modifications and coaching:

* Perform the action single-handed using a smaller ball
* Perform a *plyometric chest pass* by catching the ball at chest height with your arms straight (reach for the ball) and then throwing it back to your training partner using a chest press/basketball chest pass action.
* Perform a *power drop* by lying on the ground with your head at the base of a plyometric box, your partner standing on the box. Reach your arms straight (vertical) and catch a ball dropped by your partner. Absorb its load by flexing your arms and then throw the ball vertically into the air for your partner to catch again.

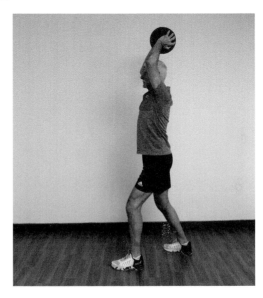

45° sit-up

Starting position:

Begin lying on the floor with your knees and hips bent to 90° (crook lying). Have your training partner stand close (1–1.5 m) to your feet. Sit up so that your trunk is at 45° to the ground.

Method:

Have your training partner throw a ball (light medicine ball or soft ball) towards your chest. Catch the ball with your arms straight. Absorb its movement by flexing through your arms and then throw the ball back.

Points to note:

- Throughout the movement maintain your 45° sit-up position, to provide *static* work to your abdominal muscles and hip flexors.

Modifications and coaching:

- To work the abdominal muscles *dynamically*, catch the ball with your arms straight and absorb the motion by curling back until your trunk touches the floor. Sit back to the 45° position again to throw the ball using the power from your trunk muscles.

> **Definition:**
>
> *Static* muscle work (isometric) involves contracting a muscle and keeping its length the same. *Dynamic* muscle work (isotonic) involves contracting a muscle to change its length. The length change may be by shortening (concentric) or lengthening (eccentric).

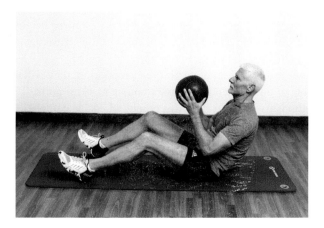

Advanced S&C techniques

Several advanced strength and conditioning (S&C) techniques may be adapted for rehabilitation and used in the resilience phase (R3) of the 3Rs approach. *Unilateral loading* involves lifting an asymmetrical weight, for example, squatting with a barbell with 20kg on one side and 15kg on the other, or lunging holding two different weight dumbbells. The effect is to challenge whole body balance by knocking the user off centre, so they have to compensate continually for a shifting weight as they move. *Time under tension* (TUT), the amount of time load is handled, may be increased by performing the same number of reps with the same weight, but slowing the reps down. Performing 10 reps with each lasting 2 seconds gives a TUT of 20 seconds, while performing the same 10 reps but slowing each down to 5 seconds gives a TUT of 50 seconds, more than double with relatively little change to set-up.

In most exercises we aim at working through a full ROM, however, when using *partial reps*, the aim is to restrict movement to a portion of the ROM only. A typical example of this is a quarter squat where only a small portion of the squat range is used. This can be useful when the range used matches the functional requirements of a task, for example, or to work on a range which targets the sticking point of a movement.

> **Definition:**
>
> The *sticking point* in a lift is the point in the motion range where upward movement reduces or stops because the lifer cannot produce enough force.

Another method of reducing motion range is to use *blocks or pin lifts*. When lifting a weight from the ground (e.g., deadlift or clean) the first part of the motion may be difficult. Raising the weight onto blocks (Olympic jerk blocks) lifts the bar off the ground meaning that the user effectively lifts from mid-shin or knee level depending on block height. When using a rack (power rack of half rack), the pins (spotters) of the rack may be adjusted to the required height and the bar lifted from the pins rather than J-hooks. In this way, the bar is again lifted from a higher point reducing the range of motion.

Where a user reaches the sticking point in a repetition, they will usually fail as they are unable to produce enough force to move past this point. There are two common methods to work through this point and enable completion of the rep. The first is to work with a training partner and use *forced reps*. Here, the partner helps the user through the sticking point, gently unloading the bar by lifting it slightly (called a touch). Once through the sticking point the user lowers the weight themselves as the eccentric phase of a lift is typically stronger than the concentric phase. If we take an example of a dumbbell arm curl, the sticking point is usually as the user's forearm approaches the horizontal position. At this point, their partner lightly lifts the bar past the horizontal to allow the user to flex their elbow maximally and lower the weight unassisted. The second method is a more specialised bodybuilding technique called a *cheating rep*. This is a deliberate modification in strict exercise form to change leverage and enable the user to move through the sticking point. Taking the arm curl above as an example, the user can dip his/her knees and swing the barbell past the horizontal using bodyweight to provide momentum and compensate for the lack of force production from the arm flexors.

Two further advanced techniques which can be useful are negatives and supersets. *Negatives* use an eccentric contraction which is generally stronger than either Concentrics or Isometrics. To perform a negative, you would first lift a weight using assistance (training partner or band, for example) and then lower under control. If we take a chin exercise as an example, a user may find it difficult to lift themselves up to the bar. To perform negative reps, they grip the bar and step on a bench to raise themselves, lowering themselves using their arm strength alone. *Supersets* use two exercises back-to-back. Rather than performing 3 sets of 10 reps on muscle A and then 3×10 on muscle B, instead using a superset the user would perform 1 set of 10 on muscle A and then 1 set of 10 on muscle B and repeat this sequence 3 times. Alternating in this way allows one muscle to rest while working another. Several sequences are used, for example, opposing muscle groups (e.g., triceps and biceps), upper body and lower body (e.g., squats and shoulder press), same muscle group with different exercise (e.g., shoulder press and cable lateral raise).

High Intensity Functional Training

High intensity interval training (HIIT) is a contemporary exercise programme which grew out of traditional circuit training popular in the military and youth sports (Morgan and Adamson 1962) and adapted for rehabilitation (Norris 1993). HIIT training involves short burst of vigorous activity interspaced with periods of lighter actions (relative rest). Its advantage is a reduction in both required space and total exercise time, and as such has become a popular fitness trend. Popular forms of HIIT often focus on aerobic activity and this has been adapted to incorporate a wider variety of actions and to include movements which are used in manual occupations and daily living. This type of training has been labelled *High Intensity Functional Training* (HIFT) (Heinrich et al. 2015, Feito et al. 2018).

HIFT has been popularised with the Crossfit type commercial model (Glassman 2007) using a combination of aerobic training (e.g., running, rowing), anaerobic activities (e.g., throwing, climbing, pulling) bodyweight movements (e.g., squat push-ups, jumps) and weightlifting derivatives (e.g., clean, snatch, press).

Comparing HIIT with HIFT, the former focusses more on aerobic exercise with pre-defined periods of rest while the later incorporates a wider variety of movements with rest periods which are taken as needed, the aim often being to complete the circuit in a specific time (Feito et al. 2018). Where this is used for fitness training, there may be a competitive element to the exercise which is not standard in early rehabilitation (R1) but may be useful in later stages (R2 and R3).

HIFT may has also been adapted to reflect actions used in uniformed services (tactical athletes) such as military, fire service, and law enforcement, for example, and may be extended to reflect any manually focussed occupation such as building, farming, or gardening in each case to improve operational readiness. As such HIFT is useful to build resilience (R3) as it uses drills which reflect the actual actions used in an occupation which may have been causal in an original injury. Such training as we have seen can prepare an individual physically (graded exercise) and psychologically (graded exposure).

HIFT has been proposed to reduce training volume and injury risk and to improve fitness across multiple domains ('S' factors). In addition, variability of training, improved adherence and use of occupation similar actions may lead to better preparedness for real world situations (Haddock et al. 2016).

Example HIFT circuit in R3 stage

Any exercise used in previous stages (R1 and R2) may be used in a HIFT programme, the difference being that the action would be performed more intensely and in a less controlled manner. However, rather than putting a HIFT circuit together by combining several individual exercises, the movements can be taken from an individual's job (occupation) and adapted as an exercise. Using elements of movement analysis and need analysis, the circuit can closely reflect a subject's requirements.

> **Definition:**
>
> *Movement analysis* assesses a single body action, *needs analysis* assesses an individual's wider requirements.

An example circuit is shown in Table 9.4. It includes typical whole-body actions used in a variety of high-level manual occupations, and alternates bodyparts to provide relative rest. The circuit may be introduced in a cut down form using exercises 1–7 initially and then adding exercises as fitness and performance improves. In addition, timing for the circuit may be progressed, with 30 second exercise bouts and 30 second rest periods to begin. As performance improves, this can be progressed to 15 repetitions for each exercise with rest-as-required (RAR) between actions. The aim being circuit completion in the shortest time to introduce a competitive element between users.

TABLE 9.4 High Intensity Functional Training (HIFT) circuit example

	Action	Movement feature
1	Bag lift floor to box	Freestyle lift
2	Sled push	Power production from legs, stability to trunk
3	Rope pull	Leg power production and arm retraction strength
4	Hurdle duck under	Agility
5	Overhead press	Trunk stability, shoulder strength
6	Deadlift	Low and trunk strength
7	Plank	Isometric trunk stability
8	Walking lunge	Leg power and whole-body balance
9	Hanging leg raise	Abdominal muscle strength
10	Overhead ball throw	Arm, leg, trunk power
11	Crawl	Quadruped action
12	Walking recovery	Slow reduction in BP & HR to resting values, EPOC recover

BP—blood pressure. HR—heart rate. EPOC—excess post-exercise oxygen consumption.

References

Alaranta, H., Hurri, H., Heliövaara, M., et al. (1994). Non-dynamometric trunk performance tests: Reliability and normative data. *Scandinavian Journal of Rehabilitation Medicine* 26(4): 211–215.

Biering–Sorensen, F. (1984). Physical measurements as risk indicators for low-back trouble over a one-year period. *Spine* 9: 106–119.

Davis, B., Bull, R., Roscoe, J., et al. (2004). *Physical education and the study of sport* (4th ed). London: Harcourt Publishers.

Demoulin, C., Vanderthommen, M., Duysens, C., et al. (2006). Spinal muscle evaluation using the Sorensen test: A critical appraisal of the literature. *Joint Bone Spine* 73(1): 43–50.

Dietz, V. (2011). Quadrupedal coordination of bipedal gait: Implications for movement disorders. *Journal of Neurology* 258: 1406.

Feito, Y., Heinrich, K.M., Butcher, S.J., and Poston, W. (2018). High-intensity functional training (HIFT): Definition and research implications for improved fitness. *Sports (Basel, Switzerland)* 6(3): 76. https://doi.org/10.3390/sports6030076

Glassman, G. (2007). Understanding CrossFit. *CrossFit Journal* 56: 1–2.

Haddock, C.K., Poston, W.S., Heinrich, K.M., et al. (2016). The benefits of high-intensity functional training fitness programs for military personnel. *Military Medicine* 181: e1508–e1514.

Heinrich, K.M., Becker, C., Carlisle, T., et al. (2015). High-intensity functional training improves functional movement and body composition among cancer survivors: A pilot study. *European Journal of Cancer Care* 24: 812–817.

Kim, S.H., Kim, M., Ahn, Y.B., et al. (2011). Effect of dance exercise on cognitive function in elderly people with metabolic syndrome: A pilot study. *Journal of Sports Science Medicine* 10(4): 671–678.

Matthews, M.J., Yusuf, M., Doyle, C., et al. (2016). Quadrupedal movement training improves markers of cognition and joint repositioning. *Human Movement Science* 47: 70–80.

McGill, S.M., Childs, A., and Liebenson, C. (1999). Endurance times for low back stabilization exercises: Clinical targets for testing and training from a normal database. *Archives of Physical Medicine and Rehabilitation* 80(8): 941–944.

Momma, H., Kawakami, R., Honda, T., et al. (2022). Muscle-strengthening activities are associated with lower risk and mortality in major non-communicable diseases: A systematic review and meta-analysis of cohort studies. *British Journal of Sports Medicine* 56: 755–763.

Morgan, R.E., and Adamson, G.T. (1962). *Circuit training.* London: G. Bell.

Norris, C.M. (1993). *Sports injuries. Diagnosis and management for physiotherapists* (4th ed). Oxford: Elsevier, 107–109.

Reid, H., Ridout, A.J., Tomaz, S.A., On Behalf of the Physical Activity Risk Consensus Group, et al. (2022). Benefits outweigh the risks: A consensus statement on the risks of physical activity for people living with long-term conditions. *British Journal of Sports Medicine* 56: 427–438.

Suchomel, T.J., McKeever, S.M., and Comfort, P. (2020). Training with weightlifting derivatives: The effects of force and velocity overload stimuli. *Journal of Strength, and Conditioning Research* 34(7): 1808–1818.

10
CASE ILLUSTRATIONS

In this chapter, we will look at examples of patients with low back pain (LBP) managed with the 3Rs approach. The case illustrations show patient history, assessment, clinical reasoning, and interventions. The full patient notes are not detailed, but outlines are given to show essential points. More detailed examination and intervention records were made in the clinic, and the outlines below are extracted from them as a learning tool.

Subject 1

History

A 31-year-old female equestrian developed spinal pain following a fall from a horse. She had not previously been a back pain sufferer and was a gym member attending classes once a week. She stated that she fell onto her right side and presented with right-sided back and hip pain. At the time (two weeks prior to assessment) she had extensive bruising to the hip and thigh, but none to the back. Her sleep was uninterrupted, but her back felt stiff on rising and eased following a shower and general movements. She looked after her horse and noticed her back pain at the end of the day when she had been carrying and lifting.

Assessment

On examination, there was residual bruising to the hip around the greater trochanter. She had full range painless hip motion with some trochanteric pain to palpation in a hip-adducted position. Motion range to the spine was full, with painful (5/10) tightness to end range flexion and side flexion but not extension. The patient's movements were guarded, and she appeared fearful. When

DOI: 10.4324/9781003366188-10

encouraged to continue moving, pain eased to 3/10 with repetition. Straight leg raise (SLR) and prone knee bend (PKB) was full and painless.

Clinical reasoning and impression

As the patient had a history of injury to the hip and side of the body, full examination was carried out to exclude hip pathology. Motion range to the spine was limited but increased with repetition indicating stiffness. SLR and PKB was full and painless and there was no morning stiffness, indicating the likelihood of simple LBP related to the fall. It is likely that the pain and bruising to the right side (primary condition) had led to a change in movement quality (secondary condition) and this was the main driver of her current pain. The treatment aims were therefore: (i) to restore free movement to the spine (ii) to enhance post-trauma recovery (iii) to build spinal resilience to lifting and carrying (iv) to restore optimal lumbo-pelvic function related to horse riding.

Intervention

Initial treatment was education concerning healing timescale and the need for exercise post-trauma. The patient was given basic spinal mobility actions (spinal flexion using chair support and side bending with thigh support). These were to be practised daily and could also be used as a warm-up prior to work in the stable yard.

On her second visit three days later, the patient stated that she was pain free. A rehab programme was planned, beginning with a needs analysis which showed the requirement for lifting weight (buckets of water) from the ground, mucking out, and making up feeds (sweeping and lifting), handling tack (awkward lifts), checking horses and putting them out (varied body movement at different heights). A functional circuit was designed involving similar movements to be used in the gym (kettlebell deadlift, zigzag walking between cones, lifting from floor to high point, seated row, core work on a gym ball). When she had no time to attend the gym, alternative actions were discussed which could be used in the yard.

Keypoints:

- Exercise therapy was used initially for pain reduction and to begin the recovery phase (R1).
- A need analysis was used to plan exercise requirements matching her lifestyle choices.
- Rehab progressed to general training taking into account patient choice.
- Resilience was built (R3) using full movements to guard against kinesiophobia to flexion (her original pain limited action).

On her third visit, the patient reported that she had used the circuit (modified) in the gym and had attended two circuit classes. She felt stronger when working in the stable yard and was keen to continue her circuit class which she enjoyed. She was encouraged to do so and given education on the need to include a variety of movements and not to avoid spinal flexion, but to train with it in her circuit.

Subject 2

History

A 45-year-old male sales representative developed low back pain of gradual onset. He had no pain on rising, but pain and stiffness occurred following three hours driving. He had no history of weight loss or bladder and bowel changes. He reported no leg pain, but occasional buttock pain. He had no other health concerns but was generally inactive. On further questioning, the patient stated that his pain was lessened or not present on the days he did not drive and when not working at weekends. Since lockdown and home working, his bodyweight had increased from 70 kgs to 85 kgs. He freely admitted that his diet was poor, and he lived on convenience foods and snacks when out on the road. He was generally inactive, occasionally gardening but stated that his work schedule precluded exercise. He considered he was "getting old and fat" and lamented the fact that 15 years ago he had run a half marathon but could not even jog now. He queried whether a back support in his car seat and office chair may help.

Assessment

In standing, the patient had limited range flexion which was painless. Motion range increased with repetition moving from fingertips to mid-thigh to fingertips to knees. Spinal extension and side flexion were again painless, but the patient described them as "feeling tight". Palpation (prone lying) revealed local lumbar tenderness with no referral into the buttocks. SLR was bilaterally painless and 45° to range. Hip movements were full, with bilateral hip flexion giving local pain to the lumbar spine at end range.

Clinical reasoning and impression

The patient was overweight and inactive but had no described red flags (see Chapter 5). Pain built up with continued flexion (sitting) but was not present first thing in the morning or at weekends. The patient was deconditioned but aware of this and had a history of previous exercise practice. Aims of treatment were: (i) enable the patient to self-manage his pain (ii) use patient education to explain the condition and focus on the importance of active care (iii) develop a fitness programme which fits in with the patient lifestyle.

Intervention

Initially patient education was used to explain the need for regular spinal movement and the likelihood of stiffness and inactivity driving symptoms. Manual therapy was used to give short-term pain reduction and to enhance therapeutic alliance. The patient was shown passive extension in both lying and standing as a self-management approach when he was travelling away from home and advised to begin a walking programme. He performed both actions in the clinic and exercise technique was coached, and response monitored. Range of motion to extension increased with repetition, and the patient stated that he felt tightness but no pain. Initially, it was agreed that the patient would drive for a maximum of two hours before getting out of the car and then he would walk around the carpark of the motorway services until his back stiffness eased, or for a minimum of five minutes. Instead of a back support, the patient was advised to use a rolled towel behind his back in the car if he felt benefit from it.

On his second visit, the patient reported no pain in day-to-day activities and stated that his back pain could be eased with walking. He had one instance where he drove for three hours and experienced mild pain, but this eased when he got out of the car and walked. He had used the passive spinal extension action on a semi-regular basis, at least every other day. In conversation, he stated that he was keen to begin an exercise programme but had very little time. We agreed on a two-pronged approach. Where time and/or facilities were limited, he would build up his walking to increase the time to 15 minutes, or 10 minutes at a faster pace. He should aim to feel breathless but not exhausted and should be able to hold a conversation throughout the exercise period (talk test, Chapter 7). Where he had more opportunity to exercise, he would use a high intensity exercise programme consisting of a variety of movements in the sequence arm/trunk/legs. We discussed several exercises and agreed on sit-to-stand, side bend, and lateral raise using two books. He would practise the movement for 30 seconds, progressing to 60 seconds and perform two circuits, progressing to three. Alternative exercises could be substituted to increase variety and examples were given and he was directed to exercise websites and YouTube videos as general resources.

On the third meeting, the patient was pain free and had a good understanding of his back pain cause and management. The rehabilitation progressed from R2 to R3, and we agreed on a gradual return to running with the aim of entering his local park run with his oldest son (aged 19) in three months' time. We progressed his walking programme to walk/run (scout pace) over a 20–30-minute period. Initially, the walk periods were longer than the run periods, but as he felt able the run timing was to increase and walk reduce. He used this training three times per week and performed his circuit on two of his 'off' days. The circuit was progressed as he had purchased a set of dumbbells and an exercise mat. He would now perform dumbbell shoulder press, lunge, bent dumbbell row, single arm dumbbell side bend, and trunk curl as a circuit each for 30–60 seconds with rest-as-required for two circuits in total. The patient was discharged with the opportunity to review via Zoom link if required.

Keypoints:

- Although general deconditioning with postural stiffness could have been deter-mined from onset (fast thinking, see Chapter 5) a full physical examination was stiff carried out.
- Use of a back support was raised by the patient but discouraged to avoid reli-ance, a temporary rolled towel to be used for short-term pain relief as required.
- Passive extension actions were used to target prolonged flexion used when sitting.
- As the patient had exercised previously, a graduated walk-run programme was chosen with a stated temporal aim (park run in three months).
- A high intensity circuit was designed in consultation with the patient for use at home or in hotels when travelling for business.

Subject 3

History

A 78-year-old female presented with low back pain following a prolonged drive. She went on holiday with her daughter and grandchildren and was in the passen-ger seat of the car for five hours. She stated that she was very stiff when getting out of the car and next morning woke with pain in her back and an inability to stand straight on rising. Her pain eased through the day, but she was stiff again the next morning. She queried whether she needed an x-ray to check if she had arthritis as her friend had been told her back had 'severe degeneration' and the joints were now 'bone-on-bone'.

Assessment

Subjective examination revealed that the patient had attended line dancing classes for five years but stopped due to lockdown and although the classes had re-started, she had not returned. She stated that her back was stiff on rising and took 30–60 minutes to ease and by breakfast time felt relatively normal. She got up in the night to visit the toilet, but there had been no change to her sleep pattern. She had had a total hip replacement eight years ago and had no problems with her hip and had had surgery for Hallux Valgus three years since. Her general health was good.

Objective assessment showed full lumbar motion range for her age with some feeling of stiffness to the low back on flexion. The stiffness eased with repeti-tion and began to lessen after five reps. She had no referred pain and was able to dress and undress normally and perform an unaided sit-to-stand action. Her gait entering the treatment room was normal and she did not use a stick.

The patient had no history of leg pain, and hip motion range was full and painless. SLR was painless and pelvic pain provocation tests were clear.

Clinical reasoning and impression

As stiffness was easing with movement during the morning and there was no history of injury, overload to flexion was likely causing an inflammatory reaction from the spinal soft tissues. No pain was referred into the legs and SLR was full indicating no likelihood of radiculopathy. A history of flexion stress and short-term pain indicates rheumatological factors are unlikely. The treatment aims were therefore: (i) reassurance of the diagnosis and explanation that x-ray is not required (ii) provide short-term pain reduction and self-management advice (iii) begin rehabilitation integrated with patient choice.

Intervention

Short-term pain reduction was given using massage and soft tissue mobilisation to the low back. Although unlikely to affect the tissues significantly, this approach was reassuring to the patient and simple education was given at the same time concerning normal ageing of joints and the spine and the need to use exercise to maintain the tissue condition. As the patient was beginning to recover (R1 moving to R2) mobility exercises were given to be practised twice daily (sitting trunk rotation, kneeling or standing arch and hollow). It was suggested that the patient begin a graduated walking programme, however she lives on a busy road and was not confident to do this. Instead, I had the patient demonstrate three of the simple movements she had used in her line dancing classes some time ago and we strung these together to use them as a simple two-minute exercise programme to be repeated three times throughout the day.

At the second treatment episode three days later, the patient reported less stiffness in the morning but noticed some LBP later in the day and stiffness on rising from prolonged sitting. Exercises were continued, and the line dancing actions were increased in intensity. The normal healing timescale was reinforced to the patient using a 'sore but safe' approach. The patient was encouraged to re-start her line dancing and was to investigate class times.

Keypoints:

- Full examination was given due to the age of the patient as a risk factor (red flag) for non-mechanical conditions.
- Massage was given for short-term pain reduction and to enhance therapeutic alliance.
- Exercise was begun early on to enhance self-efficacy.
- Exercise choice was designed to fit in with patient choice and availability of equipment.
- Rehab was continued using a simple circuit after pain had gone to target sarcopenia due to the patient's age.

Strength training was discussed with the patient to increase muscle strength and build both mental and physical resilience (R3). A simple circuit of three exercises was used (bag lift from floor/overhead push using unopened box of washing powder/sit-to-stand holding bag) this circuit was to be practised twice, on two days each week.

Subject 4

History

A 42-year-old man presented for treatment with a history of persistent low back pain over a 2-year period. He worked on an industrial production line, and was about 25 kg overweight, with a marked lordotic posture and prominent abdominal contour. His 24-hour pattern was one of pain less in the morning, scoring 3/10 and increasing throughout the day peaking in the late afternoon to 8/10. He had no problem sleeping and was comfortable lying and sitting and reported no altered sensation or change in bladder or bowel habits. Lower limb strength was symmetrical with no signs of wasting or weakness. The patient had no co-morbidities except obesity and deconditioning.

Assessment

From standing, flexion was painless with the subject able to reach his fingertips to his knees. Repeated flexion (5 reps) did not produce pain and enabled him to reach below his knees. Extension created local LBP which increased marginally to repetition but neither action produced pain referral into the buttocks or legs. Side flexion actions were free and painless. SLR was to 45° and painless. Examination of the hips and pelvis was unremarkable.

Passive spinal extension (extension in lying, see Chapter 7) gave local LBP and flexion in lying (knees to chest) began to ease his LBP after three repetitions and he was pain free after eight repetitions.

It was noticeable that the patient demonstrated central abdominal bulging when he attempted to sit up from supine lying suggesting lack of deep abdominal muscle control, diastasis recti, or an early ventral abdominal hernia. This had produced no symptoms and disappeared at rest.

Clinical reasoning and impression

The postural alignment of the patient and his history suggested overload to the lumbar spine in extension. Reproduction of his familiar symptoms with extension (standing and lying) supported this hypothesis. Repeated flexion in lying reversed his lumbar lordosis and obliterated pain confirming the hypothesis of postural overload rather than mechanical injury. His obesity, deconditioning and exercise history indicated that his back pain was part of an overall lifestyle which was driving his symptoms. The treatment aims were therefore (i) to give short-term pain relief using repeated flexion actions (ii) to support the patient to use this action as a self-management technique (iii) to increase his activity (iv) to link activity to dietary advice and onward referral (v) to introduce work on abdominal muscle strength and control.

Intervention

Initially passive lumbar flexion was used as a manual therapy technique to demonstrate the effect of repeated movements to the patient and emphasise that not all movements would harm his spine. This was considered important as the patient had repeated stated in conversation (subjective examination) that he had rested his spine and was aware that his job was probably working his back too hard. The action was coached and given as a home exercise technique to be used twice daily (a.m. and p.m.) for two sets of five repetitions with the aim of combating pain driven by postural extension loading. In addition, the effect of obesity and deconditioned were discussed as this had come up in conversation. When the patient stated "I know my weight does not help my back" empathy was shown and reflective listening (a motivational interviewing technique, see Chapter 6) used to introduce the possibility of weight loss. The patient stated that he had successfully lost weight before, and that a slimming club had helped. It was suggested that he consider re-joining the club which he liked, and we could begin a walking programme to help him. Due to the patient shift pattern at work (four days on, three days off) we agreed that he would begin a progressive walking programme each of his off days, beginning at 10 minutes and progressing to 20 minutes as he felt able. The flexion exercise and graduated walking programme were the only two home techniques given during the first treatment episode.

On the second treatment session (one week later), that patient presented with less pain (worst 4/10 and best 0/10) and was encouraged that when he had pain, the flexion exercise eased it. The passive flexion technique was progressed to an active technique to begin abdominal muscle strengthening. As the patient demonstration abdominal bulging with likely visceroptosis, a wall support starting position was chosen (see Chapter 8). The patient stood with his back against a wall with his feet forwards by 30 cms to allow his bodyweight to be taken by the wall. He was coached in an abdominal hollowing action, drawing this abdominal wall inwards and away from the waistband of his trousers without holding his breath. As the exercise was coached, a pelvic floor action was encouraged, and the patient mentioned for the first time that he sometimes suffered from urinary incontinence. The abdominal hollowing action was then linked to a pelvic floor action (penis drawing in an up) and education about the action was given. A little and often approach was taken using the wall support standing action twice daily but using a pelvic floor contraction for five reps after urinating whenever he visited the toilet at work. The patient stated that he had re-joined his weight loss club and received dietary advice and goals. He was now able to walk for 15 minutes without becoming breathless (see talk test, Chapter 7).

On the third treatment session (two weeks later due to the patient's work shift pattern), the patient reported that he was pain free. It was emphasised that the treatment should now change focus from reducing pain (the original aim) to increasing his overall fitness (primary aim) and the condition of his trunk musculature (secondary aim). Education was given about the 3Rs approach and the need to continue recovery of the low back (R2) and build resilience (R3).

A functional circuit was developed in consultation with the patient, choosing exercises which were readily available and appealing to him to reduce barriers to compliance. The walking exercise was progressed to 20 minutes at speed 5 times each week. On the day of the circuit (three days per week), he used the standing abdominal exercise progressed to back flattening (posterior pelvic tilt) holding inner range for 5 s. He also performed sit-to-stand from a firm dining chair and a shoulder press action using two heavy objects from his house.

This circuit was practised for one month and then progressed to a trunk curl (from crook lying), shoulder press using a resistance band, bag lift from the floor to a kitchen work surface, sit-to-stand with a weighted bag, and a pulling action using the resistance band (single arm rowing action). The patient stated that he was happy to continue this circuit on a regular basis and had built it into his lifestyle.

Keypoints:

- Obesity and diet were only mentioned at the first treatment session as the patient volunteered this himself.
- A standing exercise was chosen as it did not require equipment and was easily practised throughout the day.
- Pelvic floor action was an additional benefit for a co-morbidity that the patient did not mention initially.
- A walking programme was chosen as it was easy to do and less time consuming than an exercise class, gym, or swimming, for example.
- Treatment was not stopped when the patient was pain free but changed emphasis to re-conditioning (R2 leading to R3).
- A high intensity functional circuit was developed using simple actions from around the house of the patients choosing, and built into the patient's regular weekly lifestyle.

Subject 5

History

A 26-year-old regular gym user presented with low back pain on rising on the day after her gym workouts. Her training consisted of daily workouts in a gym,

using either weight-training apparatus (40 minutes) plus cardiopulmonary apparatus (20 minutes), or an exercise class (60 minutes). She had been referred for
an X-ray of the low back and pelvic joints which showed no abnormality, and
blood tests were normal. She was referred for physiotherapy three months after
the onset of pain, and stated that she thought her 'SIJ was out'.

Assessment

On examination, her lumbar spine had full painless range of motion. Examination
of the pelvis revealed no pain or reproduction of any symptoms on Sacroiliac
pain provocation tests. Movement screening tests (Chapter 5) were established
to mimic the actions she used commonly in the gym. Following discussion, she
stated that shoulder press actions, hip extension using a pulley, and kick back
actions in exercise classes would often result in pain the next day. When performing a shoulder press action her spine became hyper lordotic, as was the case
with lying hip extension and standing hip extension actions. In general conversation, she mentioned that she sat at work with a lumbar support and had used
McKenzie extension exercises which she had seen in a magazine article.

Clinical reasoning and impression

All tests for a mechanical lesion or tissue pathology were negative, suggesting
that a non-mechanical source of symptoms may be present. Subjective examination had revealed slow onset pain (day after training) brought on by extension
actions. Movement screening had demonstrated hyperlordosis on spinal and hip
extension actions. It was hypothesised that extension overload was occurring
during gym training which resulted in a tissue reaction most likely a slow onset
inflammatory response. The treatment aims were (i) to use education to establish
an understanding of the link between lumbar and hip actions (ii) to enhance
movement control of the lumbo-pelvic region (iii) to develop movement confidence as part of mental resilience (iv) to reduce kinesiophobia to spinal actions.

Intervention

The concept of neutral position of the lumbar spine was introduced to the
patient, and drills established to move between full anterior and then full posterior tilt and stop mid-way. The action was practised in several starting positions
including kneeling prone lying and standing. Resisted hip extension using a
pulley machine was then practised with video feedback provided using a tablet
computer. The aim in each case was to avoid end range lumbar extension but to
use free movement as much as possible. Pain neuroscience education (PNE) was
also used to establish the link between pain and slow onset inflammation and
to introduce the concepts of hurt and harm, and sore but safe. The patient was
instructed to modify her gym training taking on board the concepts which had

been introduced and attempting to regain movement control of the lumbo-pelvic region. She was to monitor her body reaction subsequent to training and to record this in her training diary.

The patient was reviewed two weeks later and reported no pain on rising and an increased understanding of her body movements. Exercises were progressed with load, and lumbo-pelvic control remained good. Education was used to gradually increase understanding of the need for varied load on the spine and avoiding overprotecting the area. The patient was encouraged to move away from the neutral position and use controlled full range motions.

A training plan was agreed with the patient, and she was discharged with the opportunity to review through an online session if required.

Keypoints:

- Although it is unlikely that the patient would present with positive findings after an X-ray and blood tests, full physical examination was still carried out (see priming—clinical reasoning error, Table 5.11).
- The subjective history (patient story) gave more meaningful information than the objective examination (special tests and palpation).
- Movement screening tests were designed to reflect the training information the patient had offered.
- Rather than injury, this case reflected overreaching/training of a bodypart hence training modification rather than treatment intervention was chosen.
- Neutral position was used temporarily for short-term pain reduction. Once pain had reduced, full range spinal movement was begun.

Subject 6

History

A 34-year-old male presented with acute low back pain. On entry into the treatment room, he demonstrated a semi-flexed posture bracing himself with one hand on his thigh. He stated that he had injured his back bending and lifting in the garden two days ago. The first night he had been unable to climb the house stairs, so had slept intermittently in a lounge chair.

Assessment

On examination, the patient stated that his pain radiated into his right leg as far as his knee and he had LBP which gave spasms of pain if he tried to change positions. When he attempted to stand upright, he demonstrated a left shift and his back pain intensified. On closer questioning, his leg pain centralised to mid-thigh. Due to the intense pain and suffering demonstrated by the patient, no further physical examination was attempted at this stage. Closer question suggested an absence of red flags (no change to bladder or bowel habits, no saddle anaesthesia, a positive history of injury, younger age, mechanical nature of symptoms).

Clinical reasoning and impression

Due to intense pain and suffering, treatment was begun immediately targeting the pain and attempting to centralise the pain. The hypothesis at this stage was of acute onset mechanical LBP probably non-specific. Treatment aims initially were (i) to reduced pain intensity (ii) to centralise pain (iii) to reassure the patient and reduce fear and anxiety.

Intervention

A side glide passive mobilisation was used which begun to centralise the patient's pain and he was given a side glide exercise against the wall. He performed two sets of ten repetitions of this action and the leg pain reduced and then eased completely leaving localised LBP, greater on the right side. The intervention confirmed the presence of mechanical LBP.

The patient was then able to lie prone on the treatment couch and palpation revealed marked muscle tension in the spinal extensors. He was given general soft tissue massage and mobilisations using PA (posteroanterior) and transverse low-grade movement. Muscle tension (assessed as tissue tension to palpation) reduced and the patient reported a reduction in pain intensity. The couch end was raised to lift the patient's chest and move him into lumbar extension and the manual therapy techniques were repeated.

In addition to the side glide action, the patient was begun on a simple walking programme in the gym, attempting to walk with even steps and to stand tall (lengthening through the spine). He was to use this action at home walking along the hallway/corridor or outside along the garden path.

The patient attended for a second visit the next day and reported that he had slept in his bed but had woken two or three times when he turned over. He had used the side glide exercise and had leg pain only twice over a 24-hour period. He found his back pain intensity eased by 20–30% with walking. The patient's home exercise was changed from wall supported side glide to prone lying passive extension or standing supported active extension (see Chapter 7). Walking distance was increased, and a sitting rotation exercise was given to build free movement.

The patient was seen for a third treatment four days later (seven days following pain onset) and reported that he was sleeping normally and his back pain eased considerably. He felt occasional pain with prolonged bending and general tightness across the lumbar region confirming that he had progressed from the reactive phase (R1) to the recovery phase (R2) of rehabilitation. Controlled flexion and extension was introduced in kneeling, and spinal re-strengthening begun using the kneeling single leg lift (birddog legs). Bending (spinal flexion) to chair seat level was introduced and as confidence increased, a light bag lift to chair level was introduced to reduce the fear of flexion demonstrating the beginning of the resilience phase (R3).

The patient showed interest in joining a local gym, so advice was given on a progressive fitness programme to be supervised by a personal trainer at the gym. The patient was encouraged to participate in a variety of exercise types to improve confidence in movement. Education was given concerning spinal resilience and the need to practise all movements including flexion. An initial programme was agreed on and the patient was monitored one month later to check progress.

Keypoints:
- Physical examination was curtailed as the patient demonstrated intense pain and suffering.
- The intervention also gave information to confirm the treatment hypothesis.
- A simple home technique was begun immediately to enable the patient to self-manage over a 24-hour period.
- Manual therapy was used for short-term pain relief, to reassure the patient and to strengthen the therapeutic alliance.
- Flexion was introduced as soon as pain allowed to reduce fear of this movement.

Subject 7

History

A 32-year-old office worker in her second trimester of pregnancy, presented for treatment. She had right-sided back pain which was made worse by prolonged sitting. Her pain travelled into her buttock and occasionally into her leg, and she complained that her leg often felt weak, and she stated it was "as though it can't support me," but it had never actually given way. When she was lying in bed on her back, she occasionally felt pain spreading into her pubic region. She had seen her physician and midwife and was assured that her pregnancy was normal and her pain of musculoskeletal (MSK) origin.

Assessment

In standing, the patient demonstrated a lordotic posture, with an anteriorly tilted pelvis, but exhibited some swayback tendencies, standing with her weight predominantly on her right leg. When questioned, she confirmed that she had always stood like this and often noticed her right knee aching if she stood all day at an exhibition as part of her job. Lumbar flexion was full range for her condition, but extension gave local pain and was pain limited. Side flexion movement felt tight, the patient stated. SLR was full, with pain in the right leg at end of range (EOR). Hip motion was full range with minimal right-sided lumbo-pelvic pain to full hip flexion.

Local palpation of the lumbo–pelvic region revealed tenderness over the right posterior superior iliac spine (PSIS) and local tenderness into the region of the sacroiliac joint (SIJ). There was no tenderness to palpation of the public bone or pubic symphysis. Pain provocation test cluster (femoral thrust, distraction & compression, and pelvic torsion) recreated the patient familiar symptoms. Pain was exacerbated when she performed an active straight leg raise (ASLR) movement with the right leg but not the left. Fixation of the pelvis using manual pressure removed all pain to a repeat test using the ASLR.

Clinical reasoning and impression

Positive SIJ cluster tests and history suggested pain from the SIJ region. A positive ASLR (pain diminished with pelvic stabilisation) suggested that stability exercise to the lumbo-pelvic region may provide simple patient self-management over a 24-hour period. Treatment aims were: (i) to provide short-term pain reduction using resting positions and self-applied movement techniques (ii) to enhance lumbo-pelvic stability (iii) to prevent exacerbation of symptoms as pregnancy progressed (iv) to lay the foundation for return to regular exercise following childbirth.

Intervention

The patient had been taught pelvic floor muscle contractions as part of her antenatal care but had not practised these regularly. I emphasised the importance of these exercises and combined pelvic floor contraction with abdominal hollowing in a crook-lying position to begin rehabilitation. Initially, her lumbo-pelvic control was poor and she was not able to perform a heel slide action without tipping her pelvis. To emphasise the abdominal hollowing action, the patient was taught to self-palpate. Once she had performed the exercise several times and was able to self-monitor effectively, the ASLR action was retested first without abdominal muscle contraction and then with contraction. She was surprised that the hollowing action took away her pain and was determined to practise the exercise between treatment sessions.

I fitted the patient with an SIJ support belt around the rims of her pelvis, but below her abdomen, and taught her to stand with her weight taken equally on both legs. In addition, she was shown a side lying resting position with knees and hips flexed to reduce her lumbar lordosis, and a pillow between her knees.

At the next treatment session (3 days later), the patient reported that her pain had lessened. If she forgot to wear her support belt, pain returned after 10 minutes standing, but with the belt she could stand pain free for 30 minutes. The heel slide action was repeated, and lumbo-pelvic control had improved considerably.

Abdominal muscle contraction was more forceful and normal lumbo-pelvic alignment was maintained as the heel slide action was performed for 10 reps. Lumbo-pelvic control was progressed using sitting and standing actions (knee raise and hip abduction). Education was given concerning setbacks and flare ups and the actions to take when these occurred.

On the third treatment session (5 days later), the patient reported that her pain was only occasional now and limited to the SIJ region, not referred into the buttock. Her pain only occurred through prolonged sitting and was easily removed by changing her sitting posture. Exercises were progressed to the supported hip hinge action (tabletop) and a bag lift from chair seat height. These actions replaced the heel slide, but if she had pain or felt the exercises too demanding, she could regress them back to the heel slide when required.

On the fourth treatment session (2 weeks after initial evaluation), the patient was pain free during day-to-day activities and did not require her support belt. We agreed that she should keep the belt because she may need it later due to the changing mechanics of the pelvic region as her pregnancy progressed. We arranged for a review one month after childbirth when guidance on a gradual return to exercise would be considered.

Keypoints:

- The patient had no pregnancy complications and had been screened by her physician and midwife before commencing an exercise programme.
- The patient's lumbo-pelvic pain was reduced when her pelvis was stabilised passively.
- Abdominal muscle contraction was demonstrated to take the patient's pain away, increasing compliance and providing motivation to use self-management.
- Abdominal muscle action was combined with pelvic floor contraction.
- As the patient was in pain, a support belt was used until she had regained active control of the lumbo-pelvic region.
- Resting positions were given as part of self-management.

Subject 8

History

A 56-year-old female sought treatment for persistent low back pain. She was currently undergoing chemotherapy (intravenous) which consisted of a 14-day course involving sitting for 3-hour periods. Her pain built up with prolonged sitting or when she was a car passenger on a long journey. Her chemotherapy cycle was completed in four days time after which she had a 6-week gap before beginning a second cycle. As a result of her chemotherapy, she reported general tiredness and fatigue, occasional bouts of nausea, poor concentration, and numbness in her feet. She had discussed her back pain with her oncology nurse who had confirmed that it was unrelated to her cancer, and that scans had shown no spinal secondaries.

Assessment

On assessment, the patient demonstrated full spinal movements in standing with minimal tightness and discomfort (3/10) to end range flexion. Hip movements were full and painless as was SLR and PKB. In lying (prone) there was general tenderness to the lumbar spinal extensor muscles with some tenderness to the upper buttocks. Central vertebral pressure (PA mob grade 2–3) did not give referred pain and caused only mild discomfort (4/10).

Clinical reasoning and impression

The patient history suggested that prolonged sitting in the presence of a fatigue (mental and physical) inducing treatment was the likely cause of low backs symptoms. Minimal pain to examination (active movements and palpation), full SLR and RKB, and the report of a clear scan suggested a mechanical driver. However, the nature of the case meant that symptom behaviour was closely monitored.

Intervention

On the first treatment, the patient received low back massage and was given a single simple spinal exercise (seated spinal rotation) to target stiffness and pain over a 24-hour period. She was advised on resting positions and the use of local warmth or cooling (hot water bottle or cold pack) to ease LBP. She would try both and keep the one which was most effective for her.

On her second visit five days later, she had completed her current chemotherapy cycle and had been using her exercises and hot pack. She reported her back to be less painful (intensity) and the pain to occur less often (frequency) and last a shorter time (duration). We discussed beginning an exercise programme to be built up as she felt capable, and the likelihood of flare-ups and setbacks (Chapter 6) was noted.

The initial programme (R1 to R2) consisted of the spinal rotation exercise already used, alternate dumbbell shoulder press (patient had 2 kg dumbbells) and a walking programme of 10–15 minutes which she was keen to do with her daughter who was staying with her. She was to practise this daily but was free to do more or less as she felt able.

On her third visit the patient's back pain was no longer present, and she felt more positive and wanted to increase her exercise. Her walking programme was increased to 30–40 minutes over fields with her daughter and grandchild. At home she started a resistance programme using her dumbbells and a resistance band she had bought. The programme consisted of simple sit-to-stand, dumbbell shoulder press as before, dumbbell side-bend, and resistance band pull (row) from waist height. The circuit would be practised twice or three times through depending on fatigue level and used three times per week. The patient was also offered holistic therapy (aromatherapy massage, reflexology), if she required it.

Keypoints:

- The patient had consulted her oncology nurse who had confirmed her back pain was unrelated to her cancer.
- The patient reported view above would not rule out the presence of red flags and the patient's symptom behaviour was closely monitored.
- Massage was chosen to target local pain and enhance wellness (ease suffering).
- The patient was free to choose which pain targeting therapy worked best for her.
- Exercise therapy and treatment was kept simple and progressed once the current chemotherapy cycle had ended.
- Exercise was chosen to reflect available apparatus and opportunities (walking with daughter, dumbbells, and resistance band).

INDEX

Note: **Bold** page numbers refer to tables; *italic* page numbers refer to figures.

For Product Safety Concerns and Information please contact our
EU representative GPSR@taylorandfrancis.com Taylor & Francis
Verlag GmbH, Kaufingerstraße 24, 80331 München, Germany